Laboratory Exercises in HUMAN PHYSIOLOGY

Laboratory Exercises in HUMAN PHYSIOLOGY

Gerard J. Tortora

Bergen Community College
Paramus, NJ

Hope H. Adams

Sacred Heart University
Bridgeport, CT

MACMILLAN PUBLISHING COMPANY
New York
COLLIER MACMILLAN PUBLISHERS
London

Printed in the United States of America

Macmillan Publishing Company
866 Third Avenue, New York, New York 10022

Collier Macmillan Canada, Inc.

ISBN 0-02-421203-2

Printing: 1 2 3 4 5 6 7 8 Year: 9 0 1 2 3 4 5 6 7 8

To Bruce Howlett Adams, who always believed,
and to Stephen D. Parker, Jr., who never doubted.

CONTENTS

1 INTRODUCTION 1

EXERCISE 1. Laboratory Procedures and Safety Precautions 2
EXERCISE 2. Scientific Method 4

2 SCIENTIFIC MEASUREMENT 11

EXERCISE 1. Linear Measurement 11
EXERCISE 2. Volumetric Measurement 13
EXERCISE 3. Weight (Mass) Measurement 14
EXERCISE 4. Temperature Measurement 14
EXERCISE 5. Measurement of Specific Gravity 15

3 CHEMICAL PRINCIPLES 21

EXERCISE 1. Chemical Reactions 21
A. Synthesis Reactions 21
B. Decomposition Reactions 22
C. Exchange Reactions 22
D. Reversible Reactions 23
EXERCISE 2. Acid-Base Balance 24

4 MICROSCOPY 31

EXERCISE 1. Use of the Compound Microscope 32
A. Parts of the Microscope and Rules of Microscopy 32
B. Techniques of Microscopy 34
1. The Dry Mount 35
2. Perceiving Depth 37
3. The Wet Mount 37
EXERCISE 2. Microscopic Measurement 38
A. Magnification 38
B. Field Size 38

5 TRANSPORT ACROSS PLASMA MEMBRANES 45

EXERCISE 1. Brownian Movement 46
EXERCISE 2. Diffusion: A Passive Process 46
A. Diffusion of a Solid in a Liquid 47
B. Diffusion through a Solid 47
C. Diffusion through a Membrane 48
EXERCISE 3. Dialysis: A Passive Process 49
EXERCISE 4. Osmosis: A Passive Process 51
A. Osmosis through an Artificial Membrane 51
B. Osmosis through a Natural Membrane 52
C. Osmosis through a Living Membrane 52
EXERCISE 5. Filtration: A Passive Process 54
EXERCISE 6. Active Transport: An Active Process 55
EXERCISE 7. Endocytosis: An Active Process 56

6 NUCLEAR DIRECTED ACTIVITIES 63

EXERCISE 1. Structure of DNA 63
EXERCISE 2. Protein Synthesis 66
A. Transcription 66
B. Translation 66
EXERCISE 3. Mitotic Cell Division 72
A. Observation of Mitotic Stages 73
B. Relative Frequency of Mitotic Stages 75

7 THE NERVE IMPULSE 81

EXERCISE 1. Recording the Nerve Impulse 83
EXERCISE 2. Characteristics of a Nerve Impulse 86

8 PHYSIOLOGY OF THE NERVOUS SYSTEM 93

EXERCISE 1. Brain Function 93
A. Tests for Cerebellar Function 94
B. Cranial Nerve Function 94
EXERCISE 2. Reflexes 99
A. Somatic Reflexes in the Human 101
1. Stretch reflexes 101
2. Babinski reflex 102
B. Visceral Reflexes in the Human 102
1. Ciliospinal reflex 103
2. Salivary reflex 103
3. Pupillary reflexes 103
C. Reflexes in the Frog 103

9 MUSCLE PHYSIOLOGY 115

EXERCISE 1. Biochemistry of Muscle Contraction 118
EXERCISE 2. Physiology of Muscle Contraction 120
A. Use of Recording Equipment 122
B. Measurement of Muscle Contraction 125
1. Threshold stimulus 125
2. Single muscle twitch 125
3. Effect of fatigue on a single muscle twitch 126
4. Muscle response to variation in stimulus frequency 127
5. Effect of resting length on contraction strength 127
3. Ergographic Measurement of Human Muscle Contraction 128

10 SENSORY PHYSIOLOGY: GENERAL SENSES, OLFACTION, AND GUSTATION 137

EXERCISE 1. Cutaneous Receptors 138
A. Touch Receptors 138
1. Identifying touch receptors 138
2. Localization of the touch sensation 139
3. Two-point discrimination 139
B. Pressure Receptors 140
C. Thermoreceptors 140
1. Localization of heat and cold receptors 140
2. Adaptation of temperature receptors 141
D. Pain Receptors 141
EXERCISE 2. Proprioceptive Receptors 141
EXERCISE 3. Olfactory and Gustatory Receptors 142
A. Olfactory Adaptation 143
B. Association of Smell and Taste 143

11 SENSORY PHYSIOLOGY: VISION 151

EXERCISE 1. Ophthalmoscopy 153
EXERCISE 2. Errors of Refraction 155
A. Measurement of Visual Acuity 155
B. Test for Astigmatism 157
EXERCISE 3. The Blind Spot 157
EXERCISE 4. Accommodation 158
EXERCISE 5. Visual Reflexes 158
A. Photopupillary Reflex 159
B. Accommodation Reflex 159
C. Convergence Reflexes 159
EXERCISE 6. Binocular Vision 159
EXERCISE 7. Photoreceptors 160
A. Formation of an Afterimage 160
B. Test for Color Blindness 161
C. Color Perception 161

12 SENSORY PHYSIOLOGY: HEARING 167

EXERCISE 1. Otoscopy 169
EXERCISE 2. Tests of Auditory Acuity 170
A. Sound Localization 170
B. Weber's Test 170
C. Rinne's Test 170
D. Audiometry 171
EXERCISE 3. Tests of Equilibrium 172
A. Balance Test 172
B. Barany Test 173

13 ENDOCRINE PHYSIOLOGY 179

EXERCISE 1. Endocrine Glands: Location and Hormones 180
A. Pituitary Gland (Hypophysis) and Hypothalamus 180
1. Adenohypophysis 180
2. Neurohypophysis 180
B. Thyroid Gland 184
C. Parathyroid Glands 184

D. Adrenal (Suprarenal) Glands 184
1. Adrenal cortex 184
2. Adrenal medulla 184
E. Pancreas 185
F. Gonads 185
1. Testes 185
2. Ovaries 186
G. Pineal Gland (Epiphysis Cerebri) 186
H. Thymus 187
I. Other Endocrine Tissues 187
EXERCISE 2. Hyperinsulinism in the Fish 188

14 REPRODUCTION AND DEVELOPMENT 195

EXERCISE 1. Gametogenesis 195
A. Meiosis 196
B. Spermatogenesis 201
C. Oogenesis 203
EXERCISE 2. The Female Cycle 205
EXERCISE 3. Fertilization 207
EXERCISE 4. HCG and Pregnancy Testing 208
EXERCISE 5. Development 208

15 GENETICS 219

EXERCISE 1. The Human Karyotype 220
EXERCISE 2. Sex Inheritance 222
EXERCISE 3. Punnett Squares 226
EXERCISE 4. Inherited Traits 226
EXERCISE 5. The Hardy-Weinberg Principle 228
EXERCISE 6. Monohybrid and Dihybrid Crosses 229
EXERCISE 7. Incomplete Dominance 229
EXERCISE 8. Multiple Alleles 230
EXERCISE 9. X-Linked Inheritance 230
EXERCISE 10. Probability 231

16 HEMATOLOGY 241

EXERCISE 1. Blood Plasma 242
EXERCISE 2. Blood Cell Counts 244
EXERCISE 3. Hematocrit 245
EXERCISE 4. Hemoglobin Determination 247
A. Tallqvist Method 248
B. Use of the Hemoglobinometer 248
EXERCISE 5. Sedimentation Rate 248
EXERCISE 6. Blood Clotting 250
EXERCISE 7. Blood Typing 251
A. ABO typing 251
B. Rh typing 254
EXERCISE 8. Blood Pathology 255

17 CARDIOVASCULAR PHYSIOLOGY 261

EXERCISE 1. The Conduction System of the Heart 263
A. The Electrocardiogram 263
EXERCISE 2. The Cardiac Cycle 266
A. Observation of the Normal Cardiac Cycle 268
B. Recording the Cardiac Cycle 268
C. Intrinsic Control of the Cardiac Cycle 270
D. Extrinsic Control of the Cardiac Cycle 270
1. Effect of vagal stimulation 270
2. Effect of acetylcholine 271
3. Effect of atropine sulfate 271
4. Effect of epinephrine 271
E. Demonstration of the Refractory Period 271
EXERCISE 3. Auscultation of the Heart 272
EXERCISE 4. Pulse Rate 272
EXERCISE 5. Blood Pressure 274
EXERCISE 6. Vascular Physiology 275

18 RESPIRATORY PHYSIOLOGY 283

EXERCISE 1. Mechanics of Respiration 283
A. Artificial Thorax 283
B. Chest and Abdominal Measurement 285
EXERCISE 2. Respiratory Sounds 285
EXERCISE 3. Use of Pneumograph 287
EXERCISE 4. Measurement of Respiratory Volumes 288
A. Use of Wet Spirometer 289
B. Use of Handheld Spirometer 291
C. Use of Collins Respirometer 294
EXERCISE 5. Chemical Regulation of Respiration 297

19 EXERCISE PHYSIOLOGY 303

EXERCISE 1. Muscular Flexibility 303
A. Toe Touch 304
B. Flexibility 304
C. Effect of Warm-up 304

EXERCISE 2. Muscular Strength 304
EXERCISE 3. Muscular Endurance and Aerobic Fitness 305

20 DIGESTION 311

EXERCISE 1. Deglutition 312
EXERCISE 2. Observation of the Rat Gastrointestinal Tract 314
EXERCISE 3. Physiology of Intestinal Smooth Muscle 317
A. Inherent Contractile Activity 317
B. Effect of Oxygen 318
C. Effect of Temperature 318
D. Effect of Norepinephrine 318
E. Effect of Acetycholine 318
F. Effect of Atropine 319
G. Effect of Atropine and Acetylcholine 319
H. Effect of Atropine, Acetylcholine, and Norepinephrine 320
I. Effect of Calcium Removal 320
EXERCISE 4. Enzymatic (Chemical) Digestion 320
A. Digestion of Proteins 320
B. Digestion of Fats 320
1. Emulsification 321
2. Action of lipase on fats 322
C. Digestion of Carbohydrates 322
1. Benedict's test for sugar 322
2. Lugol's test for starch 323
3. Digestion of starch 323
4. Effect of temperature on starch digestion 324
5. Effect of pH on starch digestion 324

21 METABOLISM 333

EXERCISE 1. Body Fat Determination 334
EXERCISE 2. Indirect Calorimetry 335

22 RENAL PHYSIOLOGY 347

EXERCISE 1. Urine Formation 347
EXERCISE 2. Physical Urinalysis 352
A. Color and Transparency 352
B. pH 352
C. Specific Gravity 353
EXERCISE 3. Chemical Urinalysis 353
A. Chloride and Sodium Chloride 354
B. Glucose 354
C. Protein 355
D. Ketone Bodies 356
E. Bile Pigments 356
F. Hemoglobin and Myoglobin 357
EXERCISE 4. Microscopic Urinalysis 357

APPENDIX A PITHING OF FROGS 365

FIGURE CREDITS 367

INDEX 369

PREFACE

Laboratory Exercises in Human Physiology is designed for use in one or two semester courses in human physiology and was written to accompany most of the leading human physiology textbooks.

The exercises cover virtually all aspects of human physiology and have been selected to demonstrate physiological concepts. The exercises range from simple classic experiments to those requiring specialized equipment. The manual is designed to give the instructor considerable latitude in selecting the exercises to be assigned, the sequence in which the material is to be studied, and the amount of work that is practical for the particular course.

Each chapter contains the following elements:

1. An outline of the exercises that provides an overview and sequence of the topics to be studied.
2. Word roots to help promote the understanding of selected anatomical and physiological terms.
3. A general discussion of relevant anatomy.
4. Learning objectives for each exercise.
5. Questions to promote understanding and reinforce objectives at the end of each exercise.
6. Sufficient background information for each exercise.
7. Key terms indicated in boldface.
8. Phonetic pronunciations for many terms.
9. Precise and simple procedures for each exercise.
10. Appropriate laboratory safety precautions.
11. Laboratory report results at the end of each chapter for recording and interpreting data.
12. Laboratory report questions at the end of each chapter that test knowledge of chapter contents.

ACKNOWLEDGMENTS

We wish to thank the following reviewers for their comments and suggestions: John M. Wakeman, Louisiana Tech University; Kenneth P. Kinsey, Rhode Island College; Robert Thomas, College of the Redwoods; Claranne M. Bush, University of South Carolina; James L. Hanegan, Eastern Washington University; T. Daniel Kimbrough, Virginia Commonwealth University; and Lowell Neudeck, Northern Michigan University. We also wish to thank Mary Dersch, whose outstanding medical illustrations have greatly improved the pedagogy and visual appeal of the manual.

Readers and users of this laboratory manual are invited to send their reactions and suggestions to us so that plans can be formulated for future editions.

Gerard J. Tortora
Natural Sciences and Math, S229
Bergen Community College
400 Paramus Road
Paramus, NJ 07652

Hope H. Adams
120 Sigourney Street
Hartford, CT 06105

NOTE TO THE STUDENT

Part of Exercise 1 contains a listing of laboratory safety precautions. It is essential that you read them carefully before you perform any exercises in this manual. Should you have difficulty in understanding any of the precautions, please ask your instructor to explain them to you.

INTRODUCTION 1

EXERCISE 1. Laboratory Procedures and Safety Precautions
EXERCISE 2. Scientific Method

WORD ROOTS

a- = without
hypo- = under
-septic, *-sepsis* = decay
-thesis = placing

Therefore I have uttered what I did not understand, things too wonderful for me, which I did not know.

Job 42:3

Thus the story of Job recounts the awe we experience in observing the world about us. The discipline of human physiology studies the wonderful complexity of the body and also aims to generate a yearning to understand that which is still unknown.

This chapter introduces the format of the laboratory manual. Part of your work will involve reporting data in a way that can be understood by other people working in this field. This communication requires that you use scientific vocabulary accurately. At the beginning of each chapter, roots of words used in the chapter are listed. Learning these roots will enable you to know the meaning of other words in which the roots occur. For example, *hypo-* means *under;* the same prefix is used in hypodermic (under the skin) and hypothermia (under normal temperature). The pronunciation of many terms is given in parentheses immediately following the word, using the following key:

1. The syllable with the strongest accent appears in capital letters, for example, hī-POTH-e-sis.
2. Secondary accents are denoted by a single quote mark ('), for example, hī'-pō-DERM-ic.
3. Long vowel sounds are marked with a line above the vowel and are pronounced:

ā as in make	ī as in ivy
ē as in be	ō as in pole

4. Short vowel sounds are unmarked and are pronounced:

a as in above	o as in not
e as in bet	u as in bud
i as in sip	

5. Other phonetic symbols are used to indicate:

oo as in sue	yoo as in cute
oy as in oil	

Throughout the manual, each exercise is preceded by a box that states its learning objectives. The objectives give reasons for doing the procedures. Questions to promote understanding are located at the end of each exercise, and observations are made in the LABORATORY REPORT RESULTS at the end of each chapter. A section of LABORATORY REPORT QUESTIONS also at the end of each chapter will test your understanding of the material. You can see a simplified form of this pattern in the following exercises.

EXERCISE 1. Laboratory Procedures and Safety Precautions

OBJECTIVES

To describe the laboratory procedures to be followed in this course

To understand and implement mandatory safety precautions to be followed in this course

Attention to basic laboratory procedures and safety precautions is essential. Although specific procedures and safety precautions are indicated throughout the laboratory manual, you should read the following *BEFORE* performing any experiments.

A. General Procedures and Safety Precautions

1. Read all experiments *before* coming to the laboratory to be sure that you understand all the procedures and safety precautions. This practice will allow you to use your time efficiently and help you to understand the principles involved. Ask your instructor if you do not understand exactly what has to be done.

2. Arrive promptly for the laboratory session. Your instructor will usually give verbal instructions at the beginning of each session. Since each laboratory is different, materials or procedures recommended in this manual may be changed in ways appropriate to your own laboratory setting. Take careful written notes of any changes *as well as any special precautions to be taken*.

3. *Bring* your laboratory manual, textbook, and several pencils to each session.

4. *Do not bring* any unnecessary items to the laboratory and do not place any personal items (pocketbooks, bookbags, coats, umbrellas, etc.) on the laboratory table or at your feet. Place them in a designated location.

5. *Follow directions carefully* and do not attempt any procedure unless you fully understand the techniques involved. *Do not perform any unauthorized experiments* and *do not improvise* any procedures.

6. *Tie back long hair* to prevent accidents.

7. *Do not put anything in your mouth* in the laboratory. Never eat, drink, taste chemicals, lick labels, smoke, or store food in the laboratory.

8. *Handle laboratory equipment carefully* and do not operate any equipment until you are instructed in its proper use.

9. *Protective eyewear and laboratory coats or aprons must be worn* by all students performing or observing experiments.

10. *Never remove* equipment, chemicals, biological materials, or any other materials from the laboratory.

11. Make sure all apparatus is supported squarely on the laboratory table.

12. When working with living specimens, treat them *humanely*.

13. Record your laboratory seating assignment in the LABORATORY REPORT RESULTS at the end of the chapter.

14. Record data promptly in the LABORATORY REPORT RESULTS. Information written on scraps of paper can get lost. Data that does not agree with expected results is important. Understanding why an exercise "went wrong" can reveal errors in technique or can open new areas of investigation. Much scientific advance has stemmed from an analysis of unexpected results.

15. A few exercises in the laboratory manual are designed to induce some degree of cardiovascular stress. Students should not participate in these exercises if they are pregnant or have hypertension or any other known or suspected condition that might compromise health. *Before you perform any of these exercises, check with your physician.*

16. Clean your equipment and laboratory table according to the directions of your instructor.

17. Your instructor will show you the location of various pieces of emergency equipment. *Memorize their locations and know how to use them.* Record the location of the fire blanket, fire extinguisher, first aid kit, and the eye wash station in the LABORATORY REPORT RESULTS at the end of the chapter.

18. Wash your hands before leaving the laboratory and remove protective clothing, such as laboratory coats or aprons and protective eyewear.

B. Precautions Related to Working with Blood, Other Body Fluids, or Blood Products

On August 21, 1987, the Centers for Disease Control (CDC) published a supplement to the *Morbidity and Mortality Weekly Report* (Vol. 36, no. 2S), entitled "Recommendations for Prevention of HIV Transmission in Health-Care Settings." The CDC guidelines recommend precautions to protect health-care workers from exposure to human immunodeficiency virus (HIV), the causative agent of acquired immune deficiency syndrome (AIDS). These guidelines reaffirm the basic principles involved in the transmission of not only the AIDS virus, but also other disease-producing organisms. Based on the CDC guidelines, the following precautions should be taken.

1. *Gloves must be worn* to handle all specimens or contaminated instruments or to clean up blood or other fluid spills.

2. Masks and protective eyewear or face shields should be worn during procedures that are likely to generate droplets of blood or other body fluids to prevent exposure of mucous membranes of the mouth, nose, and eyes.

3. Laboratory coats or aprons should be worn during procedures that are likely to generate splashes of blood or other body fluids.

4. Hands and other skin surfaces should be washed immediately and thoroughly if contaminated with blood or other body fluids. Hands should be washed immediately after gloves are removed.

5. Only single-use, disposable lancets and needles should be used. Never recap, bend, or break the lancet once it has been used. Place used lancets and needles in a *fresh* 1:10 dilution of household bleach (sodium hypochlorite) or commercially available disinfectant with tuberculocidal activity and then dispose of the instruments in a puncture-proof container. The bleach solution should be prepared fresh for *each* laboratory session.

6. A laboratory disinfectant should be used to clean laboratory surfaces *before* and *after* procedures and should be available for quick cleanup of any blood spills. A *fresh* 1:10 dilution of household bleach or a commercially prepared disinfectant with tuberculocidal activity can be used.

7. All reusable instruments such as hemocytometers, well slides, and reusable pipettes should be disinfected with a *fresh* 1:10 solution of household bleach or a commercially prepared disinfectant with tuberculocidal activity and thoroughly washed with soap and hot water.

8. Mouth pipetting should *never* be done. Mechanical pipetting devices should be used to manipulate all liquids in the laboratory.

9. All procedures that have a high potential for creating infectious droplets (such as centrifuging and blending) should be performed carefully. In such instances, a biological safety cabinet or other primary containment device is required.

C. Precautions Related to Working with Reagents

1. *Use extreme care when working with reagents.* Should any reagents make contact with your eyes, *flush with water* for fifteen minutes or if they make contact with your skin, flush with water for five minutes. *Notify your instructor immediately* and *seek immediate medical attention.*

2. *Report all accidents* to your instructor, no matter how minor they may appear to be.

3. The room in which you are working should be *well-ventilated* when you are working with chemicals or preserved specimens. *Avoid breathing fumes* for any extended period of time.

4. *Never point the opening of a test tube* containing a reacting mixture (especially when heating) toward yourself or another person.

5. *Do not force glass tubing or a thermometer into rubber stoppers.* Lubricate the glass and introduce it gradually and gently into the stopper. Protect your hands with toweling when inserting glass into the stopper.

6. *Never heat a flammable liquid over or near an open flame.*

7. *Do not heat any glassware unless it is marked Pyrex or Kimex.* Other glassware may shatter when heated. Handle hot glassware with test tube holders.

8. If you have to dilute an acid, *always add acid (AAA) to water.*

9. *Do not use your fingers as a stopper* for a test tube or bottle when shaking the tube.

10. Read the label on any chemical *twice* before using it.

11. Immediately after use, replace caps or stoppers on bottles and return spatulas to their correct place. *Do not move reagent bottles* from the supply location.

12. *Do not wear contact lenses when working with reagents.*

13. Mouth pipetting should *never* be done. Mechanical pipetting devices should be used to manipulate all liquids in the laboratory.

14. Dispose of chemicals, biological materials, used apparatus, and waste materials according to the directions of your instructor. Not all liquids are to be disposed of in the sink.

15. Wash your hands *carefully* before you leave the laboratory.

D. Precautions Related to Dissection

1. The room in which you are working should be *well-ventilated* when you are working with chemicals or preserved specimens. *Avoid breathing fumes* for any extended period of time.

2. It is recommended that you use specimens that have been preserved in formalin, rinsed, and held in a non-toxic fluid such as "Ward-Safe" or "Carosafe." In order to *reduce the irritating effects* of chemical preservatives to your skin, eyes, and nose, hold your specimen under running water for several minutes to wash away excess preservative and dilute the remaining preservative.

3. *Gloves should be worn when performing dissections* and *laboratory coats or aprons should be worn* to protect your skin and clothing.

4. When dissecting, there is always the possibility of skin cuts or punctures from dissecting equipment or the teeth or claws of animal specimens. *Should you sustain a wound* in this manner, wash your hands with a disinfectant soap, notify your instructor, and *seek immediate medical attention.*

5. When cleaning dissecting instruments, always *hold the sharp edges away from you.*

Sign the statement in the LABORATORY REPORT RESULTS after you have read these precautions. Your instructor may wish to initial your signature.

EXERCISE 2. Scientific Method

OBJECTIVES

To define scientific method
To list the steps in the scientific method
To distinguish dependent from independent variables

Scientific research consists of making deductions based on observations. To be valid, these deductions must be *testable* and *repeatable* in other laboratories in order to verify the findings. The ***scientific method*** is the process through which these deductions are made. It allows researchers to weigh the evidence that supports their deductions and to communicate with others about their methods and results.

The scientific method can be subdivided into the six steps listed in this exercise. Along with the description is a brief and simplified summary of the work of Christiaan Eijkman, a Dutch scientist who sought the cause of beriberi (a potentially fatal disease that affects the nervous and cardiovascular systems).

Step One: Observation of Phenomena

Observations must be *systematic* and *objective,* that is, we must observe in an organized manner what we see, not what we want to see or what we think we should see. We make the assumption that the laws governing the universe are not occasional, are the same today as yesterday and tomorrow, and that we are capable of understanding those laws.

Eijkman observed the frequency of beriberi in the Indonesian population and in experimental chickens. He noted that the chickens fed on kitchen scraps contracted the disease.

Step Two: Proposal of a Question

Scientific questions are questions of causality such as "What causes this disease?" They are not teleological questions like "Why is there disease in this world?" Such questions are appropriate to the disciplines of philosophy and theology, but they are not *testable* as scientific questions must be. "Do evil spirits cause disease?" is an untestable question since an evil spirit cannot be seen or measured. However, the question "Can believers in evil spirits contract symptoms of a disease if told that they were exposed to such a spirit?" could be tested and the resulting data measured.

Christiaan Eijkman asked, "What is the cause of beriberi?"

Step Three: Formation of a Hypothesis

A hypothesis is an educated guess, a tentative answer to the question posed, or an unproven conclusion. A hypothesis must be able to be falsified.

Eijkman's work was done in the late nineteenth century, a time when bacterial causes of disease were being investigated. Eijkman's first hypothesis was "Bacteria in the kitchen scraps cause beriberi in chickens."

Step Four: Experimentation

Experimentation requires the use of a ***control***, which is a basis of comparison to the experimental organisms. Control organisms are treated identically to experimental organisms except for the one variable being investigated.

Variables are factors that affect the outcome of the experiment. The outcome is measured in terms of the ***dependent*** or ***response variables***. The investigator manipulates ***independent variables*** to determine if they affect the outcome.

Eijkman used two groups of chickens, both living in the same environment, exposed to the same air, temperature, and so forth. Both groups were fed kitchen scraps, but the experimental group received a diet of aseptically prepared scraps.

Step Five: Observation and Recording of Experimental Data

Recording must be objective and in specific terms of category or numerical measurement.

Eijkman observed that about an equal number of control and experimental chickens developed beriberi.

Step Six: Drawing Conclusions

This step ascertains whether the original hypothesis was valid. It asks whether more experimentation is necessary and if a new hypothesis must be formulated.

When Eijkman observed that aseptic preparation of food had no effect on the outcome, he formulated a new hypothesis: "Beriberi results from the absence of a substance in the kitchen scrap diet." In a new experiment, the control chickens were fed the kitchen scrap diet (mostly polished rice) while the experimental animals ate kitchen scraps plus rice bran (unpolished rice with hulls intact). Eijkman observed that the control animals eventually contracted beriberi while the experimental animals did not.

Eijkman's second hypothesis was supported by all the experimental results. After repeated investigation and the observation that prisoners who were fed polished rice were more likely to develop beriberi than those fed a balanced diet, the hypothesis was considered a *theory*. Ultimately, the theory led to the recognition that certain substances (vitamins) are essential to life, and that a diet of polished rice is deficient in thiamine (vitamin B_1). The theory is now considered a *principle*, and thiamine deficiency is identified as the cause of beriberi.

After the chickens fed on kitchen scraps and aseptically prepared kitchen scraps both developed symptoms of beriberi, Eijkman had to develop a new hypothesis. Why would/would not the following hypothesis have been appropriate? "Beriberi results from exposure to a substance in polished rice." ____________

____

What was the dependent variable in Eijkman's experiments? ____________

____

COMPLETE THE LABORATORY REPORT QUESTIONS AT THE END OF THE CHAPTER

INTRODUCTION 1

Student ______________________ **Date** ______________________

Laboratory Section ______________________ **Score/Grade** ______________________

EXERCISE 1. Laboratory Procedures and Safety Precautions

Seating assignment ______________________

Location

Fire extinguisher ______________________

Fire blanket ______________________

First aid kit ______________________

Eye wash station ______________________

I have read and understood the safety precautions in this laboratory manual. I hereby note my intent to abide by all instructions so as not to endanger myself or others in the laboratory.

Date ______________ Signature ______________________

Laboratory Instructor ______________________

INTRODUCTION 1

Student ______________________ **Date** ______________________

Laboratory Section ______________________ **Score/Grade** ______________________

MULTIPLE CHOICE

_____ 1. A scientific question must be (a) repeatable (b) testable (c) systematic (d) teleological (e) all of the above

_____ 2. An unproven conclusion is termed a (a) dependent variable (b) principle (c) theory (d) hypothesis (e) none of the above

_____ 3. If you measure the amount of sweat produced at various temperatures, the temperature is a (a) dependent variable (b) independent variable (c) control (d) deduction

SCIENTIFIC MEASUREMENT 2

EXERCISE 1. Linear Measurement
EXERCISE 2. Volumetric Measurement
EXERCISE 3. Weight (Mass) Measurement
EXERCISE 4. Temperature Measurement
EXERCISE 5. Measurement of Specific Gravity

Measurement is an essential part of any scientific work. For example, it allows precise size comparisons, the quantification of time, and accuracy in reporting observations. Measurement is also necessary so that experiments can be standardized and repeated. The fundamental units of measurement are length, mass, and time.

In the United States, nonscientific measurement and most industrial measurement use the yard and pound as the fundamental units of length and mass. Scientific measurements of length and mass are made using the ***metric system***, a decimal system of measurement in use throughout the world.

In the ***U.S. system***, units larger and smaller than the fundamental units must be converted by using a different number for each conversion. For example, to convert yards to feet, we multiply by 3; to convert yards to inches we multiply by 36; and to convert yards to miles, we divide by 1760. In the metric system, these conversions are all made by multiplying or dividing by ten or multiples of ten; in effect, they are made merely by moving a decimal point. An additional advantage of metric measurement is the ability to make a simple interconversion between units of length, volume, and mass.

The metric system is easily understood by learning the prefixes which designate the relationship of each unit to the fundamental units of measurement. The prefixes are listed in Table 2.1; their use in each fundamental measurement is given in a table within each exercise.

EXERCISE 1. Linear Measurement

OBJECTIVES

To measure length in metric units
To convert from one metric unit to another
To observe and graph biological variation
To calculate area

Linear measurement is the measurement of distances along straight lines; its basic unit is the ***meter***. Metric units of length and their U.S. equivalents are given in Table 2.2.

Area is measured by multiplying two linear measurements and is reported in units squared. Thus, the area of a rectangular space equals its length times its width; if these dimensions are measured in centimeters (cm), the area is measured in square centimeters (cm^2).

MATERIALS

Meter stick
Small metric measures

PROCEDURE

1. Stand against a chalkboard or a wall on which paper has been placed. Have your lab-

TABLE 2.1
PREFIXES DENOTING METRIC UNITS

Prefix	Meaning	Decimal Value × Standard Unit	Exponential Value × Standard Unit
Kilo-	Thousand	1000	10^3
Hecto-	Hundred	100	10^2
Deka-	Ten	10	10^1
Standard unit		1	10^0
Deci-	1/10	0.1	10^{-1}
Centi-	1/100	0.01	10^{-2}
Milli-	1/1,000	0.001	10^{-3}
Micro-	1/1,000,000	0.000001	10^{-6}
Nano-	1/1,000,000,000	0.000000001	10^{-9}
Pico-	1/1,000,000,000,000	0.000000000001	10^{-12}

oratory partner mark your height. Using the meter stick, measure your height to the nearest millimeter. Record this measurement in the LABORATORY REPORT RESULTS at the end of the chapter.

2. Using a small metric measure, measure the distance from the base of your left middle finger to the tip to the nearest millimeter. Record this measurement in the LABORATORY REPORT RESULTS at the end of the chapter and also in the place designated for the recording of class data.

3. Using the scale imposed in Figure 2.1, measure the diameter of the red blood cell in micrometers (μm). Record this measurement in the LABORATORY REPORT RESULTS at the end of the chapter.

4. Calculate the area occupied by Figure 2.1. Measure the length and width of the photomicrograph in centimeters and multiply the length by width ($A = l \times w$) to give a result in square centimeters (cm^2). Record these measurements in the LABORATORY REPORT RESULTS at the end of the chapter.

5. Use the table in LABORATORY REPORT RESULTS at the end of the chapter to organize the class data on finger length in the following ways:

   a. Calculate the mean length of the measured fingers by summing all the finger lengths and dividing by the number of fingers measured.

   b. Make a frequency distribution by grouping the finger lengths into the categories listed.

   c. Construct a bar graph to illustrate the variation in finger length.

TABLE 2.2
METRIC UNITS OF LENGTH AND U.S. SYSTEM EQUIVALENTS

Unit	Abbreviation	Metric Equivalent	U.S. Equivalent
Kilometer	km	1000 m	3,280.8 ft or .62 mi
Hectometer	hm	100 m	328 ft
Dekameter	dam	10 m	32.8 ft
Meter	m	1 (standard unit)	3.28 ft = 39.37 in = 1.09 yd
Decimeter	dm	0.1 m	3.94 in
Centimeter	cm	0.01 m	.394 in
Millimeter	mm	0.001 m	.0394 in
Micrometer (formerly micron μ)	μm	0.000001 m	3.94×10^{-5} in
Nanometer (formerly millimicron mμ)	nm	0.000000001 m	3.94×10^{-8} in
Angstrom	Å	0.0000000001 m	3.94×10^{-9} in

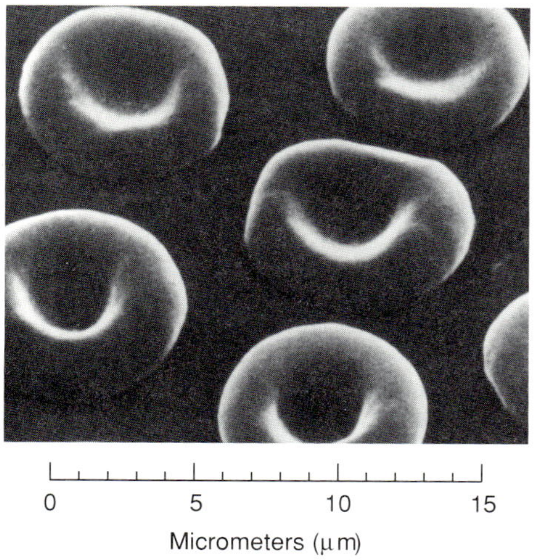

FIGURE 2.1 Scanning electron micrograph of red blood cells at a magnification of 500× with scale in micrometers (μm).

Compare the area of Figure 2.1 which you calculated in step 4 with the areas calculated by other students. Explain any discrepancies.

____

____

EXERCISE 2. Volumetric Measurement

OBJECTIVES

To measure the volume of a liquid
To measure the volume of a solid
To define the relationship between cubic centimeters (cm^3) and milliliters (ml)
To define the surface/volume ratio

Volumetric measurement measures the amount of three-dimensional space occupied by an object. The volume of a solid can be calculated by multiplying its three linear dimensions and reporting volume in cubed units. Thus, a cube with edges of 3 centimeters (cm) has a volume of 27 cubic centimeters (cm^3 or cc). Metric units of volume and their U.S. equivalents are given in Table 2.3.

The basic metric unit for measuring the volume of a liquid is the ***liter***. One milliliter (ml) of water at 4°C occupies 1 cc of space.

As a cell grows, it encounters constraints imposed by the surface/volume ratio, that is, the relationship between the cell's surface area and the amount of space it occupies. Cells need a large surface area across which nutrients and waste products can be exchanged. If a cell were 1 cm square and it grew four times its size, its volume would increase 64 times (from 1 cm^3 to 64 cm^3); cellular metabolic activity and the need for a surface to exchange water, oxygen, and so forth would increase about the same amount. Yet the cellular surface area would only increase 16 times (from 6 cm^2 to 96 cm^2). Cells and organisms have developed various modifications to cope with this problem.

MATERIALS

Eight small metal cubes
Metric ruler
100 ml graduated cylinder or displacement vessel

PROCEDURE

1. Measure the edge of one small metal cube. Calculate its surface area in cm^2 and its volume in cm^3. Record your measurements in the LABORATORY REPORT RESULTS at the end of the chapter.

2. Place eight metal cubes together to form a larger cube. Calculate the surface area and volume of the larger cube as you did in step 1; record your measurements in the LABORATORY REPORT RESULTS at the end of the chapter.

3. Fill a 100 ml graduated cylinder with 50 ml of water. Place one metal cube in the cylin-

TABLE 2.3
METRIC UNITS OF VOLUME AND U.S. SYSTEM EQUIVALENTS

Unit	Abbreviation	Metric Equivalent	U.S. Equivalent
Liter	l	Standard unit	33.81 fl oz or 1.057 qt
Milliliter	ml	0.001 l	0.0338 fl oz

der and measure the *displacement volume* of the cube. Place the other seven cubes in the cylinder and measure the total displacement volume of the eight cubes. Record your measurements in the LABORATORY REPORT RESULTS at the end of the chapter.

ALTERNATE PROCEDURE

Fill a displacement vessel with water until the water drips from the overflow spout. Place a graduated cylinder beneath the spout and add the metal cubes to the vessel. Measure the displacement volume and record as previously described.

4. In the table below, calculate the surface area and volume of cubes with edges of 1, 2, 3, 4, 5, 6, 7, and 8 cm. Determine the surface/volume ratio of these cubes by dividing the surface area of each cube by its calculated volume. Then divide the surface area by the volume to determine their ratio.

How would you measure the volume of an irregularly shaped object? ____________________

____

EXERCISE 3. Weight Measurement

> OBJECTIVES
>
> To weigh a solid and a liquid
> To define the relationship between volume and mass

Mass is the amount of matter an object contains. ***Weight*** is a force, determined by the pull of gravity on an object. Weight and mass are sometimes used synonymously because the gravitational force on the earth is nearly constant.

The ***gram (g)*** is the fundamental metric unit of mass. One cubic centimeter of water (1 ml of water) at 4°C is considered to have a mass of one gram. Metric units of mass and their U.S. equivalents are given in Table 2.4.

MATERIALS

Balance
Graduated cylinder
Weighing paper
Sodium chloride

PROCEDURE

1. Your instructor will give you instructions on the use of the balance(s) available in your laboratory.

2. Weigh a 50 ml graduated cylinder on the balance. Fill the cylinder with 50 ml of water and weigh again. Subtract the weight of the cylinder from the total weight and calculate the weight of the water. Record your measurements in the LABORATORY REPORT RESULTS at the end of the chapter.

3. Place a piece of weighing paper on the balance and record its weight. Measure out 2 g of sodium chloride (NaCl). Add the sodium chloride to the water in the graduated cylinder and weigh the cylinder again. Record your measurements in the LABORATORY REPORT RESULTS at the end of the chapter.

What is the most accurate means of obtaining 10 g of water? ____________________

____

EXERCISE 4. Temperature Measurement

> OBJECTIVES
>
> To measure temperature
> To convert from the Fahrenheit (F) scale to the Celsius (C) scale

Edge of cube in cm	1	2	3	4	5	6	7	8
Surface area of cube in cm^2		24						
Volume of cube in cm^3			27					
Surface/volume ratio				1.5				

TABLE 2.4
METRIC UNITS OF MASS AND U.S. SYSTEM EQUIVALENTS

Unit	Abbreviation	Metric Equivalent	U.S. Equivalent
Kilogram	**kg**	1000 g	2.205 lb or 35.37 oz
Hectogram	**hg**	100 g	0.205 lb
Gram	**g**	Standard unit	0.04 oz
Decigram	**dg**	0.1 g	0.004 oz
Centigram	**cg**	0.01 g	0.0004 oz
Milligram	**mg**	0.001 g	0.00004 oz
Microgram	**μg**	0.000001 g	
Nanogram	**ng**	0.000000001 g	
Picogram	**pg**	0.000000000001 g	

Temperature measurement measures the heat energy of an object. The basic metric unit of measurement is one degree Celsius (°C); the Celsius (SEL-sē-us) scale is also known as the centigrade scale. In the ***Celsius scale***, 0°C is the freezing point of water, and 100°C is the boiling point of water; normal body temperature is 37°C.

The ***Fahrenheit*** (FA-ren-hīt) ***scale*** measures temperature in the same way: it measures the degree to which a specific volume of mercury expands when heated. However, the calibrations on the scale differ so that the freezing point of water is 32°F, the boiling point of water is 212°F, and normal body temperature is 98.6°F.

To convert degrees Fahrenheit to degrees Celsius, use the following formula:

$$°C = \frac{5}{9}(°F - 32°)$$

To convert degrees Celsius to degrees Fahrenheit, use the formula:

$$°F = \frac{9}{5}(°C) + 32°$$

MATERIALS

Thermometer
Boiling water bath
Ice water bath

PROCEDURE

1. To determine temperatures, hold the thermometer without touching the bulb at the base, and read the calibrated scale. Record all measurements in the LABORATORY REPORT RESULTS at the end of the chapter.

2. Read the room temperature.

3. Measure your body temperature by holding the thermometer in the armpit.

4. Measure the temperature of hot water from the tap.

5. Measure the temperature of boiling water.

6. Measure the temperature of cold water from the tap.

7. Measure the temperature of the ice water bath.

EXERCISE 5. Measurement of Specific Gravity

OBJECTIVES

To measure the specific gravity of various substances
To understand the use of the hydrometer

The ***specific gravity*** of a substance is its density relative to water. By definition, water has a specific gravity of 1.000. Substances less dense than water have specific gravities less than 1.000; substances more dense than water have specific gravities greater than 1.000.

A device called a ***hydrometer*** (hī-DROM-e-ter) is used to measure specific gravity. A hydrometer, pictured in Figure 2.2, is a glass cylinder weighted so that it floats in water at a level marked as 1.000 on the cylinder.

Clinical uses of hydrometry include measuring the specific gravity of urine to determine its solute concentration, i.e., how dilute or concentrated it is.

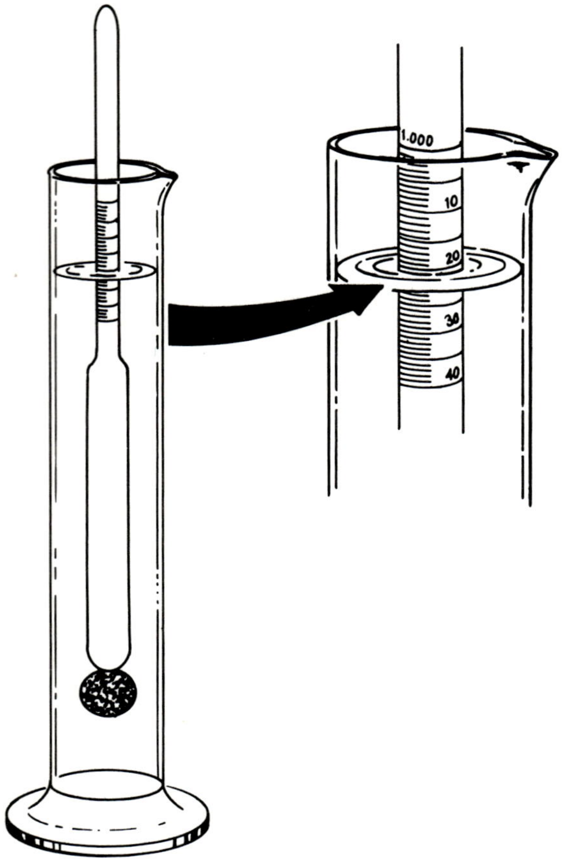

FIGURE 2.2 A hydrometer.

MATERIALS

Hydrometer jar
Light liquid and heavy liquid hydrometers
Glycerine
Alcohol
Urine

PROCEDURE

1. Obtain a hydrometer and hydrometer jar. *Carefully* study the calibrations on the scale until you understand how they are to be read.

2. Fill the hydrometer jar with one of the following substances: water, glycerine, alcohol, or urine.

3. Float the hydrometer in a liquid. If it adheres to the side of the jar, tap or spin it gently. If the level of the liquid is not on the calibration scale, use the other type of hydrometer.

4. Record the specific gravity of this substance in the LABORATORY REPORT RESULTS at the end of the chapter.

5. After washing and drying the hydrometer, repeat step 2, measuring the specific gravity of the other liquids available.

Would a substance with a specific gravity of 0.8 float on water or sink? ____ Why? ________

COMPLETE THE LABORATORY REPORT QUESTIONS AT THE END OF THE CHAPTER

SCIENTIFIC MEASUREMENT 2

Student ______________________ **Date** ______________________

Laboratory Section ______________________ **Score/Grade** ______________________

EXERCISE 1. Linear Measurement

1. Height in meters ____ in centimeters ____ in millimeters ____
2. Finger length in millimeters ____ in centimeters ____
3. Cell diameter in μm ____ in Ångstroms ____
4. Area of Figure 2.1 in cm^2 ____ in m^2 ____
5. a. Average finger length = ____ cm

   b. Frequency Distribution

	Number of Fingers	Category Symbol
< 5.9 cm		A
6.0 – 6.4 cm		B
6.5 – 6.9 cm		C
7.0 – 7.4 cm		D
7.5 – 7.9 cm		E
8.0 – 8.4 cm		F
over 8.5 cm		G

   c. Bar graph

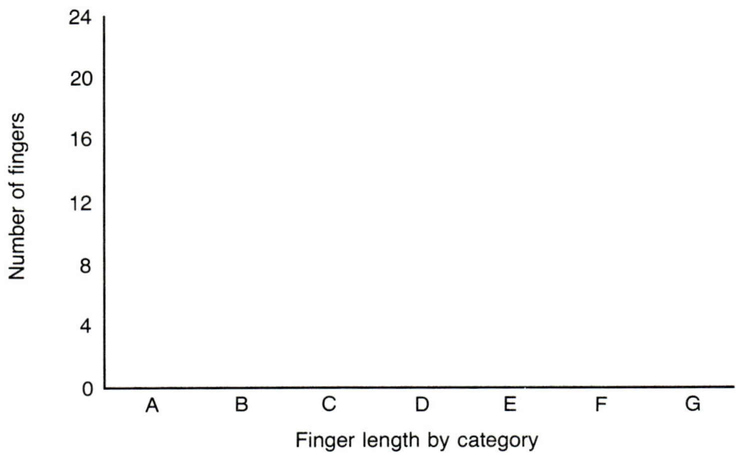

EXERCISE 2. Volumetric Measurement

1. Small cube edge = ____ cm Surface area = ____ cm^2

   Volume = ____ cm^3

2. Large cube edge = ____ cm Surface area = ____ cm^2

   Volume = ____ cm^3

3. Displacement volume of one cube = ____ ml

4. Displacement volume of eight cubes = ____ ml

EXERCISE 3. Weight Measurement

1. Weight of graduated cylinder = ____

Weight of cylinder + 50 ml of water = ____

Weight of 50 ml of water = ____

2. Weight of 50 ml water + 2 g sodium chloride (NaCl) = ____

EXERCISE 4. Temperature Measurement

	°C	°F
Room temperature		
Body temperature		
Hot water temperature		
Boiling water temperature		
Cold water temperature		
Ice water temperature		

EXERCISE 5. Measurement of Specific Gravity

Substance	Specific Gravity
Water	
Glycerine	
Alcohol	
Urine	

LABORATORY REPORT QUESTIONS

SCIENTIFIC MEASUREMENT 2

Student ______________________ **Date** ______________________

Laboratory Section ______________________ **Score/Grade** ______________________

PROBLEMS:

1. Express 2.47 meters in centimeters: ____

 in millimeters: ____

 in Ångstroms: ____

2. What is the area of a square which is 30 cm on a side?

 in cm^2 ____

 in m^2 ____

3. Visible light has a wavelength between 3.75×10^{-9} m and 8.0×10^{-9} m. Can we see light with a wavelength of 5.5×10^{-2} μm? ____

4. Express 435 cm^3 in cubic meters: ____

 in liters: ____

 in milliliters: ____

5. Will a hollow cube with sides of .3 m hold 6 liters of solution? ____ What is the capacity of this cube? ____ liters.

6. How many kg does a 100 pound person weigh? ____

7. A drug dosage is 35 μg. How many mg is this? ____

8. Convert the following temperatures:

 61°F = ____ °C

 61°C = ____ °F

 0°F = ____ °C

 100°C = ____ °F

9. Calculate the specific gravity of a given liquid from the following data, taken at 25°C:

 Weight of empty beaker: 10.589 g

 Weight of beaker + 10 ml liquid: 17.893 g

 Weight of beaker + 10 ml water: 20.636 g

Specific gravity = ____

DISCUSSION: Describe some ways in which the body might have evolved to cope with its small surface/volume ratio? Describe some stratagems which single cells may have developed to cope with this problem.

CHEMICAL PRINCIPLES 3

EXERCISE 1. Chemical Reactions
- *A. Synthesis Reactions*
- *B. Decomposition Reactions*
- *C. Exchange Reactions*
- *D. Reversible Reactions*

EXERCISE 2. Acid-Base Balance

WORD ROOTS

ana- = upward
cata- = downward
endo- = within
exo- = without
macro- = large

Each cell of the body contains thousands of different chemical compounds. Carbon (C), hydrogen (H), oxygen (O), nitrogen (N), phosphorus (P), and sulfur (S) are the principal elements in these compounds, composing over 97% of body weight. The molecules in living cells range from simple ones such as water to complex macromolecules such as proteins and nucleic acids.

All of the metabolic processes in the body involve chemical reactions; the digestion of food, the contraction of muscle, cellular growth, and division are but a few.

If these reactions require the input of energy, the reactions are termed ***endergonic,*** and the product of the reaction has more energy than the starting materials or reactants. Or the reactions may be ***exergonic,*** involving the release of energy as reactants are converted into end products. In the body, the energy is usually heat, so these reactions are referred to as ***endothermic*** and ***exothermic,*** respectively.

Even exothermic reactions may require energy to initiate them. Before molecules can react, they need to come into contact with each other. ***Activation energy*** is required to facilitate molecular collision.

EXERCISE 1. Chemical Reactions

> OBJECTIVES
>
> To observe simple chemical reactions
> To differentiate the basic types of chemical reactions
> To distinguish endergonic and exergonic reactions

CAUTION! *Please reread Section A, "General Procedures and Safety Precautions," and Section C, "Precautions Related to Working With Reagents," in Chapter 1 before you begin any of the exercises in this chapter. Be sure to read the exercises before you perform them to be certain that you understand all of the procedures and safety precautions.*

A. Synthesis Reactions

In ***synthesis (anabolic) reactions,*** two or more reactants combine to form a product. These reactions can be symbolized by the equation $A + B \rightarrow AB$.

Ammonia (NH_3) and hydrochloric acid (HCl) are colorless; they combine to form ammonium hydroxide (NH_4Cl), a white compound, according to the equation:

$$NH_3 + HCl \rightarrow NH_4Cl$$

RELEASE ENERGY (HEAT)

REQUIRE ENERGY INPUT

MATERIALS

Test tube rack
Two Pyrex or Kimex test tubes
Two droppers
Glass rod
Concentrated ammonia (NH_3) solution in a dropper bottle
Concentrated hydrochloric acid (HCl) in a dropper bottle
Safety goggles
Acid resistant or caustic resistant gloves
Laboratory apron or coat

PROCEDURE

1. Place two test tubes in a test tube rack. CAUTION! *Using extreme caution and acid resistant gloves,* carefully place a few drops of concentrated ammonia solution in one test tube and a few drops of concentrated hydrochloric acid in the other.
2. Dip a glass rod into the HCl solution and remove it slowly so that one drop remains on the rod.
3. Hold the glass rod with the drop of HCl over the mouth of the test tube containing the NH_3 solution.
4. Observe what occurs and record the nature of the reaction in the LABORATORY REPORT RESULTS at the end of the chapter.
5. *Discard the solutions and clean your materials according to the directions of your laboratory instructor.*

Synthesis reactions require energy for the formation of chemical bonds. What is the energy source in this reaction? __________

____

B. Decomposition Reactions

In ***decomposition (catabolic) reactions,*** one substance is broken down into smaller components, with a release of energy. These reactions can be symbolized by the equation $AB \rightarrow A + B$.

When heated, copper (II) carbonate, a bluish-grey compound, will decompose to yield copper (II) oxide, a black compound, and carbon dioxide, a gas, according to the equation:

$$CuCO_3 \rightarrow CuO + CO_2$$

MATERIALS

Spatula
Pyrex or Kymex test tube
Test tube holder
Test tube rack
Boiling water bath (hot plate and beaker)
Copper (II) carbonate ($CuCO_3$)
Safety goggles
Acid resistant or caustic resistant gloves
Laboratory apron or coat

PROCEDURE

1. Using a spatula, place a large pinch of copper (II) carbonate ($CuCO_3$) in a test tube and fill it about one-fourth full of water.
2. Using a test tube holder, place the test tube in a boiling water bath. CAUTION! *Be sure that the mouth of the test tube is pointing away from you and from other students.*
3. After you see a color change, use a test tube holder to remove the test tube from the water bath and note the presence or absence of gas bubbles. Record your observations in the LABORATORY REPORT RESULTS at the end of the chapter.
4. Using a test tube holder, place the test tube in the rack to cool and then *clean it according to the directions of your laboratory instructor.*

Since decomposition reactions are exothermic, why did you have to heat the $CuCO_3$? __________

____

____

C. Exchange Reactions

Exchange reactions involve the exchange of one substance for another; they can be symbolized by the equation $AB + CD \rightarrow AD + CB$.

Lead nitrate ($Pb(NO_3)_2$) will combine with hydrochloric acid (HCl) to produce lead chloride ($PbCl_2$) and nitric acid (HNO_3) in the exchange reaction:

$$Pb(NO_3)_2 + 2HCl \rightarrow PbCl_2 + 2HNO_3$$

Lead chloride can be recognized by its yellow color; nitric acid is colorless.

MATERIALS

Pyrex or Kymex test tube
Two droppers

Glass rod

Lead nitrate ($Pb(NO_3)_2$) solution in dropper bottle

Hydrochloric acid (HCl) in dropper bottle

Safety goggles

Acid resistant or caustic resistant gloves

Laboratory apron or coat

PROCEDURE

1. Add a few drops of lead nitrate solution to a test tube.

2. CAUTION! *Using extreme care and acid or caustic resistant gloves,* carefully add a few drops of hydrochloric acid to the same test tube. *Gently* agitate the mixture with a glass rod.

3. Record the color of the end product in the LABORATORY REPORT RESULTS at the end of the chapter.

4. *Dispose of the contents of the test tube and clean your materials according to the directions of your laboratory instructor.*

What are the products formed in this reaction? ______________________________

____

What exchanges are made? ______________________________

____

D. Reversible Reactions

Reversible reactions are symbolized by the equation $A + B \rightleftharpoons AB$. The double arrows in the equation indicate that the reaction can proceed in either direction, that is, toward the production of product or toward the production of reactants.

The direction and rate of the reaction are functions of several factors:

1. ***The nature of the reactants.*** Some substances are more stable than others and hence, more energy is required to elicit a chemical change. In addition, the physical nature of the substance is a significant factor; generally, the greater the surface area, the greater the reaction rate.

2. ***Temperature.*** Only molecules of high kinetic energy are capable of entering into a chemical reaction to form a product. The minimum kinetic energy required for a reaction to occur is termed ***activation energy.*** The activation energy can be increased by increasing temperature; as a general rule, increasing the temperature 10°C doubles the rate of a chemical reaction. This 10°C temperature rise increases the collision frequency of reactant molecules only about 2%, but it raises the molecules to higher energy states so that they are able to react if a molecular collision occurs.

3. ***Presence of a catalyst.*** Catalysts are substances which increase the rate of chemical reactions without themselves undergoing a chemical change. Catalysts work by reducing the activation energy requirement of a reaction. In the body, catalysts are usually enzymes which accelerate the rate of a reaction without the need for an increase in temperature. Exercises which demonstrate enzymatic reactions are found in Chapter 19.

4. ***Concentration of reactants.*** An increase in the concentration of a reactant generally increases the reaction rate.

The four factors just mentioned are considered in ***Le Chatelier's*** (leh sha-teh-lā's) ***Principle,*** which states that as long as conditions remain constant, a system at equilibrium will remain stable. If a stress, such as a change in concentration or temperature, is applied to a system at equilibrium, the equilibrium will shift in a way that tends to undo the effects of the stress.

In the following exercise, you will observe a reaction at equilibrium and see how it is affected by changes in concentration and temperature. The reaction is:

$$CuSO_4 + 4KBr + Heat \rightleftharpoons K_2(CuBr_4) + K_2SO_4$$

An aqueous solution of copper (II) sulfate ($CuSO_4$) is blue; solutions of potassium bromide (KBr) and potassium sulfate (K_2SO_4) are colorless; the copper (II) bromide complex ($K_2(CuBr_4)$) is green in solution. A shift in equilibrium is indicated by a color change.

MATERIALS

Two Pyrex or Kymex test tubes

Wax marking pencil

Test tube rack

4 10 ml graduated cylinders

0.17 M copper (II) sulfate ($CuSO_4$)

Saturated aqueous potassium bromide (KBr)

Saturated aqueous potassium sulfate (K_2SO_4)
Boiling water bath (hot plate and beaker)
Safety goggles
Laboratory apron or coat

PROCEDURE

1. Label two test tubes "1" and "2" and place them in a test tube rack; add 5 ml of 0.17M copper (II) sulfate ($CuSO_4$) to each. Record the colors in the LABORATORY REPORT RESULTS at the end of the chapter.
2. Using clean graduated cylinders, add 2 ml of saturated aqueous potassium bromide (KBr) to test tube "1"; add 2 ml of water to test tube "2" for a color comparison.
3. Record the color of the two solutions in the LABORATORY REPORT RESULTS at the end of the chapter.
4. Using a clean graduated cylinder, add 2 ml of a saturated aqueous solution of potassium sulfate (K_2SO_4) to test tube "1" and 2 ml water to test tube "2." Record the color of the solutions in the LABORATORY REPORT RESULTS at the end of the chapter.
5. Heat the solution in test tube "1" by placing it in a boiling water bath. CAUTION! *Be sure that the mouth of the test tube is pointing away from you and from other persons.*
6. In the LABORATORY REPORT RESULTS at the end of the chapter, record the color of the solution after three minutes of heating and after cooling.
7. *Discard the solutions and clean your materials according to the directions of your laboratory instructor.*

Which reaction is exergonic? COOLED SOLUTION

In which direction does the addition of K_2SO_4 drive the reaction? LEFT

NEXT WEEK

EXERCISE 2. Acid-Base Balance

> OBJECTIVES
>
> To define an acid, base, and pH
> To measure pH
> To demonstrate the effect of buffers on pH

Acids are substances which increase the concentration of hydrogen ions (H^+) in solution. Since hydrogen ions are protons, acids are also defined as ***proton donors.*** In effect, these hydrogen ions do not exist individually because they are attracted to water molecules to form hydronium ions (H_3O^+). ***Bases*** are substances that increase the concentration of hydroxyl ions (OH^-) in aqueous solution; bases are also defined as ***proton acceptors***.

The degree of acidity or alkalinity (basicity) of a solution is measured as its ***pH.*** The pH scale is based on the number of H^+ ions in a solution expressed in chemical units called moles per liter (a ***mole*** is the molecular weight of a substance expressed in grams). Pure water has 10^{-7} moles of H^+ ions per liter and the same amount (10^{-7} moles) of OH^- ions per liter. The pH of pure water reflects its H^+ ion concentration of 10^{-7} or 0.0000001 moles of H^+/liter, and it is written as the positive expression of the exponent; that is, the pH of pure water is 7. A solution with more H^+ ions is more acidic and has a pH of less than 7, reflecting a smaller exponent; basic solutions have fewer H^+ ions (and more OH^- ions), so their pH will be greater than 7, reflecting the larger exponent.

A change of one number on the pH scale represents a tenfold change from the previous number; *i.e.*, a solution of pH 5 is ten times more acidic than one of pH 6. A change of two numbers reflects a 100-fold change; *i.e.*, a solution of pH 6 is 100 times less acidic than one of pH 4, and so forth. Table 3.1 is a visual depiction of the relationship of the pH scale to H^+ and OH^- concentrations.

Acids and bases are said to be strong if they easily ionize (separate into charged particles called ***ions***) and produce many H^+ or OH^- ions; weak acids and bases do not easily ionize and therefore have less effect on the pH.

The body must maintain a narrow pH range in order for normal functions to occur. The pH of arterial blood plasma, for example, is normally 7.40, although it may vary up to 0.05 pH units without untoward effects. Yet strong acids and bases are present which could raise and lower pH drastically, sending the body into ***acidosis*** (arterial plasma pH less than 7.35) or ***alkalosis*** (arterial plasma pH greater than 7.45). The body is able to maintain the normal pH of body fluids by the use of buffer systems.

TABLE 3.1
RELATIONSHIP OF pH SCALE TO RELATIVE CONCENTRATIONS OF HYDROGEN (H^+) AND HYDROXYL (OH^-) IONS, IN MOLES PER LITER

Concentration of H^+ Ions			pH		Concentration of OH^- Ions	
1.0	10^{0}		0		10^{-14}	0.00000000000001
0.1	10^{-1}		1		10^{-13}	0.0000000000001
0.01	10^{-2}		2		10^{-12}	0.000000000001
0.001	10^{-3}		3		10^{-11}	0.00000000001
0.0001	10^{-4}		4		10^{-10}	0.0000000001
0.00001	10^{-5}		5		10^{-9}	0.000000001
0.000001	10^{-6}		6		10^{-8}	0.00000001
0.0000001	10^{-7}	(Neutrality)	7	(Neutrality)	10^{-7}	0.0000001
0.00000001	10^{-8}		8		10^{-6}	0.000001
0.000000001	10^{-9}		9		10^{-5}	0.00001
0.0000000001	10^{-10}		10		10^{-4}	0.0001
0.00000000001	10^{-11}		11		10^{-3}	0.001
0.000000000001	10^{-12}		12		10^{-2}	0.01
0.0000000000001	10^{-13}		13		10^{-1}	0.1
0.00000000000001	10^{-14}		14		10^{0}	1.0

Buffer systems consist of pairs of substances that convert strong acids or bases into neutral substances or substances that are already part of the buffer system. The members of a buffer pair are a weak acid and a weak base. In effect, buffers minimize changes in pH. An example of a buffer system is the carbonic acid-sodium bicarbonate system. Carbonic acid (H_2CO_3) is a weak acid (proton donor); sodium bicarbonate ($NaHCO_3$) acts as a weak base (proton acceptor).

If a strong acid (for example, hydrochloric acid (HCl)) is added to this system, it is buffered by sodium bicarbonate in the following reaction:

$$HCl + NaHCO_3 \rightarrow NaCl + H_2CO_3$$

HCl	$NaHCO_3$	$NaCl$	H_2CO_3
Strong acid	Buffer	Salt	Weak acid

If a strong base (for example, sodium hydroxide, NaOH) is added to the system, it is buffered by carbonic acid in the following reaction:

$$NaOH + H_2CO_3 \rightarrow NaHCO_3 + H_2O$$

$NaOH$	H_2CO_3	$NaHCO_3$	H_2O
Strong base	Buffer	Salt	Weak base

This buffer system functions in both extracellular and intracellular body fluids; it is demonstrated in the following exercise.

MATERIALS

- pH meter
- Thermometer
- Three 250 ml beakers containing pH 7.0 buffer solution
- Distilled water in squeeze bottle
- Empty beaker
- Two 250 ml beakers each containing 100 ml distilled water
- 0.1 M HCl in dropper bottle
- 0.1 M NaOH in dropper bottle
- Magnetic mixer (optional)
- Safety goggles
- Laboratory apron or coat

PROCEDURE

1. Allow the pH meter to warm up by plugging it in and turning the switch to standby. Be sure that the electrode(s) are immersed in buffer.
2. Set the temperature control knob to room temperature.
3. Calibrate the instrument by placing the electrode(s) in a prepared pH 7 buffer solution and turning the switch to pH. Adjust the pH meter until the dial or digital readout reads 7.0.
4. Return the switch to standby and carefully remove the electrode(s) from the buffer solution. Do this by raising the bar which holds

the electrode(s); do not touch the electrode(s) with your hands.

5. Rinse the electrode(s) with distilled water from a squeeze bottle directed into an empty beaker.

6. Add one drop of 0.1 M HCl to a beaker containing 100 ml of distilled water, gently swirling the beaker or using a magnetic mixing bead to stir the contents. Record the pH in the LABORATORY REPORT RESULTS at the end of the chapter.

7. If necessary, continue adding HCl, one drop at a time, until the pH is 6.0. Record the number of drops required in the LABORATORY REPORT RESULTS at the end of the chapter.

8. Turn the switch to standby and remove the electrode(s) from the solution and rinse with distilled water. Check the pH of the buffer solution to see if the electrode(s) have been properly cleaned (the pH should register 7.0).

9. Immerse the electrode(s) in a beaker containing 100 ml of pH 7 buffer solution. Turn the switch to pH. Add 0.1 M HCl drop by drop, stirring gently after each addition. Record the number of drops required to change the pH one unit in the LABORATORY REPORT RESULTS at the end of the chapter.

10. Turn the switch to standby, remove the electrode(s) from the solution and rinse them with distilled water. Check the pH of the buffer solution to see if the electrode(s) have been properly cleaned (the pH should register 7.0).

11. Transfer the electrode(s) to a beaker containing 100 ml of distilled water. Add one drop of 0.1 M NaOH to the beaker, gently swirling the beaker or using a mixing bead to stir the contents.

12. If necessary, continue adding NaOH, one drop at a time, until the pH changes one unit. Record the number of drops required in the LABORATORY REPORT RESULTS at the end of the chapter.

13. Turn the switch to standby, remove the electrode(s) from the solution, and rinse them with distilled water. Check the pH of the buffer solution to see if the electrode(s) have been properly cleaned (the pH should register 7.0).

14. Immerse the electrode(s) in a beaker containing 100 ml of pH 7 buffer solution. Turn the switch to pH. Add 0.1 M NaOH drop by drop, stirring gently after each addition. Record the number of drops required to change the pH one unit in the LABORATORY REPORT RESULTS at the end of the chapter.

15. Turn the switch to standby and clean the electrode(s) with distilled water; immerse them in the buffer solution.

ALTERNATE PROCEDURE

Use narrow range pH paper in place of the pH meter, following the instructions on the container.

What can you conclude about the effect of buffers on pH changes? ____________________

____

COMPLETE THE LABORATORY REPORT QUESTIONS AT THE END OF THE CHAPTER

LABORATORY REPORT QUESTIONS

CHEMICAL PRINCIPLES 3

Student MARK CAVE Date 1-29-92

Laboratory Section ______ Score/Grade ______

PART I. MULTIPLE CHOICE

B 1. A solution with 10^{-9} hydrogen ions per liter is (a) neutral (b) basic (c) acidic (d) none of the above

D 2. If solution A has a pH of 10. 5, and solution B is 1000 times more acidic than solution A, what is the pH of solution B? (a) 6.5 (b) 9.5 (c) 10.2 (d) 7.5 (e) none of the above

C 3. Alkalosis is the condition in which the arterial blood plasma pH is (a) below 7.35 (b) below 7.45 (c) above 7.45 (d) above 7.0

C 4. If a strong base is added to a weak acid in a buffered solution, the result is (a) a strong acid and a weak base (b) a salt and a weak acid (c) a salt and a weak base (d) a weak base and water

D 5. A strong acid is one which (a) ionizes easily in solution (b) has a large number of hydrogen ions per molecule (c) is highly concentrated (d) all of the above

D 6. Which of the following is NOT one of the principal elements in the human body? (a) carbon (b) hydrogen (c) phosphorus (d) bromine (e) nitrogen

D 7. $A + B \rightleftharpoons AB$ is a symbol for (a) a synthesis reaction (b) a decomposition reaction (c) an exchange reaction (d) a reversible reaction

D 8. Decomposition reactions (a) can be symbolized by the equation $AB \rightarrow A + B$ (b) are also called catabolic reactions (c) are exergonic reactions (d) all of the above (e) none of the above

C 9. In the reversible reaction $AB \rightleftharpoons A + B$, the addition of B would result in (a) the production of more A (b) the depletion of substance AB (c) the production of more AB (d) the accumulation of B; concentration of A and AB would stay constant

C 10. A substance which decreases the activation energy requirement of a reaction is a/an (a) reactant (b) end product (c) catalyst (d) equilibrator

PART II. FILL-INS

11. EXERGONIC reactions are those in which the reactants have more energy than the end product.

12–15. Name four factors that affect the direction and rate of a reversible reaction.

1) NATURE OF THE REACTANTS
2) TEMPERATURE
3) PRESENCE OF CATALYST.
4) CONCENTRATION OF REACTANT.

16. The minimum kinetic energy required for a reaction to occur is called ACTIVATION ENERGY.

17. A hydrogen ion donor is a/an ACID OR PROTON DONOR

DISCUSSION: How do you think LeChatelier's Principle applies to pressure changes in a gaseous system?

MICROSCOPY 4

EXERCISE 1. Use of the Compound Microscope
- *A. Parts of the Microscope and Rules of Microscopy*
- *B. Techniques of Microscopy*
  - *1. The Dry Mount*
  - *2. Perceiving Depth*
  - *3. The Wet Mount*

EXERCISE 2. Microscopic Measurement
- *A. Magnification*
- *B. Field Size*

Microscopes are used to increase the apparent size of small objects. There are two basic kinds of microscopes: light microscopes and electron microscopes. In ***light microscopy*** (mī-KROS-kō-pē), light rays are focused by lenses and can magnify specimens about 1000 times (1000×). In ***electron microscopy***, beams of electrons are focused by electromagnets; magnification can be up to 200,000 times.

The light microscope that you will use most often in this course is the ***compound light microscope***, which uses two lenses to magnify objects. Since this microscope uses light from a source below the specimen, and since light cannot pass through thick or opaque objects, the light microscope can only be used to magnify thin specimens or thin sections of a specimen. Yet, since cells are about 70% water, they have few structures to limit the passage of light rays; therefore, stains are often needed to increase the contrast in such transparent structures.

The ***dissecting microscope*** is a light microscope used to view objects in three dimensions at low magnifications (about 2–5 times). The light source is usually directed onto the top of the specimen.

While the magnifying power of a microscope is important, the real limiting power of a microscopic system is its resolving power. The ***resolving power (resolution)*** of a microscope is its ability to distinguish two points as separate objects. In effect, it is the ability to distinguish fine detail and structure. The compound light microscope, with a maximum resolving power of about 0.2 micrometers (mī-KROM-e-ters), (0.2 μm)[1], can distinguish two points as separate objects if they are at least 0.2 μm apart. Objects closer to each other than 0.2 μm are seen as a single object because the images fuse. Even if magnified hundreds of times, such a fused image is no more than a very large blur.

Resolving power is a function of the wavelength of light; that is, it depends on the ability of light waves to pass between two objects. The shorter the wavelength, the greater the resolution. Thus, since blue light has a shorter wavelength than red light (400 vs. 700 nm), most light microscopes are fitted with blue filters to improve the resolving power slightly.

In order to see objects smaller than 0.3 μm, it is necessary to use an electron microscope with a higher resolving power. Such microscopes work by focusing a beam of electrons through a vacuum tube onto a specimen. Since the wavelength of electrons is about 0.5 nm, the resolving power is much greater than that of light microscopes (about 0.1^{-1} nm). All electron microscopy requires that specimens be

[1]Metric measurement is discussed in Chapter 2.

placed in a vacuum, so the microscope cannot be used to examine living structures.

There are two types of electron microscopes. The ***transmission electron microscope*** passes electrons through an ultra-thin section (50–100 nm thick, about 1/200 the thickness of a single cell) and is useful in providing details of the interior structure of cells.

The ***scanning electron microscope*** causes electrons to be emitted from the surface of a specimen which has been coated with a heavy metal. The shape of the specimen causes variations in the angle with which electrons strike and leave the specimen, giving a three-dimensional image that is useful for studying surface features (see Figure 2.1). The resolving power of the scanning electron microscope is about one-tenth as great as that of a transmission microscope and magnifications are typically in the range of 10,000 times.

EXERCISE 1. Use of the Compound Light Microscope

A. Parts of the Microscope and Rules of Microscopy

OBJECTIVES

To learn the parts of the compound light microscope and their functions

To learn the proper use and care of the compound light microscope.

It is mandatory that you understand and follow several basic rules when you use a microscope. They will make your work more efficient and will prevent damage to these expensive instruments.

1. *Always carry the microscope with two hands*, using one hand to support the base. Never carry two microscopes at once.

2. Place the microscope on the table, as far away from the edge as is comfortable for you. Make certain that the table is free from clutter.

3. Note the manner in which the electric cord has been stored so that you can rewind it in a similar way at the end of the laboratory period.

4. Locate the following parts of the microscope and after you read about each part, label Figure 4.1 by placing the correct numbers in the spaces next to the list of terms which accompanies the figure.

Base—the bottom support on which the microscope rests.

Arm—The angular or curved part of the frame.

Body tube—The structure which holds the ocular.

Ocular (eyepiece)—A removable lens at the top of the body tube which magnifies 5× or 10×. Oculars are sometimes fitted with a pointer or a measuring scale.

Inclination joint—A movable hinge which allows some microscopes to be tilted to a comfortable viewing position.

Stage—A platform on which slides or other objects to be viewed are placed. The opening in the center, called the ***stage opening***, allows light to pass through the object being examined. Some microscopes have a ***mechanical stage*** in which adjustor knobs move the slide in four directions. Mechanical stages allow for smooth, precise movement of a slide; they also are fitted with calibrations which permit the numerical "mapping" of a slide. If a microscope does not have a mechanical stage, it will be fitted with spring clips to hold a slide in place.

Substage lamp—The source of illumination for some light microscopes with a built-in lamp. Some microscopes have variable intensity lamps; if such a device is present, keep the voltage as low as possible.

Condenser—A lens below the stage which concentrates light onto the specimen. The condenser is raised and lowered by the condenser adjustment knob; it should usually be at the highest position where light is concentrated to the greatest degree. When the condenser is lowered, the resolving power of the microscope is reduced.

Diaphragm—A device located between the condenser and the stage which regulates the intensity of the light beam. Such regulation is needed because transparent specimens cannot be seen in bright light. There are two types of diaphragms. The ***iris diaphragm*** is composed of sliding leaves which are moved by the iris diaphragm lever in

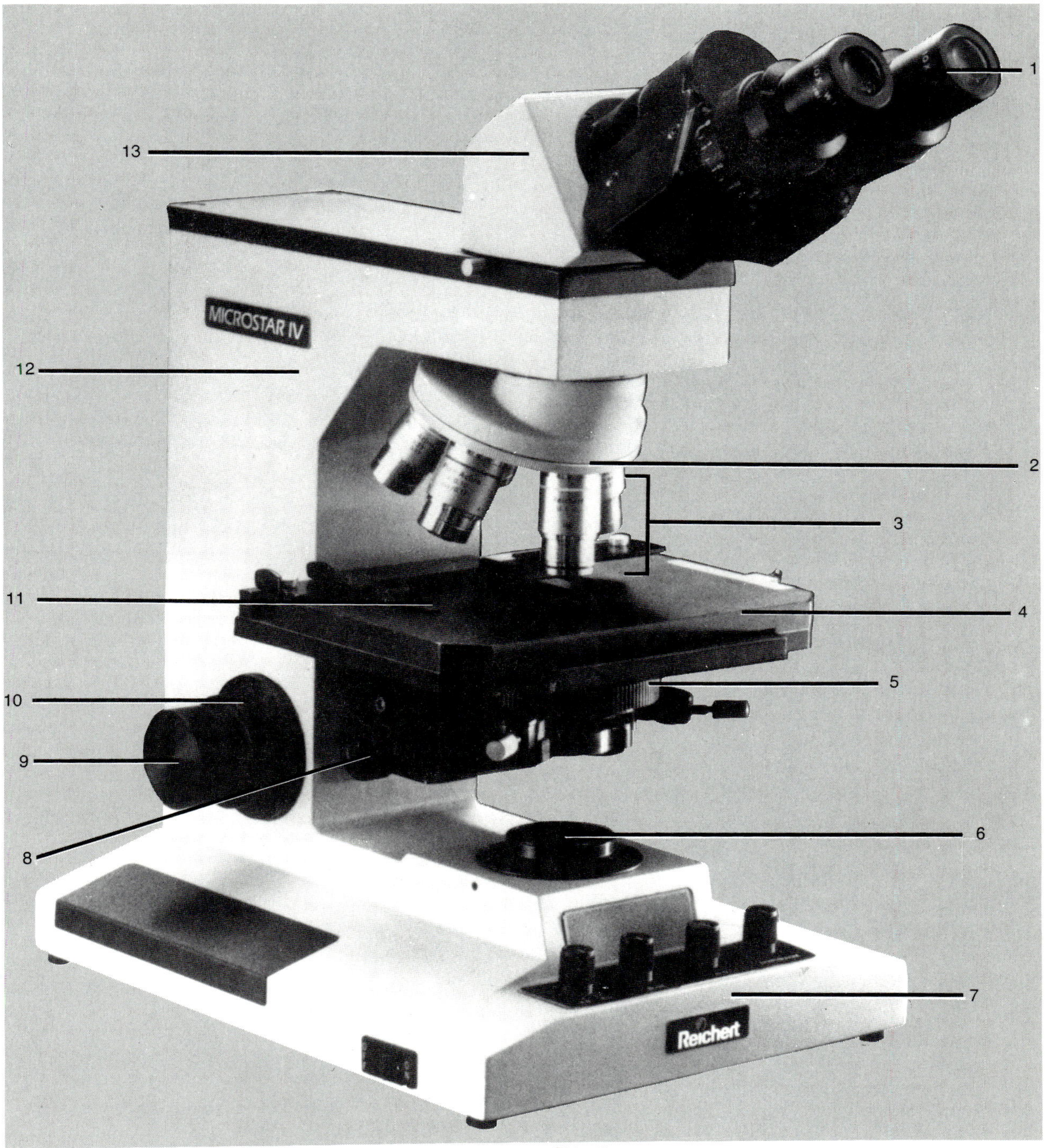

___ Arm
___ Base
___ Body tube
___ Coarse adjustment knob
___ Condenser
___ Diaphragm control lever
___ Fine adjustment knob
___ Objectives
___ Ocular
___ Revolving nosepiece
___ Stage
___ Stage clip of mechanical stage
___ Substage lamp

FIGURE 4.1 Photograph of a compound light microscope.

order to regulate the diameter of a central opening. The ***disc diaphragm*** is a plate with a series of holes of various sizes which can be rotated into position.

Coarse adjustment knob—A usually larger knob which raises and lowers the body tube to bring a specimen into view.

Fine adjustment knob—A usually smaller knob found below or external to the coarse adjustment knob which allows precise final focusing of a specimen.

Revolving nosepiece—The part of the microscope at the bottom of the body tube which contains the objectives and can be rotated to align each objective with the body tube.

Scanning objective—The shortest objective; it contains a lens, usually marked 4× or 5×. This objective is not present on all microscopes.

Low-power objective—The next shortest objective, containing a lens, usually marked 10×.

High-power objective—The second longest objective, containing a lens usually marked 43× or 45×. This is also called the ***high-dry objective***.

Oil-immersion objective—The longest objective, containing a lens usually marked 95× or 100× and distinguished by an etched colored circle.

5. Clean all parts of the microscope, especially the lenses, mirror, and condenser *with special lens paper. Never use paper towels or cloth, which will scratch the delicate glass surfaces.* When using lens paper, change the position of the paper as you wipe the lens, so as not to scratch the lens with the dust which adheres to the paper. If grease or immersion oil is present on the lens or ocular, remove it with cleaning alcohol on lens paper.

6. Do not permit the objectives to get wet, especially when observing a wet mount. *You must use a cover slip when you examine a wet mount* or the image will be distorted and the lens will become dirty.

7. Consult your instructor if any mechanical or optical difficulties arise. *Do not try to solve these problems yourself.*

8. Keep both eyes open at all times while observing objects through the microscope. This is difficult at first, but it becomes natural with practice. This important technique will help you observe and draw specimens without moving your head.

9. Always use the scanning or low-power objective first to locate an object; if necessary, then switch to a higher power.

10. *When using the high-power and oil-immersion objectives, never use the coarse adjustment knob to focus.* The distance between these objectives and the slide (the ***working distance***) is very small, and you may break the cover slip and slide and scratch the lens if you focus improperly.

11. When looking through the microscope, *never focus downward.* If downward focus is necessary, observe the slide and objective from the side while focusing to see that the objectives do not make contact with the cover slip or slide.

12. Raise the body tube before placing a slide on the stage or removing a slide.

13. When you are finished using the microscope,

a. Remove slides from the stage.

b. Clean the ocular and lenses with lens paper.

c. Align the mechanical stage so that it does not protrude.

d. Leave the scanning or low-power objective in place.

e. Wrap the cord according to your instructor's directions.

f. Replace the dust cover or place the microscope in a cabinet.

Name two parts of the microscope which affect the amount of light transmitted through the specimen. ____________ and ____________

Why must you avoid focusing downward?

____

____

B. Techniques of Microscopy

OBJECTIVE

To learn basic procedures in microscopy

To begin looking at a specimen, use the following procedure:

1. *After reviewing the rules of microscopy*, place the microscope in a comfortable position for viewing.

2. Make sure the low-power objective is positioned in line with the body tube; it will click as it moves into the proper position. Set the objective about one-quarter inch above the stage.

3. Make sure the condenser is in its highest position, and adjust the diaphragm until it admits the maximum amount of light.

4. Place your eye to the ocular and adjust the light until a uniform field (the microscopic field) appears without any shadows.

1. The Dry Mount

> OBJECTIVES
>
> To learn the techniques of scanning and changing magnification
>
> To compare the orientation of the specimen as seen with the unaided eye with the orientation of the microscopic image

MATERIALS

- Compound light microscope
- Lens paper
- Prepared slide of the letter "e"
- Xylol or other cleaning alcohol
- Immersion oil

PROCEDURE

For zoom microscopes, follow the instructions below, substituting the italicized portions for the numbered sections with asterisks (*).

1. Obtain a prepared slide of the letter "e" and observe it with the unaided eye. Draw its orientation on the slide in the sketch below.

*2. Align the low-power objective with the body tube until a click is heard. *(*Move the knurled knob to the setting with the lowest number, usually 100.)*

3. Place the slide on the stage and center the letter over the stage opening. Secure the slide with the stage clip(s).

4. While watching from the side, use the coarse adjustment knob to lower the body tube as far as it will go without touching the slide.

5. While looking through the ocular, turn the coarse adjustment counterclockwise, thereby raising the body tube. Watch for the image to appear suddenly in the microscopic field. If you have difficulty finding the specimen, move the slide to center the specimen more accurately.

6. Use the fine adjustment to complete the precise focusing.

7. Compare the orientation of the letter as originally seen with the unaided eye with its appearance under the microscope.

Has its orientation changed? ____ Draw the appearance of the letter as seen under low-power in the LABORATORY REPORT RESULTS at the end of the chapter.

8. While looking through the ocular, change the position of the slide by using the mechanical stage knobs or your thumbs.

In which direction does the letter move when you move the slide to your left? ____________

In which direction does the letter move when you move the slide toward you? ____________

9. Change your magnification from low power to high power by carrying out the following steps:

a. Place the letter in the center of the microscopic field under low power. Centering is important because field size decreases with higher magnifications. If the specimen is not centered, it will not appear in the smaller field.

b. Make sure the illumination is at its maximum. Illumination must be increased at higher magnifications because the amount of light entering the lens decreases at higher magnifications.

*c. Revolve the nosepiece so that the high-power objective clicks into place. Since most microscopes are ***parfocal*** (meaning that when clear focus has been attained with any objective, other objectives will give a change in magnification while still keeping the specimen in focus), you should be able to see a smaller portion of the specimen clearly. If it is not completely in focus, a slight turn of the fine adjustment knob should bring it into clear focus.

If your microscope is not parfocal, observe the stage from the side and carefully switch the high-power objective in line with the body tube. While still observing from the side, carefully lower the objective until it almost touches the slide by using the coarse adjustment knob. Look through the ocular and focus up slowly. Finish focusing with the fine adjustment knob. *(*Move the knurled knob up to 500 times.)*

d. In the LABORATORY REPORT RESULTS at the end of the chapter, draw the appearance of the letter as seen through the high-power objective.

*10. After reading this section, change your objective from high-dry to oil-immersion. *(*This step is not possible with zoom microscopes.)* Because the microscopic field is much smaller with the oil-immersion objective, the amount of light that enters the field is also reduced. Consequently, it is important that all available light is utilized and not lost.

When light passes from one medium to another (from water to air, for example), light rays are bent or refracted. This phenomenon is apparent when you observe the apparent bending of a straight drinking straw in a glass of water. The ***refractive index*** of a substance determines the extent to which light rays are bent. When light passes through a glass slide (and specimen) to air, the light rays are refracted so that light is lost (Figure 4.2).

Immersion oil has a refractive index similar to that of glass; you can see this by trying to find the glass rod in a full bottle of immersion oil. Because the refractive indices of glass and this oil are similar, light rays that pass from glass into immersion oil are not bent but pass directly to the objective lens (Figure 4.2).

To use the oil-immersion objective, follow these instructions:

a. After centering the specimen, move the high-dry objective to the side and place a drop of immersion oil onto the slide directly over the specimen.

b. Click the oil-immersion objective into place.

c. Use the fine adjustment knob to give precise focus. This objective is extremely close to the slide, so when it is in position, *be careful never to focus downward while you are looking through the ocular.*

d. In the LABORATORY REPORT RESULTS at the end of the chapter, draw the letter "e" as it looks under oil immersion.

e. Whenever you finish using immersion oil, blot the slide and objective with lens paper to remove most of the oil. Then apply some cleaning alcohol to a clean piece of lens paper and wipe the objective carefully. Use another piece of lens paper to wipe the lens. If oil appears on the

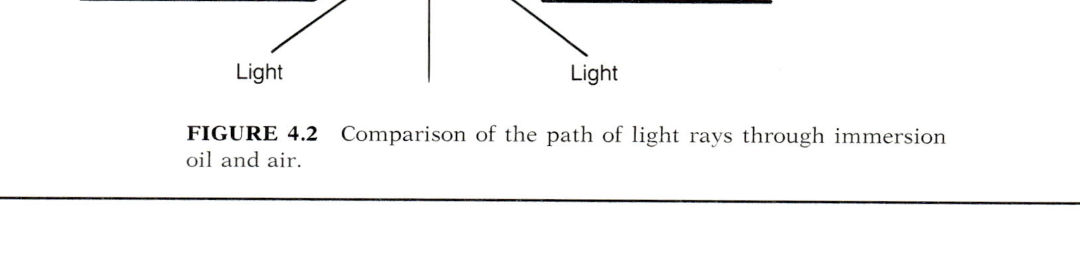

FIGURE 4.2 Comparison of the path of light rays through immersion oil and air.

lens paper, use more cleaning alcohol on a clean piece of lens paper. Clean the slide in the same manner.

Is as much of the specimen visible under high power as under low power? Explain. ________

____

2. Perceiving Depth

> OBJECTIVE
>
> To determine the relative depth of specimens on a slide

Microscopic specimens have depth as well as length and width. It is possible to focus on different depths of a specimen and determine which structures lie beneath others; this technique is important in determining the three-dimensional structure of a specimen. At lower magnifications, the amount of a specimen that is clearly in focus, that is, the depth of field, is greater than it is at higher magnifications. In this exercise, you will determine how three overlapping differently colored threads are oriented on a slide.

MATERIALS

Compound light microscope

Lens paper

Slide of three crossed differently colored threads

PROCEDURE

1. Obtain a slide of crossed threads and view them with the unaided eye. Is it possible to determine which thread lies on top, in the middle and on the bottom of the preparation? ____

2. Using the low-power objective, focus on the portion of the slide where the three threads cross.

3. Using the coarse adjustment, *slowly and carefully* focus until all three threads in the area of crossing are in blurred focus.

4. Slowly focus upward until the first thread comes into clear focus. What is its color?

____

5. Using the fine adjustment, focus upward on the middle and upper threads. Which thread comes into clear focus next? ____________
Record your results in the LABORATORY REPORT RESULTS at the end of the chapter.

6. Repeat this procedure with high-power magnification. At which magnification is it easier to determine the orientation of the threads?

____

3. The Wet Mount

> OBJECTIVES
>
> To prepare and examine a wet mount of living material
>
> To perform a simple staining procedure

The internal structures of living cells generally offer little contrast, making it difficult to view them without the use of a stain. Fortunately, various parts of a cell form complexes with specific stains, thereby differentiating them from each other and from the background material in the cell itself.

Since a liquid stain (or other solution) can damage the objective lens and also distort the image, it is necessary to cover the wet specimen with a cover slip.

MATERIALS

Two flat toothpicks

Two glass microscope slides

1% methylene blue in dropper bottle

Absorbent towel

Forceps

Cover slip

Microscope

Lens paper

PROCEDURE

1. Obtain two clean glass microscope slides; place one drop of 1% methylene blue in the center of one of them.

2. *Gently* scrape the inside of your cheek with the flat side of a toothpick. Smear the cells that you obtain onto the dry slide. Let the preparation dry as you perform steps 3 and 4.

3. Repeat the cheek scraping and mix the cells with the toothpick in the drop of methylene blue solution.

4. Hold the cover slip at a 45 degree angle to the slide as shown in Figure 4.3. Using a forceps, gently lower it into place. If there is any excess liquid on the sides of the cover slip, remove it with absorbent tissue or paper towel.

5. Examine the slide of unstained cells under low power and high-dry power. If you make a mistake and touch an objective lens to the slide, ask your instructor for the procedure to clean it. Draw the appearance of the cells in the LABORATORY REPORT RESULTS at the end of the chapter.

6. Examine the stained cells under low power and high power. It may be necessary to reduce the light. Draw the appearance of the cells in the LABORATORY REPORT RESULTS at the end of the chapter. If you see the sharp outline of a dark circle, you have trapped an air bubble beneath the cover slip.

How is the appearance of the stained cells different from that of the unstained cells? ______

______

______

EXERCISE 2: Microscopic Measurement

In all forms of microscopy it is important to be aware of the degree to which a specimen is magnified and the diameter of the microscopic field.

A. Magnification

> OBJECTIVE
>
> To calculate the magnification of various combinations of ocular and objective lenses

Magnification depends on the degree of curvature of the lens. A highly curved lens magnifies more than a flatter lens. Because the diameter of a lens decreases as it becomes more curved, lenses become smaller as their magnifying power increases. The diameter of the lens in millimeters is etched on each objective.

The total magnification of a microscope is determined by multiplying the magnification of the ocular lens by the magnification of the objective lens that is used. For example, an ocular of 10× used with an objective of 5× gives a total magnification of 50×.

Zoom microscopes bear numbers on a knurled knob which give a reading of the total magnification at any setting.

If you are not using a zoom microscope, calculate the total magnification for the use of each of the objectives on your microscope.

1. Ocular ____ × Objective ____ = ____
2. Ocular ____ × Objective ____ = ____
3. Ocular ____ × Objective ____ = ____
4. Ocular ____ × Objective ____ = ____

B. Field Size

> OBJECTIVE
>
> To measure the field size at various magnifications

In Exercise 1, you saw that the size of the microscopic field decreases with higher magnification. It is important to determine the exact size of each field so that you can estimate the size of the structures that occupy that field.

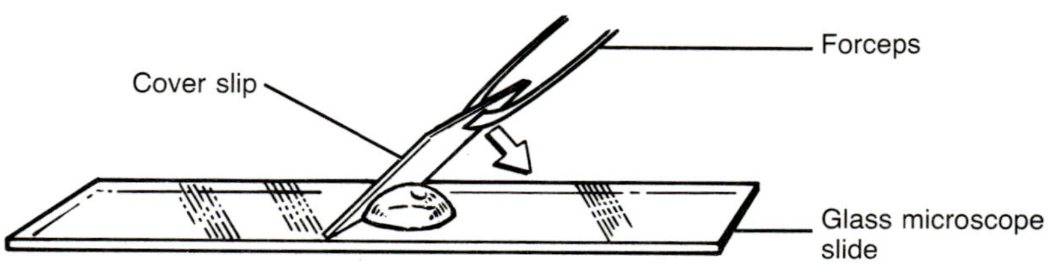

FIGURE 4.3 Placement of a cover slip on a wet mount.

MATERIALS

Measuring device
Compound light microscope
Lens paper

PROCEDURE

1. Obtain one of the following items:

   a. A micrometer slide or stage micrometer that has lines etched 0.01 mm apart.

   b. A millimeter ruler.

   c. A slide of graph paper that has been ruled in millimeters.

2. Using low power, focus on the measure so that one line abuts the left-hand side of the field.
3. Count the lines visible on the diameter of the field. Estimate any portion of a division seen at the right-hand side of the field.
4. Record this distance in the LABORATORY REPORT RESULTS at the end of the chapter.
5. Calculate the diameter of the microscopic fields using the other objectives by the following formula:

$$\frac{\text{Magnification of high-power objective}}{\text{Magnification of low-power objective}} = \text{Differential value}$$

$$\frac{\text{Diameter of low-power field}}{\text{Differential value}} = \text{Diameter of high-power field}$$

EXAMPLE: If high-power magnification is 500× and low-power magnification is 100× and the diameter of the low-power field is 2.5 mm, then:

$$\frac{500\times}{100\times} = 5$$

$$\frac{2.5\text{ mm}}{5} = 0.5\text{ mm (diameter of 500× field)}$$

Record your calculations in the LABORATORY REPORT RESULTS at the end of the chapter.

If an object occupies one-quarter the diameter of the low-power field described in the example above, what is its actual width? ________

Could you see all of this object at 500×? ____

COMPLETE THE LABORATORY REPORT QUESTIONS AT THE END OF THE CHAPTER

TRANSPORT ACROSS PLASMA MEMBRANES 5

EX. 2 A) DO ALL
B) DO ALL
C) DEMOSTRATION!

(NOTE) TURN IN QUESTIONS.

EX. 4 A) DEMONSTATION!
B) DEMONSTRATION
C) DO ALL

EXERCISE 1. Brownian Movement
EXERCISE 2. Diffusion: A Passive Process
A. Diffusion of a Solid in a Liquid
B. Diffusion through a Solid
C. Diffusion through a Membrane
EXERCISE 3. Dialysis: A Passive Process
EXERCISE 4. Osmosis: A Passive Process
A. Osmosis through an Artificial Membrane
B. Osmosis through a Natural Membrane
C. Osmosis through a Living Membrane
EXERCISE 5. Filtration: A Passive Process
EXERCISE 6. Active Transport: An Active Process
EXERCISE 7. Endocytosis: An Active Process

WORD ROOTS

cyto- = cell
diffus- = spreading
hyper- = greater than
hypo- = less than
iso- = same
phago- = eating
pseudo- = false
-lysis = breaking
-osis = condition of
-podium, -pod = foot

In order for an organism to grow and maintain a relatively constant cellular environment, various materials must be transported into and out of cells across the plasma membrane. This transport can occur only if the substances are dissolved in a fluid medium. In the human body, this medium is water. Substances that dissolve (form a homogeneous dispersion) in water are termed ***soluble***; those that do not dissolve are referred to as ***insoluble***. The dispersion medium (water) is called the ***solvent***; the dissolved substance is known as the ***solute***.

Body water, which constitutes 45–75% of body weight, is located in two compartments: (1) within cells, where it is called ***intracellular fluid (ICF)***, and (2) outside cells, where it is known as ***extracellular fluid (ECF)***. These two fluid compartments contain very different concentrations of most solutes. Some of these differences in ionic concentration, expressed in milliequivalents (meq) per liter, are:

		Extracellular fluid	Intracellular fluid
Na^+	(sodium)	142 meq/liter	10 meq/liter
K^+	(potassium)	4 meq/liter	140 meq/liter
Mg^{2+}	(magnesium)	3 meq/liter	58 meq/liter
Cl^-	(chloride)	103 meq/liter	4 meq/liter

The maintenance of the differences in the solute concentrations of intracellular and extracellular fluid requires both energy and a means of moving substances across the plasma membrane.

Since the phospholipid bilayer and proteins that constitute the plasma membrane allow only some substances to pass through it, the membrane is called ***selectively (differentially) permeable***.

Substances move across plasma membranes by two major types of processes: passive and active. In ***passive (physical) processes*** substances move because of differences in concentration or pressure from an area of higher concentration or pressure to an area of lower concentration or pressure. The movement usually continues until an ***equilibrium*** or equal distribution of substances is reached. Passive processes are the result of the kinetic energy (energy of motion) of the substances themselves, and the cell does not have to expend energy (ATP) to move the substances. Examples of passive processes are filtration, diffusion, dialysis, and osmosis.

In ***active (physiological) processes*** substances may move against their concentration gradient, from areas of lower concentration to areas of higher concentration. In order to do so, cells must expend energy (ATP). Examples of active processes are active transport and endocytosis.

CAUTION! *Please reread Section A. "General Procedures and Safety Precautions" and Section C. "Precautions Related to Working With Reagents" in Chapter 1 before you begin any of the exercises in this chapter. Be sure to read the exercises before you perform them to be certain that you understand all of the procedures and safety precautions.*

EXERCISE 1. Brownian Movement

OBJECTIVE

To observe Brownian movement

At temperatures above absolute zero (−273°C or −460°F), all molecules are in constant random movement because of their inherent kinetic energy. This phenomenon, first noted by the botanist Robert Brown, is termed ***Brownian movement***. It requires less energy to move small molecules or particles than large ones. Thus, since all molecules are constantly bombarded by the molecules surrounding them, the smaller the particle, the greater its random motion in terms of speed and distance. Brownian movement is the key to understanding the principles involved in passive transport.

MATERIALS

Dropper bottle of dilute detergent solution
Dropper bottle of India ink diluted 1:10 with water
Depression slide
Cover slip
Forceps
Microscope
Toothpick
Hot plate
Safety goggles
Laboratory apron or coat

PROCEDURE

1. Place a drop of dilute detergent solution in the depression slide. Add a drop of dilute India ink.
2. Stir with a toothpick and cover with a cover slip. Place this preparation on the microscope stage and allow it to stand undisturbed for about ten minutes before observing it.
3. Observe under high power.
4. Using forceps, place the slide on a hot plate and warm it for 15 seconds. Remove the slide with forceps and observe again under high power.
5. Record your observations in the LABORATORY REPORT RESULTS at the end of the chapter.

Detergent reduces the surface tension of water.

Why was it used in this exercise? ____________

____

____

EXERCISE 2. Diffusion: A Passive Process

OBJECTIVES

To demonstrate diffusion through a liquid and through a solid
To demonstrate diffusion through membranes
To identify factors that affect the rate of diffusion

Diffusion is the movement of particles from an area of higher concentration to an area of lower concentration. It involves movement of both solute and solvent; it can occur through living membranes or artificial membranes or without membranes. The particles move randomly due to their kinetic energy (Brownian movement). ***Net diffusion*** occurs when there is a concentration difference within a system (a ***concentration gradient***), and it continues until an equilibrium is reached. After equilibration, diffusion continues because the particles are always in motion, but there is no net diffusion (change in concentration) when a concentration gradient does not exist.

The rate of diffusion is affected by the molecular size and concentration of the solute, the nature of the solvent, and the temperature. Gases, liquids, and solids may diffuse into gases, liquids, and solids. An example of diffusion in the body is the exchange of carbon dioxide (CO_2) and oxygen (O_2) between blood and other body tissues.

A. Diffusion of a Solid in a Liquid

MATERIALS

Petri dish or graduated cylinder
$KMnO_4$ (potassium permanganate) crystals
Forceps
Millimeter ruler
Safety goggles
Laboratory apron or coat

PROCEDURE

1. CAUTION! *Avoid contact of $KMnO_4$ with your skin. Using forceps, carefully* place a large crystal of $KMnO_4$ (potassium permanganate) into a petri dish or graduated cylinder filled with cold water.

2. Place the container against a light background where it will not be disturbed.

3. Measure the extent of diffusion with a millimeter ruler at 30 minute intervals. Calculate the diffusion of the crystal into the water in millimeters per minute.

4. Record these measurements and calculations in the LABORATORY REPORT RESULTS at the end of the chapter.

5. Repeat this procedure with hot water. Record these measurements and calculations in the LABORATORY REPORT RESULTS at the end of the chapter.

B. Diffusion through a Solid

MATERIALS

Petri dish filled with 1.5% agar
Cork borer
Four medicine droppers
Opaque cover
Millimeter rule
1M $AgNO_3$ (silver nitrate)
1M $K_3Fe(CN)_6$ (potassium ferricyanide)
1M NaCl (sodium chloride)
1M KBr (potassium bromide)
Safety goggles
Laboratory apron or coat

PROCEDURE

1. Take a petri dish filled with 1.5% agar. Using a cork borer, make four holes in the agar as indicated in Figure 5.1. Make each hole the same size and take care to avoid disturbing the agar. The distance from hole #1 to each of the other three holes must be indentical.

2. Select a portion of your laboratory table which will not be disturbed for the duration of the laboratory period and place the petri dish there. Do not move it from this point until the end of the laboratory period.

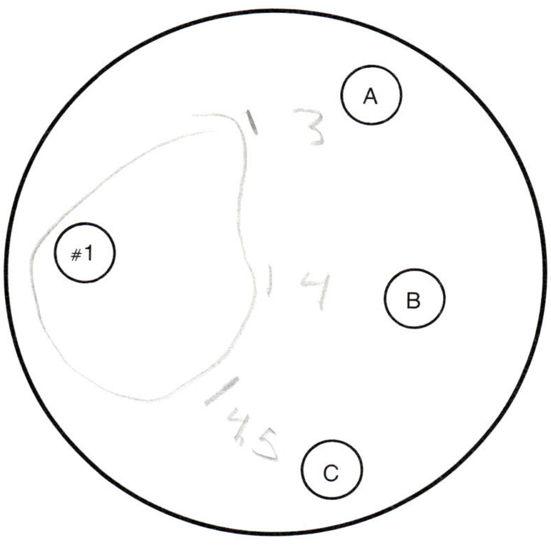

FIGURE 5.1 Diffusion through a solid (agar).

3. CAUTION! *Working carefully to avoid spilling or touching the solutions*, fill each hole to a level just below the surface of the agar with the following solutions. Use a *separate* medicine dropper for each solution.

Hole #1: 1M $AgNO_3$ (silver nitrate)

Hole A: 1M $K_3Fe(CN)_6$ (potassium ferricyanide)

Hole B: 1M NaCl (sodium chloride)

Hole C: 1M KBr (potassium bromide)

4. Cover the petri dish with an opaque box top or with aluminum foil to avoid the destruction of the products by light. Check it every half hour until you can see colored precipitates.

5. Silver ions are precipitated by cyanide, chloride, and bromide ions to yield products that are white and yellow. Measure the distance between holes A, B, and C and the colored precipitate which has formed in the space between these holes and hole #1.

6. Record these distances in the LABORATORY REPORT RESULTS at the end of the chapter.

Given the following molecular weights (KI [potassium iodide] = 166, KBr [potassium bromide] = 109), would you expect silver iodide to precipitate nearer to or farther from hole #1 than the region where silver bromide precipitates? ______________________

C. Diffusion through a Membrane

MATERIALS

Beaker
Distilled water
Five 7" pieces of dialysis tubing
Dialysis clamps or twist ties
Sponge
Basin
Medicine dropper
Dropper bottle of .05M $K_4Fe(CN)_6$ (potassium ferrocyanide)
Dropper bottle of .05M $FeCl_3$ (ferric chloride)
Lamp
Disposable gloves
Graduated cylinder less than 1" in diameter
Safety goggles
Laboratory apron or coat

PROCEDURE

1. Immerse five pieces of cellophane dialysis tubing about seven inches long in a beaker of distilled water for one to two minutes.

2. Tie *one* end of each tube tightly.

3. Wet a flat sponge or other absorbent material of light color and place it in a laboratory basin. Locate the basin so that it will not be disturbed for the remainder of the laboratory period.

4. Open three dialysis tubes by rubbing the open end between the thumb and forefinger.

5. Fill the tubes two-thirds full with distilled water using the following method: place the tied end of the tubing into a graduated cylinder; fold the open end around the top of the graduated cylinder and hold it in place while you fill the tubing with a medicine dropper; leave about one and a half inches of the tubing unfilled.

6. Close the dialysis tubing by forcing the air out of it and fastening the end with a dialysis clamp or a twist tie.

7. As indicated in Figure 5.2, place the three tubes adjacent to each other in the center of the sponge. Make sure that the tubes touch each other along their lengths.

8. CAUTION! *Wear disposable gloves while performing this step*. Using the method given in step 5, fill another prepared tube with .05M $K_4Fe(CN)_6$ (potassium ferrocyanide), a poison. Rinse the tube in running water and place it immediately next to the tube of water on the right.

9. *NOTE*: *Wash your hands thoroughly before proceeding*.

10. Using the method given in step 5, fill the last tube with .05M $FeCl_3$ (ferric chloride) and place it immediately next to the tube of water on the left.

11. Make sure that all five tubes are adjacent to each other along their lengths. If they tend to separate, brace them with beakers filled with water.

12. One half of the class should leave the setup undisturbed and observe it after one hour.

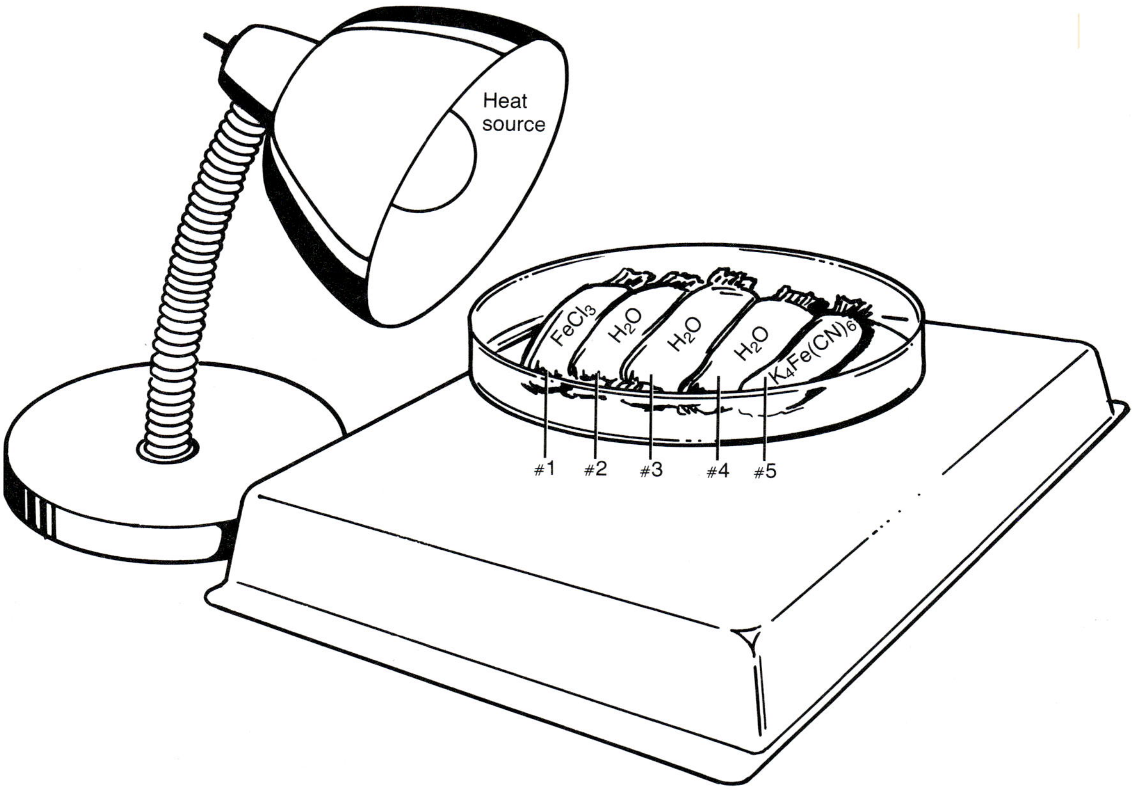

FIGURE 5.2 Diffusion through adjacent membranes.

The other half of the class should place a heat source, such as a lamp, at the left side of the set-up and also observe it after one hour. Each student should observe both versions of this exercise.

13. Ferric ions react with hexacyanoferrate ions to form an insoluble precipitate, Prussian blue. Note where this precipitate is formed and record your results in the LABORATORY REPORT RESULTS at the end of the chapter.

14. CAUTION! *When you are finished, rinse the basin and absorbent material and follow your instructor's directions for the disposal of the potassium ferrocyanide.*

In which bag would the precipitate form if the heat source were on the top or bottom of the set-up? ______________________

Why doesn't the Prussian blue diffuse into the adjacent bags? ______________________

____

EXERCISE 3. Dialysis: A Passive Process

OBJECTIVE

To demonstrate dialysis
To determine which of a group of substances is capable of dialysis

Dialysis (dī-AL-i-sis) is the separation of smaller molecules from larger ones through a selectively (differentially) permeable membrane that permits diffusion of the smaller molecules but not the larger ones. The principle of dialysis is employed in artificial kidneys.

MATERIALS

One piece of dialysis tubing
Two beakers
Distilled water

Two dialysis clamps (optional)
Beaker of starch, NaCl, glucose, and albumin solution
Glass rod
String
Dropper bottle of concentrated nitric acid
Beaker of Benedict's solution
Dropper bottle of Lugol's solution
Dropper bottle of 1% silver nitrate
Five graduated cylinders
Four Pyrex or Kimex test tubes
Test tube holder
Test tube rack
Boiling water bath (hot plate and beaker)
Caustic or acid resistant gloves
Safety goggles
Laboratory apron or coat

PROCEDURE

1. Refer to the dialysis apparatus shown in Figure 5.3.

2. Soak a piece of dialysis tubing in water for one to two minutes. Tie off one end of the tubing tightly or use a dialysis clamp to close it.

3. Open the other end of the tubing by rubbing it between the thumb and forefinger and pour into it a prepared solution containing starch, NaCl, glucose, and albumin until it is about two-thirds full.

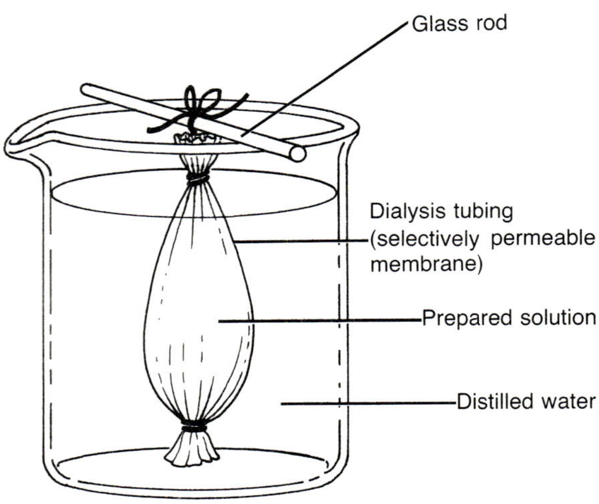

FIGURE 5.3 Dialysis apparatatus.

4. Close the tubing with a dialysis clamp or press out the air and tie it tightly.

5. Tie the tubing to a glass rod and immerse the tubing in a beaker of distilled water.

6. After one hour, test the solution in the beaker for the presence of each of the substances in the tubing, as follows:

a. ***Albumin***—Using a graduated cylinder, place about 2 ml of the solution in the beaker into a test tube. CAUTION! *Using caustic or acid resistant gloves, carefully* add several drops of concentrated nitric acid. A white coagulate is positive for the presence of albumin. *Be careful using nitric acid; it can damage the skin severely. If it does touch your skin or eyes, immediately flush the area with cold water for several minutes and then seek immediate medical attention.*

b. ***Sugar***—Using a graduated cylinder, place about 5 ml of the solution in the beaker into a test tube and add about 5 ml of Benedict's solution. Using a test tube holder, place the test tube into a boiling water bath for three minutes. CAUTION! *Make sure the mouth of the test tube is pointed away from you and all persons in the area.* A green, yellow, orange, or red precipitate is positive for the presence of sugar.

c. ***Starch***—Using a graduated cylinder, place about 2 ml of the solution in the beaker into a test tube and add several drops of Lugol's solution. A blue-black color is positive for the presence of starch.

d. ***Sodium chloride***—Using a graduated cylinder, place about 2 ml of the solution in the beaker into a test tube and add several drops of 1% silver nitrate. If sodium chloride is present in the beaker solution, a white precipitate of silver chloride will be apparent in the test tube.

7. Record your results in the LABORATORY REPORT RESULTS at the end of the chapter.

What can you conclude about the comparative particle size of the substances in the dialysis tubing? ______________________________

____

____

____

EXERCISE 4. Osmosis: A Passive Process

OBJECTIVES

To demonstrate osmosis and osmotic pressure

To determine the characteristics of a solute which affect the rate of osmosis

In the body, ***osmosis*** is the net movement of water through a selectively permeable membrane from an area of higher water (lower solute) concentration to an area of lower water (higher solute) concentration. The force of the water movement across the membrane is called ***osmotic pressure***. Water moves in and out of cells by osmosis.

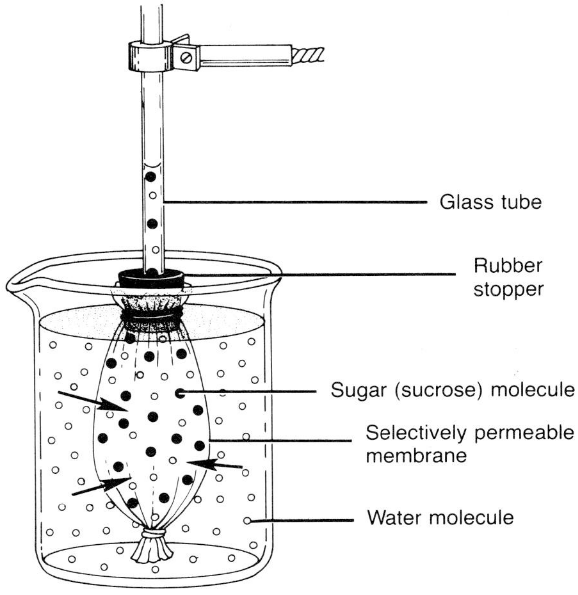

FIGURE 5.4 Osmosis apparatus.

A. Osmosis through an Artificial Membrane

MATERIALS

- Ring stand and clamp
- Glass tube
- Rubber stopper
- Dialysis tubing
- Dialysis clamp (optional)
- 500 ml beaker
- String
- 20% sucrose solution
- 5% sucrose solution
- Congo red
- Graduated cylinder
- Wax pencil
- Millimeter rule
- Safety goggles
- Laboratory apron or coat

PROCEDURE

1. Refer to the apparatus shown in Figure 5.4.
2. Tie a tight knot at one end of a piece of dialysis tubing (or use a dialysis clamp) which has been soaking in water for a few minutes.
3. One-half the class should fill the dialysis tubing with a 20% sucrose solution which has been colored with Congo red (or with food coloring). The other half of the class should fill the dialysis tubing with a 5% sucrose solution which has also been colored in the same manner.
4. Obtain a one-hole rubber stopper into which a glass tube has already been inserted by a laboratory assistant or your instructor.

CAUTION! *Do not attempt to insert the glass tube yourself since it may break and result in serious injury.*

5. Secure the filled dialysis tubing to the rubber stopper by tying it tightly with string.
6. Secure and suspend the glass tube by means of a clamp attached to a ring stand.
7. Immerse the dialysis tubing in a beaker of water until the water is at the level of the bottom of the rubber stopper.
8. As soon as the colored solution becomes visible in the glass tube, note the time. TIME: __________
9. With a wax pencil, mark the height of the liquid on the glass tube at 15, 30, 45, 60, 75, and 90 minutes.
10. Measure the distances and record them in the LABORATORY REPORT RESULTS at

the end of the chapter. Each student should observe both variations of this exercise.

Since the solution within the dialysis tubing will always contain more solute than water, why won't 100% of the water leave the beaker? (Hint: the weight of the water in the glass tube exerts hydrostatic pressure.) ______________

____

____

____

Would you have obtained the same results with 20% and 5% NaCl solutions? Explain.

____

____

____

B. Osmosis through a Natural Membrane*

Soaking eggs in vinegar (which is 4% by volume acetic acid) for 48–72 hours decalcifies the shells by removing the minerals. However, this process leaves the collagen fibers of the shell intact. Beneath the soft shell remains a selectively permeable membrane (the chorion) which encases the egg white.

MATERIALS

- Five decalcified eggs
- Paper towels
- Balance
- Four beakers
- 0.5M glucose solution
- 1.0M glucose solution
- 1.5M glucose solution
- 2.5M glucose solution
- Safety goggles
- Laboratory apron or coat

PROCEDURE

1. Wash the eggs and blot them on a paper towel. Handle them carefully and record their initial weights in the LABORATORY REPORT RESULTS at the end of the chapter.

2. Submerge one egg in distilled water, one in 0.5M glucose, one in 1.0M glucose, one in 1.5M glucose, and one in 2.5M glucose.

3. After 60–90 minutes, gently blot the eggs on paper toweling and reweigh them. Record the weights in the LABORATORY REPORT RESULTS at the end of the chapter.

4. Calculate the percent weight change for each egg by the following formula:

percent weight change =

$$\frac{(\text{post-immersion wt.} - \text{initial wt.})}{\text{initial weight}} \times 100$$

If water has entered the egg, the percent weight change will be positive; if water has left the egg, the percent weight change will be negative. A percent weight change of zero indicates that no *net* flow of water has occurred.

5. Record the percent weight change in the LABORATORY REPORT RESULTS at the end of the chapter.

At approximately what molarity do you think the percent weight change would be zero? Why? ______________

____

____

C. Osmosis through a Living Membrane

Osmosis can be demonstrated through the plasma membranes which surround red blood cells. The solution within red blood cells has an osmotic pressure which is the same as that of a solution of 0.90% NaCl. 0.90% NaCl is said to be ***isotonic*** to red blood cells, meaning that the two solutions have the same osmotic pressure. When placed in an isotonic solution, red blood cells retain their shape because there is no concentration gradient and thus, no net movement of water.

If red blood cells are placed in a ***hypotonic solution*** (one with a solute concentration which is less than that of 0.90% NaCl), a net movement of water into the cells occurs, causing them to swell or even to burst, since the plasma membranes are fragile. This rupture of red blood cells and the consequent liberation of hemoglobin is called ***hemolysis*** (hē-MOL-i-sis).

If red blood cells are placed in a ***hypertonic solution*** (one with a solute concentration

*This exercise was suggested by Barbara Cocanour and Alease S. Bruce, "Osmosis and the Marvelous Membrane," *Journal of College Science Teaching*, 1985, 15(2): 127–130.

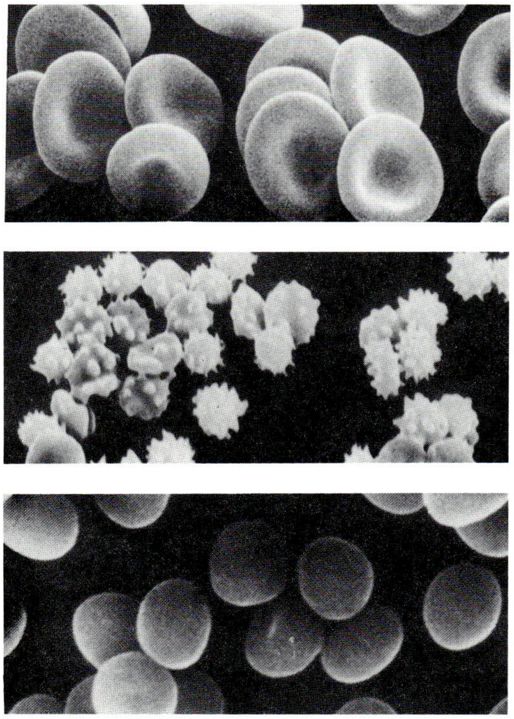

FIGURE 5.5 Scanning micrographs of red blood cells in: (a) An isotonic solution; (b) A hypertonic solution causing crenation; (c) A hypotonic solution causing the cells to swell.

greater than that of 0.90% NaCl), a net movement of water out of the cells occurs, causing them to shrink. This shrinkage is called ***crenation*** (krē-NĀ-shun). Scanning micrographs of red blood cells in solutions of different osmotic pressures are shown in Figure 5.5.

MATERIALS

Four microscope slides
Wax marking pencil
Fresh uncoagulated ox blood
Microscope
Three cover slips
Medicine dropper
Distilled water
0.90% NaCl solution in dropper bottle
5.0% NaCl solution in dropper bottle
Distilled water
Three toothpicks
Fresh 10% solution of household bleach
Safety goggles
Laboratory apron or coat
Latex gloves

PROCEDURE

CAUTION! *Please reread Section B, "Precautions Related to Working With Blood, Other Body Fluids, or Blood Products," in Chapter 1 before you begin the following exercise.*

1. When working with blood in this experiment, wear latex gloves. With a wax marking pencil, mark three microscope slides "DW" (distilled water), "0.90%," and "5%."
2. On the appropriately marked slides, place one drop of distilled water, one drop of 0.90% NaCl, and one drop of 5.0% NaCl.
3. Using a medicine dropper, place one small drop of fresh uncoagulated ox blood on each of the three microscope slides.
4. Dip a toothpick in the blood and quickly swirl it in the 5% NaCl solution. Mix gently and thoroughly. Repeat *with a clean toothpick* and swirl in the 0.90% NaCl. Repeat *with another clean toothpick* and swirl in the distilled water.
5. Cover each of the preparations with a cover slip.
6. Examine the slide marked "DW" under high power on the microscope. Reduce the illumination for clarity.
7. Examine the slide marked "0.90%" next, and then examine the slide marked "5%."
8. Record your observations in the LABORATORY REPORT RESULTS at the end of the chapter.
9. *When you finish this part of the exercise, place the toothpicks, microscope slides, and cover slips in a fresh bleach solution.*

Do you think the rate of osmosis would be increased if the surface area of the cell were increased? ______________________

Why? ______________________

____

____

Osmotic pressure is generated by the number of solute particles in solution. In water, electrolytes such as NaCl dissociate into two charged particles (ions). Nonelectrolytes such as glucose do not dissociate in water. Would a concentration of glucose isotonic to red blood cells be greater or less than 0.90%? ________

EXERCISE 5. Filtration: A Passive Process

OBJECTIVES
To demonstrate filtration To determine the factors which affect filtration

Filtration is the movement of solutes and solvent across a selectively permeable membrane from an area of higher mechanical pressure to an area of lower mechanical pressure. In the body, the solvent is water, and the pressure is the result of two forces. The first is the hydrostatic pressure of blood and body fluids; the second is the hydrostatic pressure due to gravity and blood pressure.

The rate of filtration is a function of the particle size of the solvent and solute, the pore size of the membrane, and the pore density (number of pores per unit area of the membrane). Filtration is one mechanism by which the kidneys regulate the chemical composition of blood. Urine is produced when water and solutes are filtered out of small blood vessels in the kidney into kidney tubules. This process is largely the result of the difference between the hydrostatic pressure of the blood and that of the tubules.

In this exercise, three solutes will be used: copper sulfate ($CuSO_4$), starch, and charcoal. Copper sulfate is a crystalloid (particle size with diameter <.001 micra); starch is a colloid (particle diameter from .001 to 0.1 micra); charcoal is in suspension (particle size too large to dissolve).

MATERIALS

Ring stand, ring clamp, and beaker OR graduated cylinder
Mixture of $CuSO_4$, starch, and powdered charcoal in water
Filter paper
Funnel
Pyrex or Kymex test tube
Lugol's solution
Medicine dropper
Stop watch or watch with second hand
Safety goggles
Laboratory apron or coat

PROCEDURE

1. Set up a filtration apparatus as illustrated in Figure 5.6 or place a funnel in a graduated cylinder.
2. Fold a piece of filter paper in quarters. Open the filter paper into a cone and wet it; place the filter paper in the funnel.
3. Shake the mixture of powdered charcoal (black), copper sulfate (blue), and starch (colorless) and pour it into the funnel until the mixture almost reaches the top of the filter paper.
4. Observe the rate of filtration by counting the number of drops which pass through the funnel in the first 20 seconds and then in 20 second intervals until 100 seconds have elapsed.
5. Record your counts in the LABORATORY REPORT RESULTS at the end of the chapter.
6. Examine the filter paper to determine whether any substances were not filtered.
7. Check for the presence of copper sulfate and charcoal in the filtrate by examining its color.
8. To determine if starch is present in the filtrate, use a medicine dropper to place about 5 ml of the filtrate in a test tube and add a few

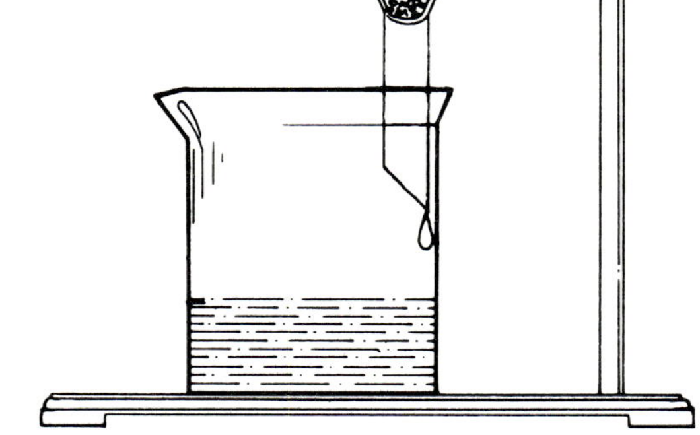

FIGURE 5.6 Filtration apparatus.

drops of Lugol's solution. A blue-black color indicates the presence of starch.

What can you conclude about the particle size of the substance(s) in the filtrate relative to the pore size of the filter paper you used? ________

____

How did the rate of filtration vary over time?

____

Why did this rate change occur? ____________

____

EXERCISE 6. Active Transport: An Active Process

> OBJECTIVE
>
> To demonstrate facilitated transport in living cells

Active transport requires the expenditure of energy (ATP) to move substances across plasma membranes. The energy expenditure is required because these substances cannot move by diffusion, since they may be: (1) transported against their concentration gradient, that is, from an area of lower solute concentration to an area of higher solute concentration; (2) insoluble in the lipid core of the plasma membrane; or (3) too large to pass through the membrane pores. Since active transport systems are complex and difficult to demonstrate and measure, in this laboratory exercise we will instead demonstrate facilitated diffusion.

In ***facilitated diffusion***, the cell actively moves nondiffusible substances down their concentration gradient. The rate depends on the concentration of the solute and the availability of carrier molecules. In this exercise, the nondiffusible substance is neutral red, an indicator that is red at pH 6–7 and yellow at pH 7–8.

MATERIALS

125 ml flask
Two large (20+ ml) test tubes (Pyrex or Kymex)
Two small (3–5 ml) test tubes (Pyrex or Kymex)
Wax pencil
Boiling water bath (hot plate and beaker)
Test tube rack
Test tube holder
Two pipettes and bulbs
Two graduated cylinders
1 g bakers' yeast
25 ml 0.75 Na_2CO_3 (sodium carbonate) solution
0.02% neutral red
0.75% acetic acid
Medicine dropper
Microscope
Two microscope slides
Two cover slips
Filter paper, funnel, and beaker
Ring stand
Safety goggles
Laboratory apron or coat

PROCEDURE

1. In a 125 ml flask, combine 1 g bakers' yeast with 25 ml of 0.75% Na_2CO_3 (sodium carbonate) solution. Swirl until the yeast is evenly suspended in the solution
2. Divide the suspension into two large test tubes marked "U1" (unboiled) and "B1" (boiled) with a wax pencil.
3. Using a test tube holder place tube "B1" in a boiling water bath for 2–3 minutes. Be sure that all the suspension is below water level so that the yeast cells will all be killed. CAUTION! *Make sure the mouth of the test tube is pointed away from you and all other persons in the area.*
4. Using a test tube holder, place both test tubes into a rack and add 7.5 ml of 0.02% neutral red to both of them.
5. Record the color of the suspensions in the LABORATORY REPORT RESULTS at the end of the chapter.
6. After 15 minutes, use a pipette to place 1 ml of each suspension into small test tubes marked "U2" and "B2."
7. Add enough drops of 0.75% acetic acid to tube "B2" to make its color identical to that of tube "U2."
8. Mark two microscope slides "U" and "B." *Using a cover slip,* examine a sample from tubes "B2" and "U2" under high power and note whether the cells are stained.

9. Record your observations in the LABORATORY REPORT RESULTS at the end of the chapter.

10. Filter half the suspension remaining in tube "B1" and examine the filtrate. Repeat for tube "U1."

11. Observe the color of the filtrate and that of the yeast cells on the filter paper. Record in the LABORATORY REPORT RESULTS at the end of the chapter.

12. To the suspension remaining in tubes "U1" and "B1" add about 9 ml 0.75% acetic acid. Filter again according to the instructions in step 10.

13. Observe the color of these "U1" and "B1" filtrates and cells and record in the LABORATORY REPORT RESULTS at the end of the chapter.

How does boiling affect the facilitated transport of neutral red by the cells? ____________

____

Describe the plasma membrane's permeability to neutral red. ____________

____

Did acetic acid enter the living cells? ________

Did sodium carbonate enter the living cells?

____

EXERCISE 7. Endocytosis: An Active Process

OBJECTIVES

To describe endocytosis
To observe phagocytosis

Large molecules and particles enter a cell through a process called ***endocytosis***, in which a segment of the plasma membrane surrounds the particle and then folds inward to bring the particle within the cell. The particle does not actually pass through the plasma membrane; rather, it is enclosed within a fragment of the membrane which detaches and moves within the cell. The reverse process, ***exocytosis***, is an important mechanism for secretory cells. There are three basic kinds of endocytosis: phagocytosis, pinocytosis, and receptor-mediated endocytosis. This exercise will demonstrate phagocytosis.

Phagocytosis (fag′-ō-sī-TŌ-sis) is the engulfment of solid particles or organisms by ***pseudopodia*** (false feet). These cytoplasmic projections surround the particle until it is completely enfolded by the plasma membranes of the pseudopodia. Then the membrane surrounding the particle pinches off from the rest of the plasma membrane and forms a vesicle around the particle. The particle is digested by enzymes secreted into the vesicle or by a union of the vesicle with a lysosome. Through phagocytosis, white blood cells engulf and destroy bacteria and other foreign substances.

Phagocytosis can be demonstrated by observing the feeding behavior of an amoeba, a unicellular organism whose movement and ingestion are similar to those of human neutrophils (a type of white blood cells).

MATERIALS

Amoeba proteus
Depression slide
Two medicine droppers
Tetrahydra pyriformis
Cover slip
Microscope

PROCEDURE

1. Place a drop of culture containing amoebae that have been starved for 48 hours into the well of a depression slide and cover the well with a cover slip.

2. Examine the amoebae under low power, being sure that your light is considerably reduced.

3. Observe the locomotion of an amoeba for several minutes. Pay particular attention to the pseudopodia that appear to flow out of the cell.

4. To observe phagocytosis, add a drop of a culture containing *Tetrahydra pyriformis* to the well in the slide.

5. Examine under low power and observe the phagocytosis of *T. pyriformis* by the amoebae. Also observe the vesicle formed around the ingested organism.

COMPLETE THE LABORATORY REPORT QUESTIONS AT THE END OF THIS CHAPTER

NUCLEAR DIRECTED ACTIVITIES 6

EXERCISE 1. Structure of DNA
EXERCISE 2. Protein Synthesis
A. Transcription
B. Translation
EXERCISE 3. Mitotic Cell Division
A. Observation of Mitotic Stages
B. Relative Frequency of Mitotic Stages

WORD ROOTS

adeno- = gland
ana- = upward
chromo- = colored
cyto- = cell
karyo- = nucleus
meta- = across, beyond
pro- = before
telo-, *tele-* = far, end
-kinesis = motion

Nucleic acids are large organic molecules containing carbon (C), hydrogen (H), oxygen (O), nitrogen (N), and phosphorus (P). Depending on their structure, nucleic acids are categorized as either ***DNA (deoxyribonucleic acid)*** or ***RNA (ribonucleic acid)***. DNA contains instructions for cell division and protein synthesis; various types of RNA carry out the steps of protein synthesis.

EXERCISE 1. Structure of DNA

OBJECTIVE

To demonstrate the structure and synthesis of DNA

The DNA molecule is a ***double helix***, a portion of which is shown in Figure 6.1a. The backbones or uprights of this spiral molecule consist of a pentose (5-carbon) sugar called ***deoxyribose***, and a ***phosphate group*** (see Figure 6.1b). The rungs of the DNA molecule are paired ***nitrogenous bases***. These bases may be ***purines***, the larger double-ring structures, ***ade-***

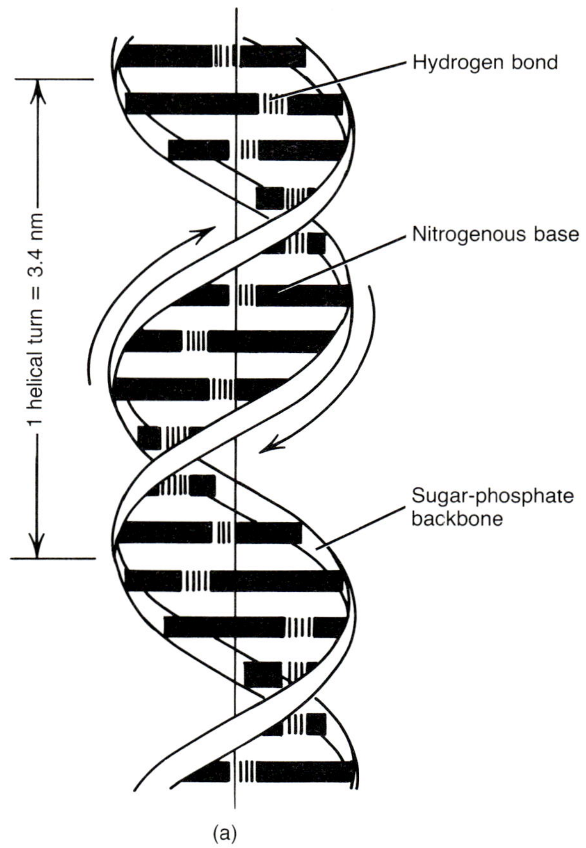

FIGURE 6.1 Structure of nucleic acids. (a) Portion of a DNA helix.

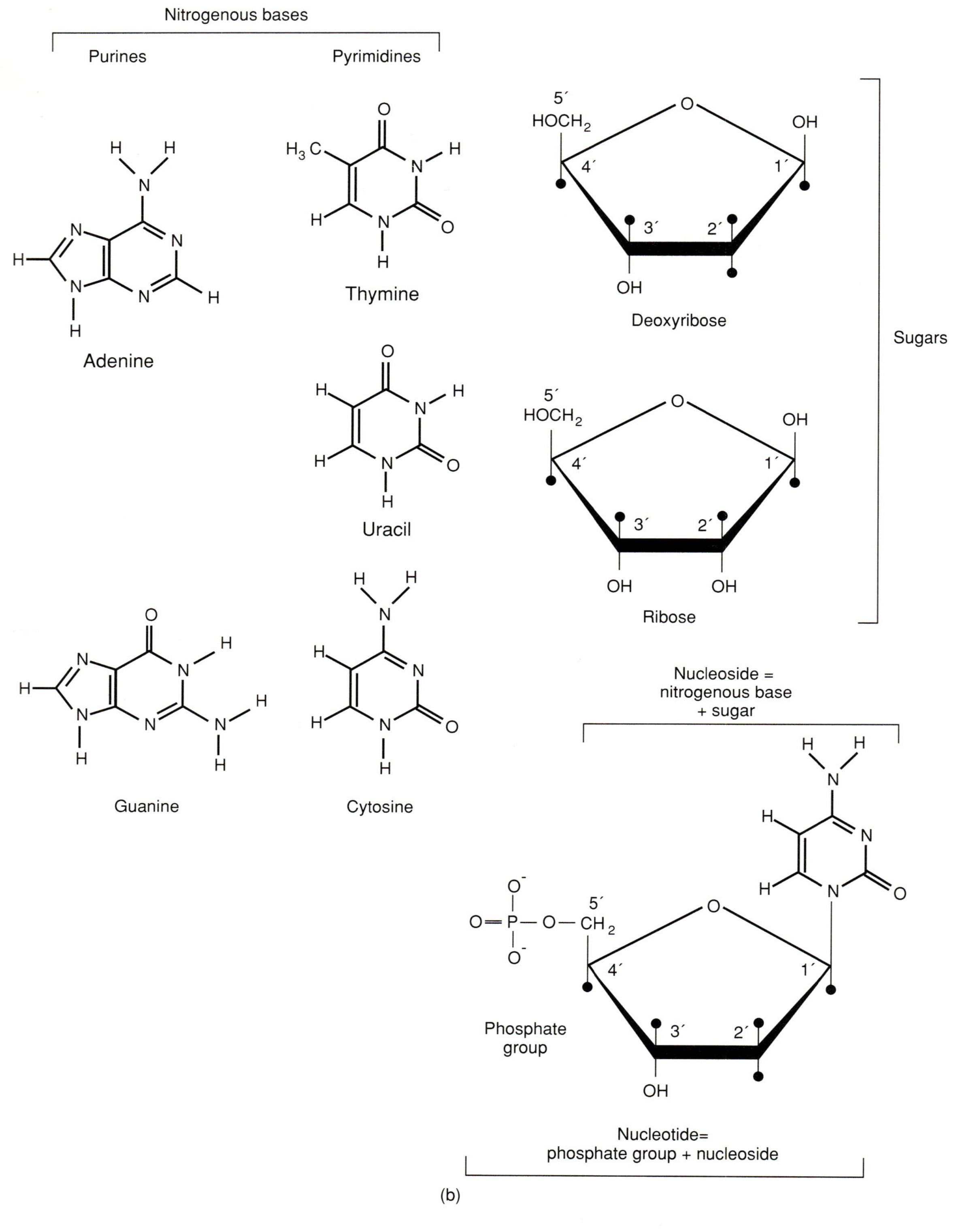

FIGURE 6.1 ***(Continued)*** Structure of nucleic acids. (b) Components of nucleic acids.

nine (A) and ***guanine*** (G), shown in Figure 6.1b, or they may be ***pyrimidines***, the smaller single-ring structures, ***thymine*** (T) and ***cytosine*** (C), also shown in Figure 6.1b. Adenine and thymine are named after the thymus gland in which they were first isolated. Cytosine is so named because it is present in all cells; guanine was first isolated in bat guano (feces). Nitrogenous bases bond with the 1′ carbon of deoxyribose to form a precursor of DNA called a ***nucleoside***. A nucleoside forms a ***nucleotide*** when the phosphate group links with the 5′ carbon of deoxyribose (Figure 6.1b). DNA is a polymer of nucleotides. The phosphate group of one nucleotide binds another nucleotide at the 3′ carbon of the deoxyribose, so that a series of 5′–3′ phosphate linkages (strong covalent bonds) holds the backbone of the molecule together. Thus, the order of the nucleotides determines the base sequence of the DNA.

The nitrogenous bases which project from the sugar-phosphate backbone form weak hydrogen bonds with the bases of free nucleotides, thereby creating a "ladder" configuration which coils into a double helix (Figure 6.1a). Because of the molecular structure of the nitrogenous bases, cytosine can pair only with guanine, and adenine can pair only with thymine. This pairing of a (large) purine with a (small) pyrimidine keeps the rung width constant throughout the molecule. Purine-purine base pairs are too large to fit; similarly, pyrimidine-pyrimidine pairs are too small.

The ***complementary base pairing*** of A-T and C-G means that the base sequence of one strand of DNA determines the sequence of bases on the other. In other words, one strand of DNA serves as a template for the formation of its complementary strand.

In this exercise, you will construct a paper model of DNA in the sequence in which this synthesis occurs *in vivo*. You will be acting as the enzymes which catalyze this process. Before you deem this a kindergarten cut-and-paste exercise, be aware that Watson and Crick worked with cardboard representations and ball-and-stick models in order to determine the arrangement of the DNA components. They received the Nobel prize for their work in 1962.

MATERIALS

Page 67, scissors, tape (optional)

PROCEDURE

1. Cut along the solid lines of page 67. You will have 24 models of deoxyribose, 22 models of phosphate, and 6 models each of adenine, cytosine, guanine, and thymine. Discard the portions of the paper marked W (waste).

2. Assemble 24 nucleosides by linking the 1′ carbon of a deoxyribose with a nitrogenous base.

3. Attach a phosphate to the 5′ carbon of each deoxyribose. You now have 24 nucleotides (deoxyribonucleotides) which should look like Figure 6.2. (In vivo, the phosphate group is a high-energy triphosphate; two phosphates are removed in this step, liberating the energy contained in their bonds to be used in this synthesis.)

4. Polymerize the nucleotides by attaching the free end of each phosphate to the 3′ carbon of the deoxyribose in another nucleotide. Make 11 of these 5′–3′ phosphate linkages, so that your DNA "polymer" is 12 nucleotides long. Place this model to your left.

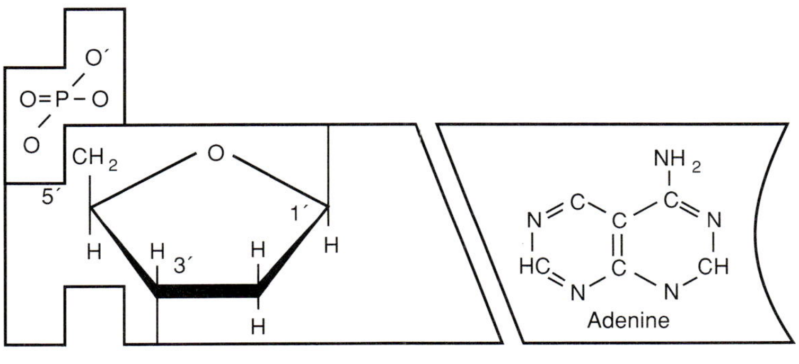

FIGURE 6.2 Model of adenine deoxyribonucleotide.

5. Using the principle of complementary base pairing, match the remaining nucleotides with those on the template strand of DNA you have just constructed. Note that the base sequence on one strand determines the base sequence of the other. Note also that the left hand strand has a 5′–3′sequence of sugar and phosphate, while the right hand strand has a 3′–5′ sequence.

6. Retain this model for use in future portions of this unit. Record the base sequence of the DNA you have constructed in the LABORATORY REPORT RESULTS at the end of the chapter.

Which bonds are most easily broken, (1) those between deoxyribose and phosphate or (2) those between the nitrogenous bases? ______

EXERCISE 2. Protein Synthesis

> OBJECTIVE
>
> To demonstrate RNA structure
> To demonstrate protein synthesis

Proteins are manufactured outside of the nucleus in association with organelles called ***ribosomes***. The information for this process is contained on the DNA within the nucleus. The first step in protein synthesis is ***transcription***, the synthesis of a messenger molecule to carry instructions about protein synthesis to the ribosomes. The second step, ***translation***, is the actual synthesis of the particular protein specified by the DNA.

Transcription and translation both require RNA (ribonucleic acid). RNA is similar to DNA with the following exceptions: (1) it is single-stranded, (2) the pentose sugar in the backbone is ribose, and (3) the pyrimidine uracil substitutes for thymine and forms a complementary base pair with adenine (see Figure 6.1b).

Refer to your textbook for a complete description of protein synthesis. A simplified overview of the process is illustrated in Figure 6.3 and described by the following steps:

A. TRANSCRIPTION

1. Separation of the complementary strands of a portion of the DNA molecule.

2. Formation of an mRNA (messenger RNA) molecule on one strand of DNA.

B. TRANSLATION

1. Movement of mRNA to the ribosomes.

2. Pairing of mRNA codons with tRNA (transfer RNA) anticodons.

3. Release and linkage of amino acids carried by tRNA.

MATERIALS

Page 69, scissors, tape (optional)

A. Transcription

PROCEDURE

1. Cut along the solid lines of page 69. You will have 24 models of ribose, 22 models of phosphate, and 6 models each of adenine, cytosine, guanine, and uracil. Discard the portions of the paper marked W (waste).

2. Assemble 24 nucleosides by linking the 1′ carbon of a ribose with a nitrogenous base.

3. Attach a phosphate to the 5′ carbon of ribose. You now have 24 nucleotides (ribonucleotides). (In vivo, the phosphate group is a high-energy triphosphate; two phosphates are removed in this step, liberating the energy contained in their bonds to be used in this synthesis.)

4. Separate the two strands of DNA you constructed in Exercise 1 by "breaking" the hydrogen bonds between base pairs. Assign one strand the role of the sense (coding) strand. The other strand will be the nonsense (noncoding) strand.

5. Beginning at the 5′ end of the DNA strand, transcribe the information on the sense strand by making complementary base pairs with ribonucleotides. The polymer you have constructed represents mRNA (messenger RNA).

6. Record the base sequence of the mRNA in the LABORATORY REPORT RESULTS at the end of the chapter. Note its similarity to the nonsense strand of DNA.

B. Translation

PROCEDURE

1. Move the strand of mRNA to an area which you have designated as representing a ribosome. Starting at the 5′ end of the RNA, read each group of three bases as a codon, a single instruction or "letter" in the genetic code.

mRNA UACGAC → RIBOSOME
CODON CODON

AMINO ACID
tRNA
AUG
ANTI CODON

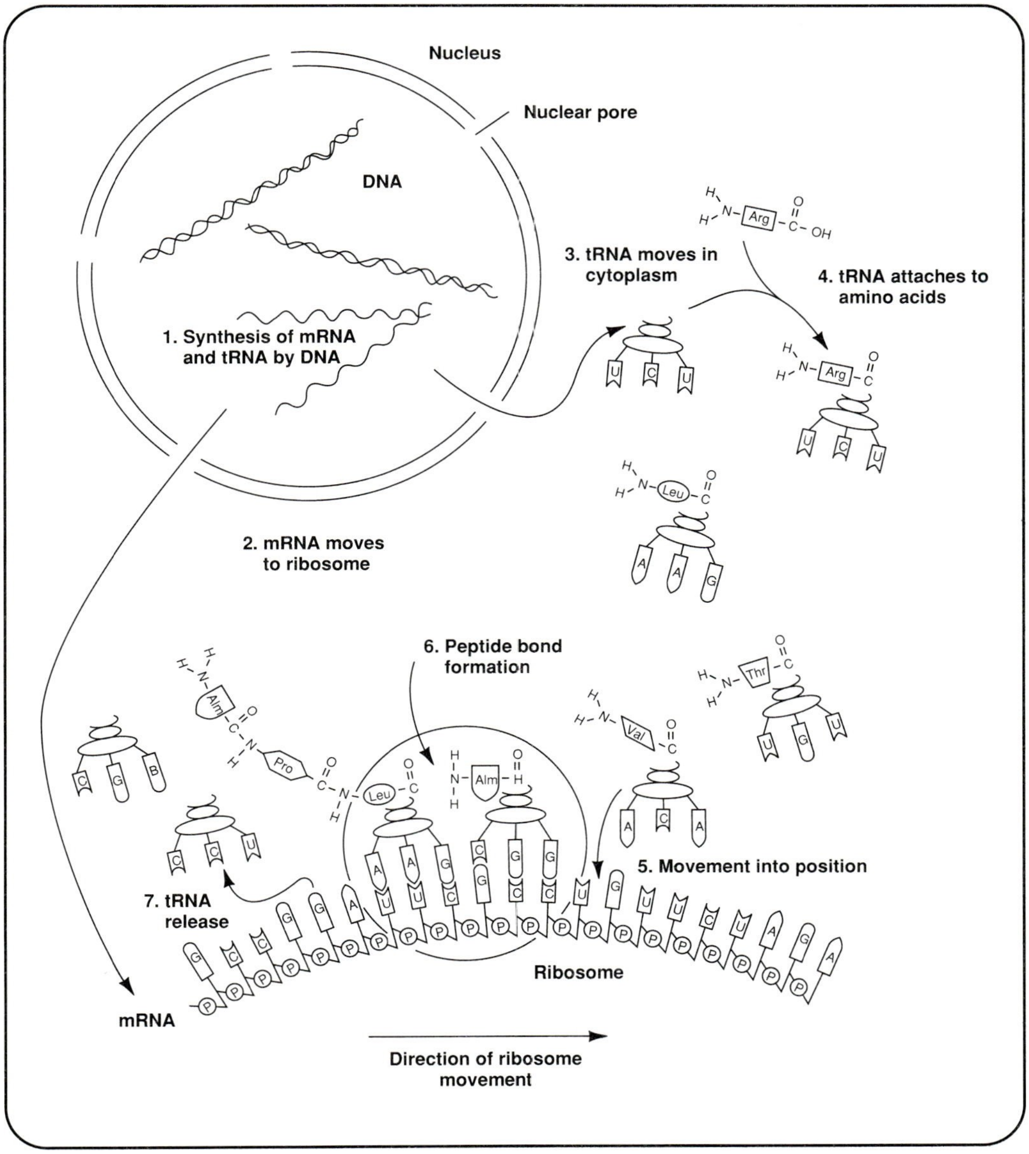

FIGURE 6.3 Protein synthesis.

2. Determine the anticodon sequence of tRNA which associates with the mRNA codons you have constructed.

3. Using the information in Figure 6.4, determine the amino acid sequence of the polypeptide specified by the DNA fragment you constructed. Note that if one mRNA codon is UAG, UAA, or UGA, then synthesis is terminated.

4. Record your conclusions in the LABORATORY REPORT RESULTS at the end of the chapter.

What is the relationship between DNA triplet codons, complementary mRNA codons, and tRNA anticodons? ______________________________

____

____

____

____

____

____

Second nucleotide

First nucleotide	DNA Codon A	RNA Codon U		DNA Codon G	RNA Codon C		DNA Codon T	RNA Codon A		DNA Codon C	RNA Codon G		Third nucleotide
A or U	AAA	UUU	Phenylalanine	AGA	UCU	Serine	ATA	UAU	Tyrosine	ACA	UGU	Cysteine	A or U
	AAG	UUC		AGG	UCC		ATG	UAC		ACG	UGC		G or C
	AAT	UUA	Leucine	ACT	UCA		ATT	UAA	"Stop"	ACT	UGA	"Stop"	T or A
	AAC	UUG		ACG	UCG		ATC	UAG		ACC	UGG	Tryptophan	C or G
G or C	GAA	CUU	Leucine	GGA	CCU	Proline	GTA	CAU	Histidine	GCA	CGU	Arginine	A or U
	GAG	CUC		GGG	CCC		GTG	CAC		GCG	CGC		G or C
	GAT	CUA		GGT	CCA		GTT	CAA	Glutamine	GCT	CGA		T or A
	GAG	CUG		GGC	CCG		GTC	CAG		GCC	CGG		C or G
T or A	TAA	AUU	Isoleucine	TGA	ACU	Threonine	TTA	AAU	Asparagine	TCA	AGU	Serine	A or U
	TAG	AUC		TGG	ACC		TTG	AAC		TCG	AGC		G or C
	TAT	AUA		TGT	ACA		TTT	AAA	Lysine	TCT	AGA	Arginine	T or A
	TAC	AUG	Methionine ("Start")	TGC	ACG		TTC	AAG		TCC	AGG		C or G
C or G	CAA	GUU	Valine	CGA	GCU	Alanine	CTA	GAU	Aspartic acid	CCA	GGU	Glycine	A or U
	CAG	GUC		CGG	GCC		CTG	GAC		CCG	GGC		G or C
	CAT	GUA		CGT	GCA		CTT	GAA	Glutamic acid	CCT	GGA		T or A
	CAC	GUG		CGC	GCG		CTC	GAG		CCC	GGG		C or G

FIGURE 6.4 The genetic code. Both DNA codons and the complementary RNA codons are shown. The 20 amino acids are specified by 61 of the 64 triplet codons. The remaining 3 codons signal "stop" or chain termination. The codon for methionine is the recognized "start" signal. All polypeptides begin with this amino acid when synthesized; it is often removed after synthesis.

Using the representational configurations of this exercise, draw the shape of the tRNA anticodons used in your polypeptide.

EXERCISE 3. Mitotic Cell Division

OBJECTIVES

To note the arrangement of the nuclear material in the various stages of mitosis

To determine the relative frequency of the stages of mitosis

Cell nuclei divide by two processes called ***meiosis*** and ***mitosis***. After nuclear division, the cytoplasm divides by ***cytokinesis*** (sīt′-ō-kin-Ē-sis).

Meiosis (mī-Ō-sis) is a specialized type of cell division which produces gametes (eggs and sperm). Meiosis results in cells which have one-half their normal chromosome complement. Each resulting cell has one member of each chromosome pair; this number is referred to as the ***haploid number***, symbolized as n. Since human gametes contain 23 chromosomes, $n = 23$. Meiosis will be studied in detail in Chapter 13.

In ***mitosis***, also called ***karyokinesis*** (kar′-ē-ō-kin-Ē-sis), nuclei divide to produce two progeny identical to the parent nucleus. Each nucleus contains both members of all chromosome pairs; this number is referred to as the ***diploid number***, symbolized as $2n$. In the human, $2n = 46$.

Although it is a continuous process, cell division is divided into stages for the purposes of study. The cycle is represented in Figure 6.5; the mitotic phases are illustrated in Figure 6.6 and described below.

1. ***Interphase*** (Figure 6.6a and 6.6f). Most of a cell's life cycle is spent in interphase. During this phase, no chromosomes are visible. Rather, the nuclear material exists as ***chromatin***, long threads of DNA complexed with protein. When stained, the chromatin appears granular because of its irregular pattern of deposition throughout the nucleus. In an inter-

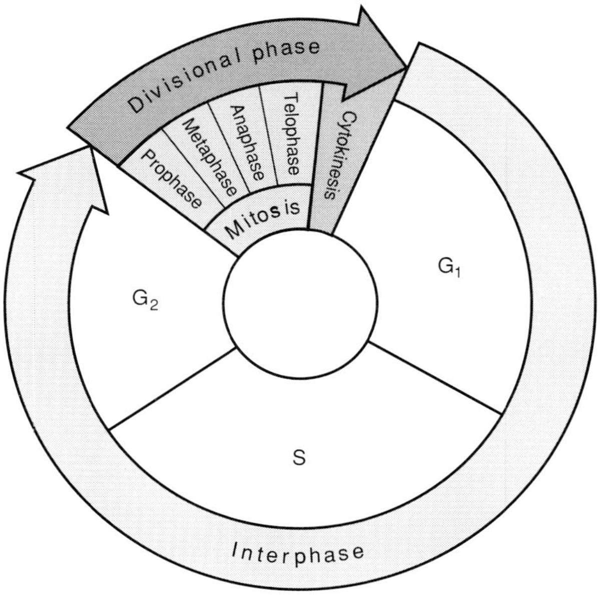

FIGURE 6.5 The cell cycle.

phase nucleus, you may see a nucleolus, an aggregate of rRNA (ribosomal RNA) and protein; just outside the nucleus, centrioles may be visible.

Interphase can be divided into three parts (see Figure 6.5). During the first part, G_1 (gap one), the cell grows extensively and synthesizes enzymes necessary for DNA synthesis. During the next part, the ***S*** phase or synthesis phase, the cell makes copies of its DNA. During the last part of interphase, G_2 (gap two), tubulin, the protein that composes spindle fibers, is synthesized.

2. ***Prophase*** (Figure 6.6b). Toward the end of G_2, the chromatin material begins to condense into distinct rod-shaped bodies called ***chromosomes***. Each prophase chromosome consists of two ***chromatids***, joined at a point called a ***centromere***. When the chromatids are visible, prophase is said to have begun. During this phase, the paired centrioles separate and move to opposite poles (ends) of the cell. Once in position, they project a series of ***continuous microtubules*** which grow toward each other, connect, and thus extend from one pole of the cell to another. As this is happening, ***chromosomal microtubules*** grow out of each centriole and extend to both poles of the cell. Together, the continuous and chromosomal microtubules constitute the ***mitotic spindle***. During the spindle formation, the nucleoli become less distinct, and the nuclear membrane disassembles into fragments. At the end of prophase, the chromatid pairs move toward the ***equatorial plane*** (center) of the cell.

3. ***Metaphase*** (Figure 6.6c). The short period during which the chromatid pairs are aligned at the equatorial plane is called metaphase. The centromere that joins each chromatid pair is attached to a continuous microtubule. When the centromeres divide, the cell enters anaphase.

4. ***Anaphase*** (Figure 6.6d). Upon the division of the centromere, the chromatids fully separate from each other and are now referred to as chromosomes. Complete sets ($2n$) of identical chromosomes move to opposite poles of the nucleus.

5. ***Telophase*** (Figure 6.6e). The final stage of mitosis consists of a series of events nearly the reverse of the events of prophase. When the chromosome sets reach their respective poles, new nuclear membranes assemble and enclose them, chromosomes uncoil and lengthen into their chromatin form, nucleoli reappear, and the mitotic spindle disappears. The formation of two nuclei identical to those in the interphase cell terminates telophase.

Cytokinesis begins in late anaphase and usually terminates in the following interphase. The first sign of cytokinesis is the formation of a ***cleavage furrow*** which extends around the cell at the equatorial plane and constricts when microfilaments in the cell bind to each other. When cleavage is complete two new progeny cells are formed.

Following cytokinesis, each progeny cell now reenters the G_1 portion of interphase during which it will grow and carry out its metabolic functions. In most tissues of the body, cells go through many divisional cycles of mitosis and cytokinesis.

How many chromosomes are present in a human anaphase cell? ____________

In a human prophase cell? ____________

A. Observation of Mitotic Stages

MATERIALS

Slide of whitefish blastula

Microscope

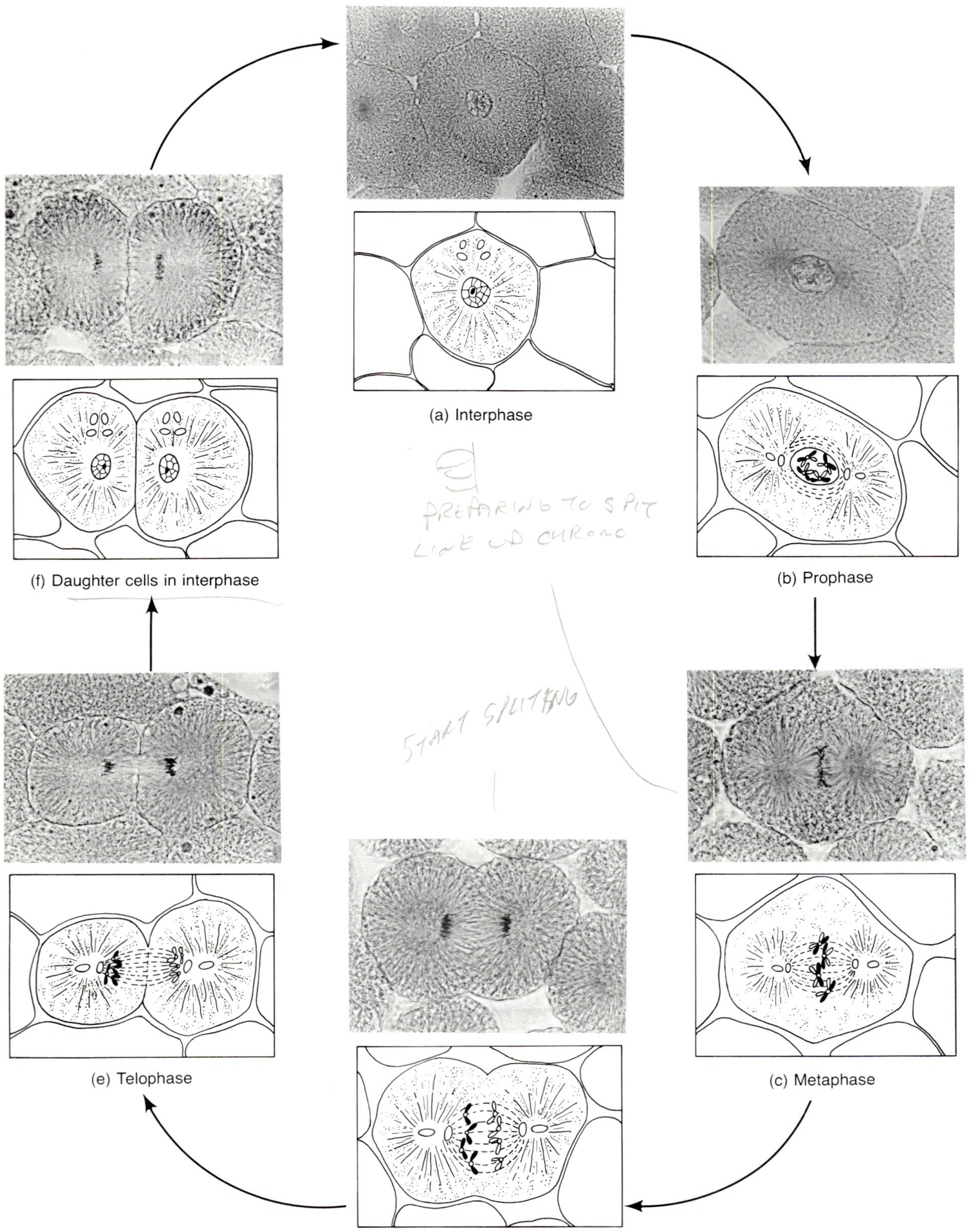

FIGURE 6.6 Mitosis and cytokinesis. Photomicrographs (1000×) and drawings of the mitotic stages in whitefish blastulae.

PROCEDURE

1. Obtain a slide of sections through a whitefish blastula.

2. Examine under high power.

3. In the LABORATORY REPORT RESULTS at the end of the chapter, make a labeled drawing of a typical cell in interphase, prophase, metaphase, anaphase, and telophase.

Why is embryonic tissue used for this exercise rather than a mature tissue? ____________

____

B. Relative Frequency of Mitotic Stages

MATERIALS

Slide of whitefish blastula
Microscope

PROCEDURE

1. Select a section of a whitefish blastula which has a large number of dividing cells visible.

2. Using high power objective and starting at the 12 o'clock position, move around the blastula and count the number of cells in each mitotic phase. It will be easier to do this if you imagine lines dividing the blastula into quadrants. Count the interphase cells in each quadrant, and then assign each dividing cell to a specific mitotic stage. It will be hard to assign some cells to a phase, e.g., to distinguish late anaphase from early telophase. If you cannot make a decision, assign one cell to the earlier of the phases in question, the next cell to the later of the phases.

3. Record your results in the LABORATORY REPORT RESULTS at the end of the chapter.

4. Divide the number of cells in each stage by the total number of cells counted and multiply by 100 to determine the percent of the cells in each mitotic stage at a given point in time.

5. Record your results in the LABORATORY REPORT RESULTS at the end of the chapter.

What percent of the cells are in interphase?

__________ %

COMPLETE THE LABORATORY REPORT QUESTIONS AT THE END OF THIS CHAPTER

12

LABORATORY REPORT QUESTIONS

NUCLEAR DIRECTED ACTIVITIES 6

Student ______________________ **Date** ______________________

Laboratory Section ______________________ **Score/Grade** ______________________

PART I. MULTIPLE CHOICE

A 1. In an interphase cell, DNA is in the form of (a) chromosomes (b) chromatin (c) chromatids

B 2. Which element is *not* contained in nucleic acids? (a) nitrogen (b) sulfur (c) carbon (d) hydrogen (e) oxygen

D 3. The "rungs" of a DNA molecule are composed of (a) nitrogenous bases (b) purines and pyrimidines (c) adenine, cytosine, guanine, and thymine (d) all of the above (e) none of the above

_____ 4. In DNA each nitrogenous base forms covalent bonds with (a) another nitrogenous base (b) a pentose sugar (c) a phosphate group (d) all of the above (e) none of the above

_____ 5. A sugar, phosphate group, and nitrogenous base form (a) a nucleotide (b) a nucleoside (c) the "uprights" of the DNA ladder (d) all of the above (e) none of the above

_____ 6. Which of the following statements is *false* regarding RNA? (a) it is a double helix (b) the bases are adenine, cytosine, guanine, and uracil (c) the pentose sugar is ribose

_____ 7. Transcription is (a) the transport of amino acids by tRNA (b) the formation of an mRNA molecule on a DNA template (c) the formation of a protein in a ribosome (d) the synthesis of tRNA

_____ 8. Mitosis (a) is also called karyokinesis (b) is a type of nuclear division (c) results in two identical progeny cell nuclei (d) all of the above (e) none of the above

_____ 9. The diploid ($2n$) number of chromosomes in the human is (a) 23 pair (b) 23 (c) 46 (d) 46 pair

_____ 10. Replication of DNA occurs during (a) G_1 phase (b) S phase (c) G_2 phase (d) prophase (e) none of the above

PART II. MATCHING

_____ 11. Mitotic spindle appears

_____ 12. Centromeres align at equatorial plane

_____ 13. Chromosomes are not visible

_____ 14. Chromatids separate fully

_____ 15. DNA is synthesized

_____ 16. Centromeres split at beginning of this phase

_____ 17. Chromosomes decondense, uncoil

_____ 18. Cleavage furrow appears

_____ 19. Centrioles move to opposite poles

_____ 20. Chromosomes move to opposite poles

A. Interphase
B. Prophase
C. Metaphase
D. Anaphase
E. Telophase

PART III. COMPARISONS. WRITE "A" OR "B" TO INDICATE WHICH MEMBER OF EACH PAIR IS GREATER.

_____ 21. A. Number of chromosomes in a prophase cell
B. Number of chromosomes in an anaphase cell

_____ 22. A. Length of interphase
B. Length of prophase

_____ 23. A. Size of DNA molecule
B. Size of RNA molecule

_____ 24. A. Size of a pyrimidine
B. Size of a purine

_____ 25. A. Diploid number
B. Haploid number

_____ 26. A. Nucleotide
B. Nitrogenous base

_____ 27. A. Number of spindle fibers in late telophase
B. Number of spindle fibers in late metaphase

_____ 28. A. Length of chromosomes in interphase
B. Length of chromosomes in prophase

_____ 29. A. Number of centromeres in an anaphase cell
B. Number of centromeres in a prophase cell

_____ 30. A. Rate of cell growth during interphase
B. Rate of cell growth during cell division

THE NERVE IMPULSE 7

EXERCISE 1. Recording the Nerve Impulse
EXERCISE 2. Characteristics of a Nerve Impulse

WORD ROOTS

limin- = threshold
oscillo- = swing

The cell membranes of all cells exhibit a differential permeability to ions in their environment. This property allows them to maintain a ***potential difference (polarity)*** in the electrical charge on the inside and outside of the cell membrane. The outside surface has a larger net concentration of positive ions, so it is positively charged, while the inside surface of the cell has a larger net concentration of negative ions and is negatively charged.

Resting neurons (nerve cells that are not conducting an impulse) are no exception. They maintain a ***membrane (resting) potential,*** the difference in charge on both sides of the cell membrane, of about 70 millivolts (mV). This means that the inside of the neuron cell membrane is about 70 mV less positive than the outside, that is, the membrane potential is -70 mV.

The neuron maintains this electrical difference or polarity by actively transporting sodium ions (Na^+) out of the cell and potassium (K^+) ions into the cell membrane by an active transport mechanism called the ***sodium-potassium pump.*** This physiological pump creates concentration gradients for these two ions; consequently Na^+ ions tend to diffuse back into the cell and K^+ ions tend to diffuse out of the cell through membrane proteins called voltage-sensitive sodium and potassium channels. Since the cell membrane is about 100 times more permeable to K^+ than to Na^+, Na^+ ions remain concentrated outside of the cell.

The polarity of the cell membrane is further maintained because the inside of the cell contains a large number of negatively charged proteins that cannot diffuse outside of the cell because of their large size.

A ***nerve impulse (nerve action potential)*** is a self-propagating wave of depolarization that spreads across the surface of the cell membrane. Nerve impulses are initiated by ***stimuli,*** changes in the environment of the cell that are of sufficient strength to cause depolarization.

A stimulus to a polarized membrane greatly increases the membrane's permeability to Na^+ ions at the point of stimulation. As a result, voltage-sensitive sodium channels open and allow Na^+ ions to diffuse inward. This influx of positive ions causes a change in the polarity of the membrane.

First the membrane potential is depolarized or reduced to 0 mV; the influx of Na^+ ions continues until the polarity is reversed and the inside of the cell becomes 30 mV positive relative to the outside.

A stimulus that evokes such a $+100$ mV change (from -70 mV to $+30$ mV) is called a ***threshold (liminal) stimulus.*** A threshold stimulus is the minimal stimulus required to elicit an action potential. Nerve cells obey what is called the ***all-or-none law,*** which states that excitable cells, under a given set of conditions, respond to a stimulus with a maximal response or no response at all. Thus, the size of the nerve impulse is never a function of the size of the stimulus.

Stimuli evoking less than a 100 mV change are called ***subthreshold (subliminal) stimuli;*** they cannot initiate a nerve impulse, although they can produce an ***excitatory postsynaptic potential (EPSP)*** that makes the nerve easier to fire. EPSPs allow the influx of some Na^+ ions thereby lowering the magnitude of the threshold stimulus required to initiate a nerve impulse. This effect is called ***facilitation,*** a state of near excitation.

Once a neuron has been depolarized, the stimulated portion of the cell membrane depolarizes the positive portion (still polarized) of the membrane adjacent to it. This reversal repeats over and over until the nerve impulse has been conducted along the length of the neuron.

As soon as a nerve impulse has traveled from one portion of the cell membrane to the next, the previous portion is repolarized, that is, its resting potential is restored. The repolarization occurs because the membrane becomes more permeable to K^+ ions and less permeable to Na^+ ions. K^+ ions diffuse out of the cell, and the outer surface of the cell becomes relatively electropositive again.

Until this repolarization has occurred, the neuron is not able to respond to a second threshold stimulus. The period of recovery is called the ***refractory period.*** The refractory period can be subdivided into the ***absolute refractory period,*** during which no stimulus can initiate a nerve impulse and the ***relative refractory period,*** during which stimuli greater than threshold stimuli (+100 mV) can initiate a nerve impulse.

The electrical changes that occur during a nerve impulse are shown in Figure 7.1.

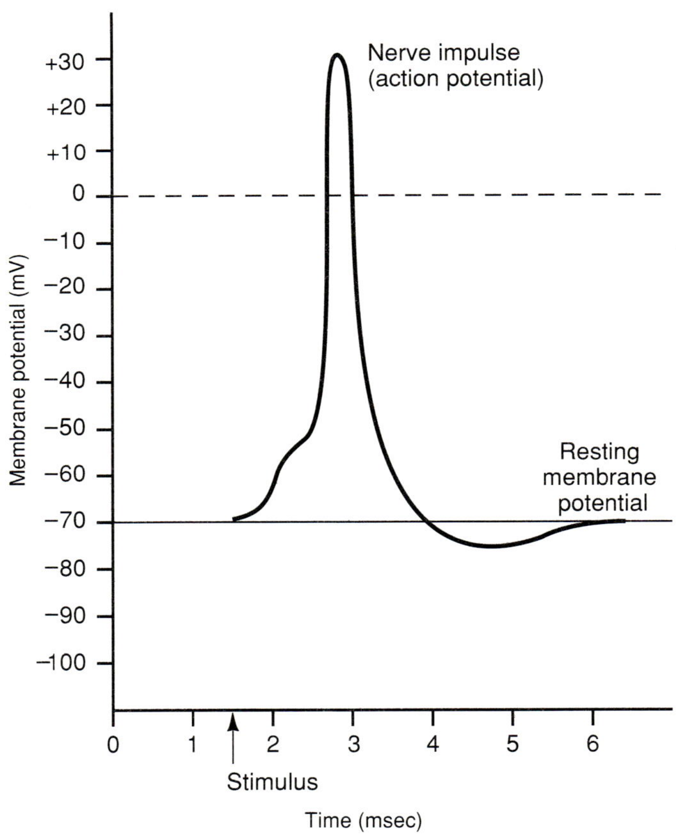

FIGURE 7.1 Changes in membrane potential during a nerve impulse.

EXERCISE 1. Recording the Nerve Impulse

> OBJECTIVES
>
> To describe the events that occur during a nerve impulse
> To record a nerve impulse in the sciatic nerve of a frog
> To measure a threshold stimulus
> To measure a refractory period
> To demonstrate the effect of cooling, heating, potassium ions, and anaesthesia on a nerve impulse

An ***oscilloscope*** is an instrument that plots variations in electric potential against time. It can amplify the small changes in electric potential during a nerve impulse and display them as a trace on the screen of the oscilloscope tube. The screen is etched in lines that represent milliseconds (msec) on the horizontal (x) axis and millivolts (mV) on the vertical (y) axis.

The recording of a nerve impulse on an oscilloscope screen (Figure 7.2) looks different from that shown in Figure 7.1 for two reasons. First, a stimulus artifact will be present as a deflection that records the strength of the stimulating voltage.

Second, the oscilloscope trace is biphasic rather than monophasic. The monophasic potential shown in Figure 7.1 represents a difference in potential between the inner and outer surfaces of a cell membrane at a single point. This type of tracing is evoked when one recording electrode is placed within the interior of the nerve cell and another recording electrode is placed outside the cell. In contrast, the oscilloscope is used in this exercise to compare the electrical potentials of two different places (biphasic) on the outside surface of a nerve.

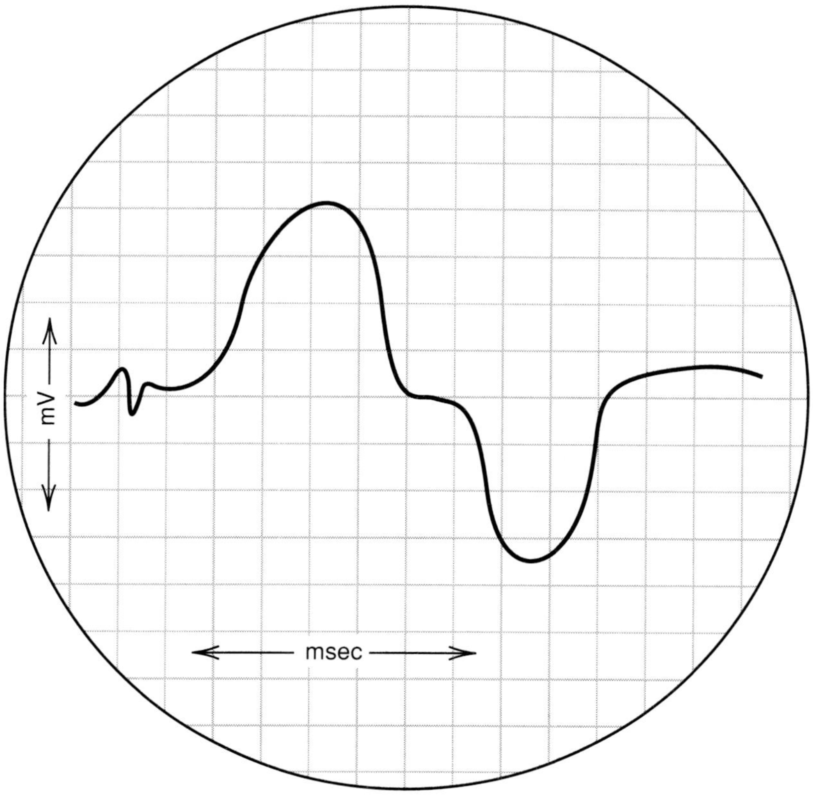

FIGURE 7.2 An oscilloscope tracing of a nerve impulse.

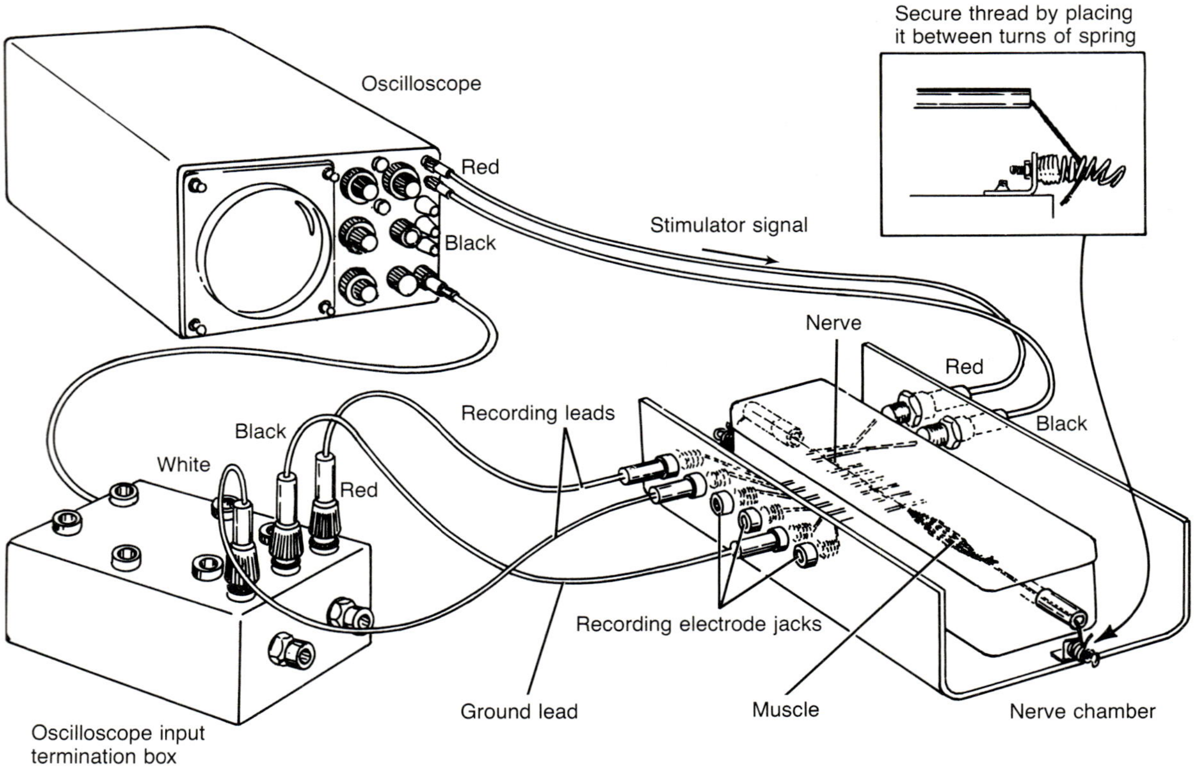

FIGURE 7.3 Oscilloscope setup. (Adapted from Sylvia L. Mader, *Biology: Evolution, Diversity, and the Environment*. Dubuque, IA: Wm. C. Brown Publishers, 1985.)

Figure 7.3 shows the oscilloscope set-up used in this exercise. Recording electrodes are placed at two different positions along the surface of a nerve. The oscilloscope records no potential difference between these two electrodes when the nerve is at rest. When a stimulating electrode generates a nerve impulse in the nerve, this electrical charge moves down the nerve cell. When it reaches the first recording electrode, this electrode becomes negative relative to the second recording electrode. The oscilloscope is connected in such a way as to record an upward deflection indicating that the second electrode is positive relative to the first, since the second recording electrode is as yet still uncharged. As the area of the nerve becomes repolarized, the deflection disappears (a return to the baseline). When the nerve impulse reaches the second recording electrode, this electrode will be negative relative to the first recording electrode, and a downward deflection is recorded. The duration of this nerve impulse is proportional to the speed of conduction of the nerve and to the distance between the two recording electrodes.

MATERIALS

Stimulator, nerve chamber, and oscilloscope
Living frog
Dissecting pan and tools
Frog Ringer's solution at room temperature, 10°C, and 37°C
Glass probes
Thread
Isotonic potassium chloride (KCl) solution
1% procaine solution
Medicine dropper
Safety goggles
Laboratory apron or coat

CAUTION! *Please reread Section C. "Precautions Related to Working With Reagents" and Section D. "Precautions Related to Dissection" in Chapter 1 before you perform any of the following exercises.*

PROCEDURE

1. Set up a stimulator, nerve chamber, and oscilloscope according to the directions of your laboratory instructor. Set the amplitude and frequency to their lowest levels.

2. Double pith a frog according to the instructions in Appendix A on page 365. Remove the skin from the left pelvis and leg. *NOTE: It is strongly suggested that either your instructor or a laboratory assistant perform the pithing procedure since it requires some practice and may prove difficult for inexperienced individuals.*

3. Place the frog on its back in a dissecting pan and moisten the leg by dropping frog Ringer's solution on it.

4. Using glass probes, isolate the sciatic nerve as shown in Figure 7.4. Using thread, tie (ligate) the nerve in two places: close to the three roots where it emerges from the spinal cord and close to the knee. Moisten with frog Ringer's solution.

5. *Being careful not to touch the nerve with your fingers,* cut it just proximal to the spinal ligature and just distal to the knee ligature. Lift the nerve with the threads and carefully free it from the connective tissue that holds it in place, *without stretching the nerve.*

6. Lay the nerve across the stimulating and recording electrodes in the nerve chamber. Moisten it with frog Ringer's solution and keep the preparation moist.

7. Set the stimulus duration at 0.1 milliseconds (msec).

8. Gradually increase the stimulator pulse amplitude until a stimulus artifact occurs. Continue to increase it until a nerve impulse appears. If the image is not stable, adjust the sweep speed. Record the threshold stimulus, *i.e.*, the voltage which evokes a response; measure the amplitude and duration of the response on the oscilloscope screen; and record these values in the LABORATORY REPORT RESULTS at the end of the chapter.

9. Increase the stimulus above threshold level until a maximal response occurs. Record the voltage that evokes a maximal response and the amplitude and duration of the response in

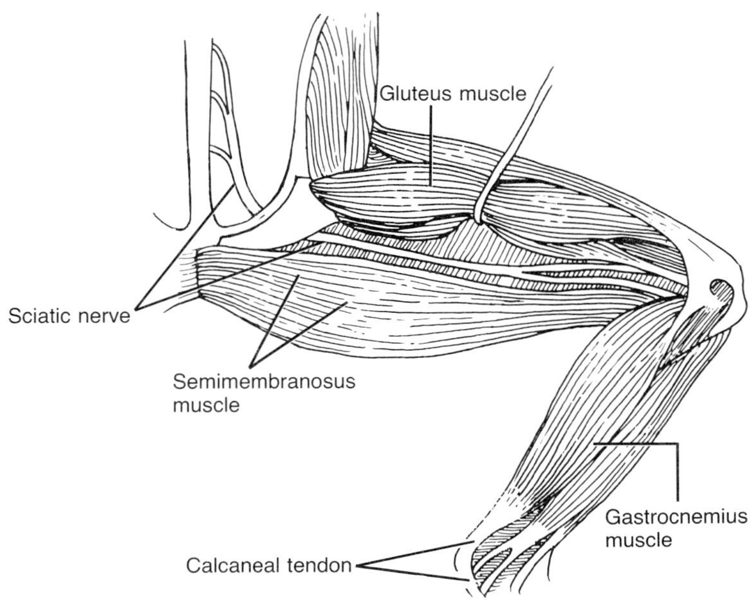

FIGURE 7.4 Isolation of frog sciatic nerve (posterior view).

the LABORATORY REPORT RESULTS at the end of the chapter.

10. At a frequency of 10 stimuli per second, stimulate the nerve with two stimuli of the maximal intensity determined in step 9. Record the results in the LABORATORY REPORT RESULTS at the end of the chapter.

11. Gradually decrease the time interval between the two stimuli. In the LABORATORY REPORT RESULTS at the end of the chapter, record the frequency when only a single nerve impulse is evoked. On the oscilloscope screen, measure the distance (representing milliseconds) from the beginning of the first nerve impulse to the disappearance of the second nerve impulse. This distance measures the refractory period of the nerve.

12. Moisten the nerve with 10°C frog Ringer's solution and stimulate it with the voltage producing maximal response. Measure the refractory period. Record the effect of cooling in the LABORATORY REPORT RESULTS at the end of the chapter.

13. Moisten the nerve with 37°C frog Ringer's solution and stimulate it with the stimulus producing maximal response. Measure the refractory period. Record the effect of warming in the LABORATORY REPORT RESULTS at the end of the chapter.

14. While the nerve is being stimulated with a stimulus of maximal intensity, moisten the neuron with an isotonic potassium chloride (KCl) solution. Record the reaction in the LABORATORY REPORT RESULTS at the end of the chapter.

15. Moisten the nerve with a 1% procaine solution, a local anaesthetic. Stimulate with a stimulus of maximal intensity and record the results in the LABORATORY REPORT RESULTS at the end of the chapter.

16. After four minutes, thoroughly wash the nerve with frog Ringer's solution. Stimulate with a stimulus of maximal intensity and record the results in the LABORATORY REPORT RESULTS at the end of the chapter.

17. Clean your equipment according to the directions of your laboratory instructor.

What is meant by a threshold stimulus? ______

____

____

EXERCISE 2. Characteristics of a Nerve Impulse

> OBJECTIVE
>
> To demonstrate factors that can elicit a nerve impulse in an isolated frog sciatic nerve

In vivo, nerves are stimulated by ***neurotransmitter substances,*** like acetylcholine (ACh), that change the membrane's permeability to sodium ions. *In vitro,* a nerve impulse can be elicited by any factor that allows an influx of sodium ions into the cell, for example, mechanical compression, chemical application, electrical stimulation, and so forth.

In this exercise, you will examine many of these factors by subjecting the sciatic nerve of a frog to various stimuli. Measurement of the nerve impulse will not be done by mechanical recording, but by noting the response of the muscle. Any nerve impulse elicited in the sciatic nerve will cause contraction of the gastrocnemius muscle.

MATERIALS

- Living frog
- Dissecting pan and tools
- Glass probes
- Electronic stimulator
- Watch glass
- Beaker
- Room temperature frog Ringer's solution
- Ice water bath
- Boiling water bath
- Filter paper
- 0.5% hydrochloric acid (HCl)
- Sodium chloride (NaCl) crystals
- Medicine dropper
- Safety goggles
- Laboratory apron or coat

PROCEDURE

1. Double pith a frog according to the instructions in Appendix A on page 365. *NOTE: It is strongly suggested that either your instructor or*

a laboratory assistant perform the pithing procedure since it requires some practice and may prove difficult for inexperienced individuals.

2. Prepare a nerve-muscle preparation according to the following instructions and the illustrations in Figure 7.5:

   a. Remove the skin from the entire lower pelvis and leg by cutting the skin around the lower trunk and pulling it down over the ankle.

   b. Cut the calcaneal (Achilles) tendon as far down over the ankle as possible and gently pull the gastrocnemius muscle free of the lower leg.

   c. On the dorsal side of the frog, gently separate the gluteus muscle from the semimembranosus muscle to expose the sciatic nerve. It will look like a silvery-white thin band.

   d. Without touching the sciatic nerve, dissect away the tissues surrounding the nerve all the way to its origin at the spinal cord, as seen in Figure 7.4.

   e. Snip the nerve as close to its origin as possible. Using glass rods, free the entire sciatic nerve from its attachments in the thigh. Scissors may be used to sever branch nerves.

   f. Using a scalpel, cut the proximal end of the gastrocnemius muscle away from its origin in the knee.

3. With glass rods, transfer the nerve-muscle preparation to a watch glass that is resting atop a beaker. Moisten the preparation with frog Ringer's solution and keep it moist throughout this exercise.

4. Move the sciatic nerve so that its proximal end hangs over the edge of the watch glass.

5. Set the electronic stimulator to administer single stimuli, and set the stimulus duration to 0.1 milliseconds (msec). Set the voltage to the lowest level.

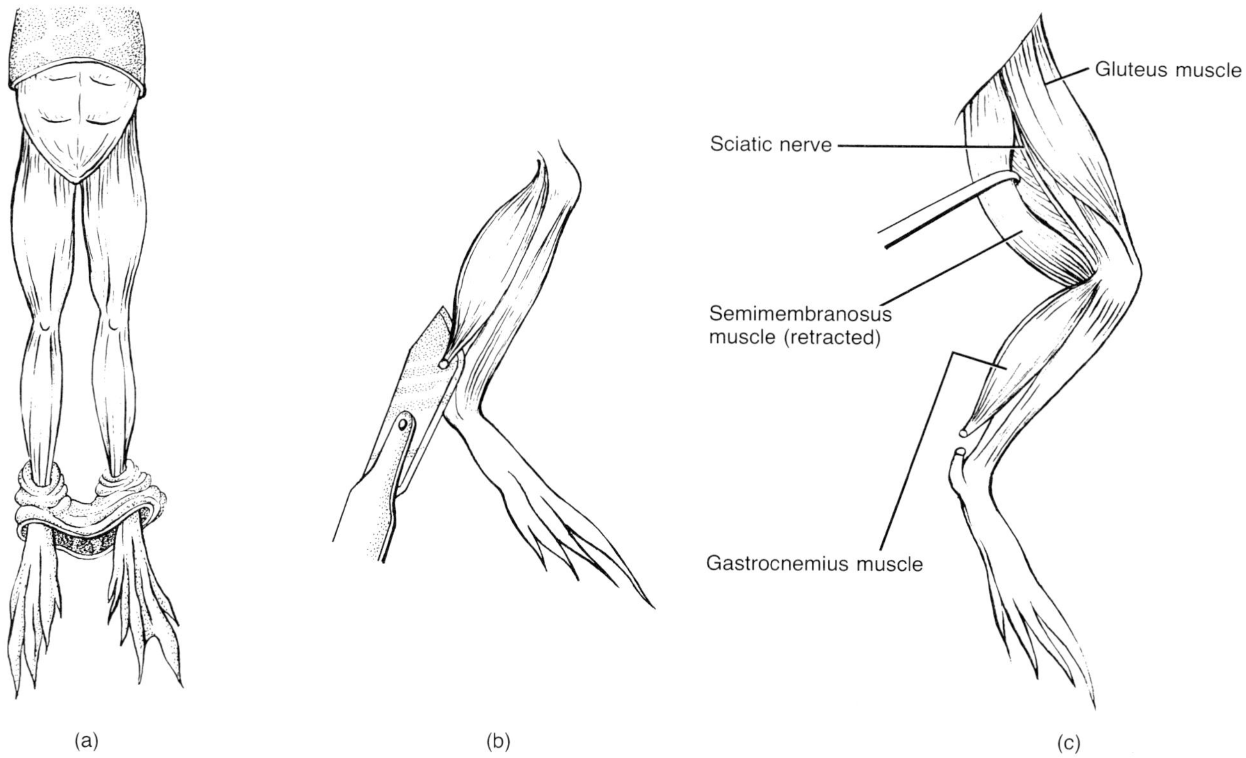

FIGURE 7.5 Nerve-muscle preparation. (a) Removal of skin. (b) Cutting the calcaneal tendon. (c) Dissection of sciatic nerve.

6. Place the electrodes of the electronic stimulator against the sciatic nerve and administer a single stimulus. Increase the voltage until a response (muscle contraction) occurs. Record this voltage in the LABORATORY REPORT RESULTS at the end of the chapter.

7. Pinch the end of the nerve with two glass rods. Record the reaction in the LABORATORY REPORT RESULTS at the end of the chapter.

8. Place a glass rod in ice water for three minutes. Touch the end of the nerve with the rod. Record your observations in the LABORATORY REPORT RESULTS at the end of the chapter.

9. Place a glass rod in boiling water for three minutes. Touch the end of the nerve with the rod. Record your observations in the LABORATORY REPORT RESULTS at the end of the chapter.

10. Saturate a small piece of filter paper with 0.5% hydrochloric acid (HCl). Touch the paper to the end of the nerve. Record your observations in the LABORATORY REPORT RESULTS at the end of the chapter. Rinse the nerve well with frog Ringer's solution.

11. Place a few grains of sodium chloride (NaCl) on the end of the nerve. Record your observations in the LABORATORY REPORT RESULTS at the end of the chapter.

What is common to all types of stimuli that evoke contraction? ______________________

____

COMPLETE THE LABORATORY REPORT QUESTIONS AT THE END OF THE CHAPTER

LABORATORY REPORT RESULTS

THE NERVE IMPULSE 7

Student ______________________ **Date** ______________________

Laboratory Section ______________________ **Score/Grade** ______________________

EXERCISE 1. Recording the Nerve Impulse

1. Threshold voltage = ____________ mV

   Amplitude of threshold response = ____________ mV

   Duration of threshold response = ____________ msec

2. Stimulus producing maximal response = ____________ mV

   Amplitude of maximal response = ____________ mV

   Duration of maximal response = ____________ msec

3. If you were working with a single neuron rather than the sciatic nerve, would you see a difference in threshold voltage and the voltage that produces a maximal response? Explain. ____________

____

____

4. Result of two maximal stimuli at 10 pulses/sec:

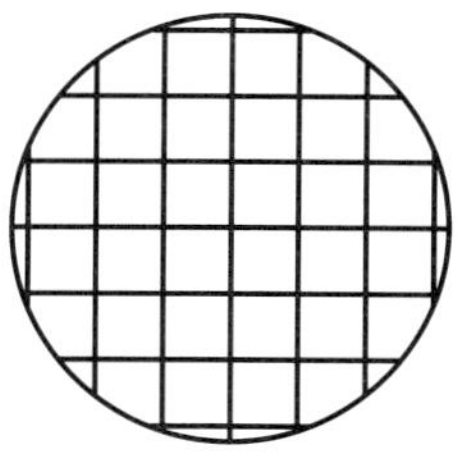

5. Frequency evoking a single nerve impulse = ____________ pulses/sec

   Length of refractory period = ____________ msec

6.

	Effect of cooling	Effect of warming
Threshold stimulus		
Size of nerve impulse		
Refractory period		

7. Effect of high potassium solution

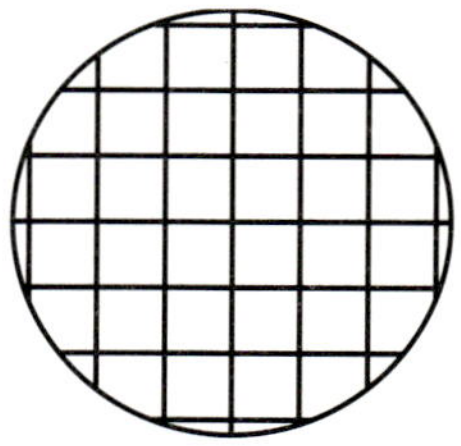

8. Effect of procaine

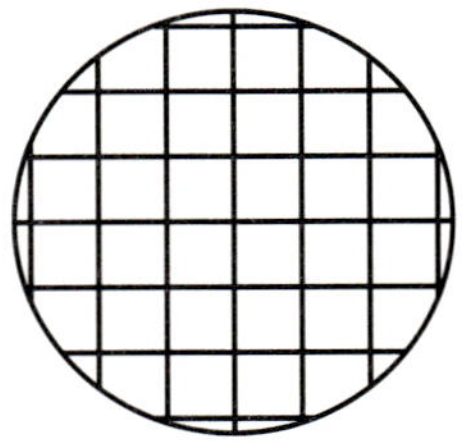

9. Was recovery from procaine complete? ____________

	Changes occurring during depolarization	Changes occurring during repolarization
In membrane potential		
In membrane permeability		

EXERCISE 2. Characteristics of a Nerve Impulse

1. Threshold stimulus = __________ mV
2.

Stimulus	Effect
Pinching	
Cooling	
Warming	
0.5% HCl	
NaCl	

3. Which of the stimuli that you applied evoked the strongest response? ____________

LABORATORY REPORT QUESTIONS

THE NERVE IMPULSE 7

Student ______________________ **Date** ______________________

Laboratory Section ______________________ **Score/Grade** ______________________

PART I. COMPLETION

1. The difference in the electrical charge on both sides of the membrane of a nerve which is not conducting a nerve impulse is called the ______________________ .
2. A wave of negative electrical current which travels along the surface of a neuron cell membrane is called a/an ______________________ .
3. A change in the environment of a cell which causes depolarization is a/an ______________________ .
4. The minimal stimulus required to evoke a response is a ______________________ or ______________________ stimulus.
5. A stimulus that makes a nerve easier to fire but does not itself evoke a nerve impulse is called a/an ______________________ .
6. The period of time during which no stimulus can initiate a nerve impulse is the ______________________ period.
7. The period of time when a nerve impulse can only be initiated by stimuli greater than a threshold stimulus is the ______________________ period.
8. During a nerve impulse, the membrane polarity reverses; this is called ______________________ .
9. The reversal of polarity is caused by the influx of ______________________ ions into the cell.
10. Ions that diffuse into the cell are removed from the cell by the action of the ______________________ .

PART II. MULTIPLE CHOICE

______ 11. The resting potential of a neuron is caused by (a) the differential permeability of the cell membrane (b) the sodium-potassium pump (c) the presence of protein within the cell (d) all of the above (e) none of the above

______ 12. The resting potential of a neuron is (a) about +70 mV (b) about −70 mV (c) about +100 mV (d) about −100 mV

______ 13. Facilitation (a) decreases the permeability of the neuron cell membrane to sodium ions (b) causes an excitatory post-synaptic potential (c) increases the permeability of the neuron cell membrane to potassium ions (d) all of the above (e) none of the above

_____ 14. Which of the following stimuli cause a response *in vitro*? (a) mechanical stimulation (b) chemical stimulation (c) electrical stimulation (d) all of the above (e) none of the above

_____ 15. The height of an oscilloscope tracing of a nerve action potential measures (a) the amplitude of the stimulus (b) the frequency of the stimuli (c) the duration of the response (d) the amplitude of the response

DISCUSSION: When you increased the voltage used to stimulate the frog sciatic nerve, the amplitude of the recorded nerve impulse increased. How do you reconcile this phenomenon with the all-or-none law?

PHYSIOLOGY OF THE NERVOUS SYSTEM 8

EXERCISE 1. Brain Function
- *A. Tests for Cerebellar Function*
- *B. Cranial Nerve Function*

EXERCISE 2. Reflexes
- *A. Somatic Reflexes in the Human*
  - *1. Stretch reflexes*
  - *2. Babinski reflex*
- *B. Visceral Reflexes in the Human*
  - *1. Ciliospinal reflex*
  - *2. Salivary reflex*
  - *3. Pupillary reflexes*
- *C. Reflexes in the Frog*

WORD ROOTS

a- = without
ab- = away from
ad-, af- = toward
encephalo- = brain
epi- = on top, above
glosso- = tongue
hypo- = below
oculo- = eye
pharyngeo- = throat
somato- = body
-taxia, -taxis = order
vago-, vagus = wandering
viscero- = internal organs

The nervous system has two principal divisions: central and peripheral. The ***central nervous system (CNS)*** consists of the brain and spinal cord and is the control and integration center of the entire nervous system. The ***peripheral nervous system (PNS)*** consists of the various processes which connect the CNS with receptors (structures sensitive to stimuli) and effectors (muscles and glands). The PNS is divided into afferent and efferent systems. The ***afferent system*** consists of sensory neurons that convey nerve impulses from receptors to the CNS. The ***efferent system*** consists of motor neurons that convey nerve impulses from the CNS to muscles and glands. Finally, the efferent system is subdivided into the somatic and the autonomic nervous system. The ***somatic nervous system (SNS)*** consists of efferent neurons that convey nerve impulses from the CNS to skeletal muscles; the SNS is under conscious control. The ***autonomic nervous system (ANS)*** consists of efferent neurons that convey nerve impulses from the CNS to smooth muscle, cardiac muscle, and glands; the ANS is usually involuntary.

This exercise examines the functions of selected parts of the nervous system and several tests of reflex function.

EXERCISE 1. Brain Function

The brain may be divided in a number of different ways. One system of division consists of the following four principal parts.

1. ***Brain stem,*** which consists of the medulla oblongata (me-DULL-la ob′-long-GA-ta), pons, and midbrain. The ***medulla oblongata*** contains the tracts that run between the spinal cord and brain, vital centers (cardiac, respiratory, and

vasomotor centers), as well as the sneezing, coughing, swallowing, hiccuping, and vomiting centers. The ***pons*** consists of tracts linking parts of the CNS as well as reflex centers for respiratory activity. The ***midbrain*** also contains tracts linking parts of the CNS, along with reflex centers for auditory and visual reflexes. All three parts of the brain stem contain nuclei of origin for cranial nerves.

2. ***Diencephalon*** (dī′-en-SEF-a-lon), which includes the ***thalamus***, a relay station and interpretive center for all sensory input except for smell; the ***epithalamus*** or pineal gland, concerned with diurnal rhythms and reproductive activity; and the ***hypothalamus.*** The hypothalamus controls and integrates the ANS with parts of the endocrine system, receives sensory impulses from the viscera, secretes regulating hormones (or factors), manufactures two hormones, controls body temperature, thirst, and appetite, and is associated with primal feelings such as rage and aggression.

3. ***Cerebellum,*** which is concerned with subconscious movement of skeletal muscles.

4. ***Cerebrum,*** which interprets sensory input, controls voluntary muscle movement, and is concerned with emotional and intellectual processes.

To review your knowledge of brain anatomy, label Figure 8.1.

A. Tests of Cerebellar Function

OBJECTIVE

To describe and test the functions of the cerebellum

Motor areas of the cerebral cortex voluntarily initiate skeletal muscle contraction. At the same time, nerve impulses are sent from the cerebrum to the cerebellum. The cerebellum then generates subconscious motor impulses that stimulate prime movers and synergists to contract and also inhibit the contraction of antagonists. The result is smooth, well-coordinated movement. The cerebellum is also required for the maintenance of posture, balance, and normal muscle tone.

Damage to the cerebellum causes a lack of muscle coordination called ***cerebellar ataxia.*** Movement is jerky and uncoordinated, resulting in disturbances of gait and speech, the inability to locate a body part with the finger, and intention tremor (shaking when making purposeful movements).

PROCEDURE

The following tests for cerebellar function should be done with a laboratory partner. Record your observations in the LABORATORY REPORT RESULTS at the end of the chapter.

1. While looking straight ahead, walk heel to toe for 20 ft without losing your balance.
2. Stand with your feet together and your eyes closed without losing your balance.
3. While looking straight ahead, move the heel of one foot down the shin of your other leg.
4. With your eyes open, touch your partner's fingers.
5. With your eyes closed, touch your nose with the index finger of one hand and then of the other.
6. Place an object an arm's length away. Place your hands at your sides and then grasp the object with a single movement.

Would damage to the cerebellum cause paralysis? _____ a loss of sensation? _____

B. Cranial Nerve Function

OBJECTIVES

To name, number, and locate the cranial nerves

To describe and test the function of the cranial nerves

Twelve pairs of ***cranial nerves*** leave the brain through foramina in the skull. All but the first two pairs arise from the brain stem; all but the vagus nerve (X), serve structures in the head and neck.

The cranial nerves are designated both by name and Roman numeral. The names indicate the function or distribution of the nerves. The Roman numerals indicate the order in which nerves arise from the brain, from front

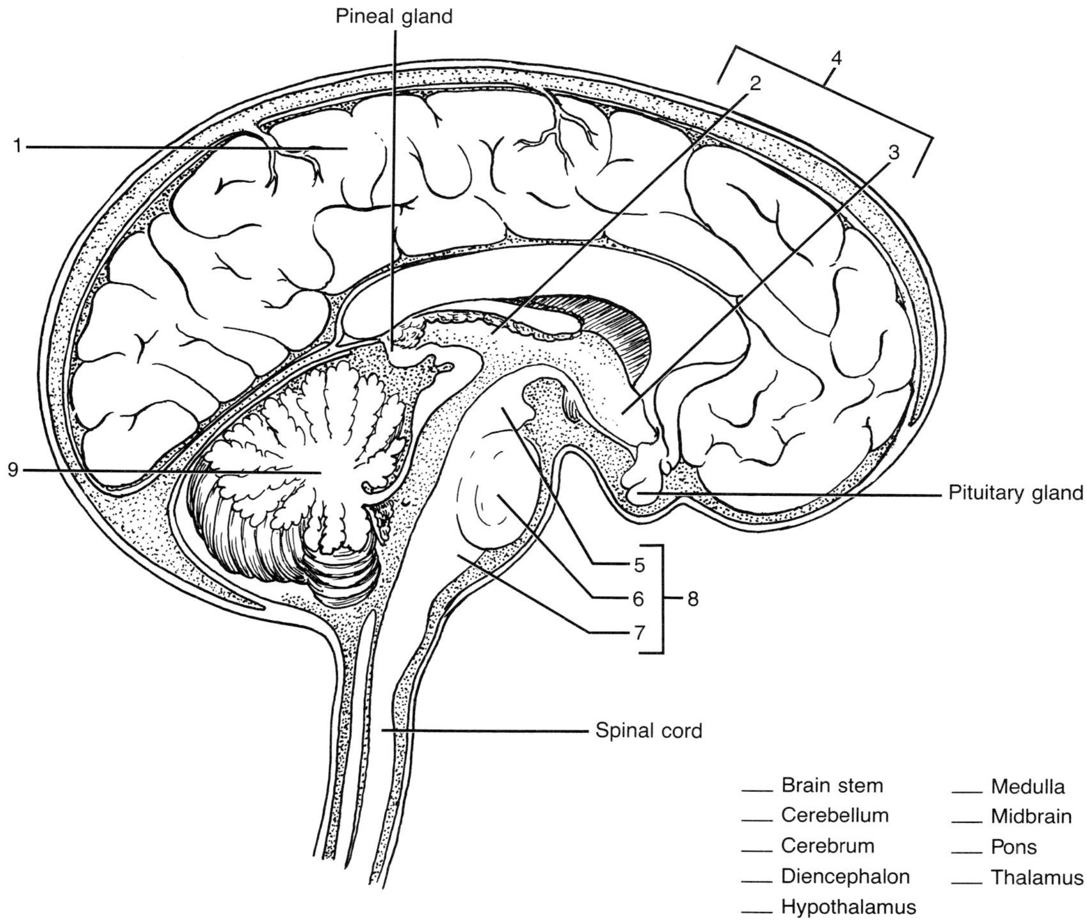

FIGURE 8.1 Midsagittal section of the human brain.

to back. A mnemonic device used to remember the names of the nerves is "On old Olympus topmost top, a Finn and German viewed a hop."[1] The initial letter of each word corresponds to the initial letter of each pair of cranial nerves.

The cranial nerves may contain sensory (afferent) fibers only, be composed primarily of motor (efferent) fibers, or have both motor and sensory fibers (mixed nerves). The nerves designated as primarily motor nerves all contain a few sensory fibers which carry nerve impulses necessary for ***proprioception,*** a sense of the body position of the organ innervated. A mnemonic device used to remember the type of cranial nerve is "Some say marry money, but my brother say 'Bad business, marry money.'" The initial letter of each word is an *S* for sensory nerve, an *M* for a nerve with a primary motor function, or a *B* for both, meaning a mixed nerve containing both motor and sensory fibers.

Review your knowledge of the anatomy and location of cranial nerves by labeling Figure 8.2.

The tests in this exercise are performed to determine cranial nerve function. Although they provide only superficial information, they will help you to understand how the vari-

[1]When this mnemonic was devised, cranial nerve VIII was called the acoustic or auditory nerve and was considered to have two branches, the vestibular and the cochlear. Hence, the eighth word begins with the letter *a*. Currently, cranial nerve VIII is known as the vestibulocochlear nerve. A mnemonic reflecting the name change is "Oh, oh, oh, to touch and feel very green vegetables—AH!"

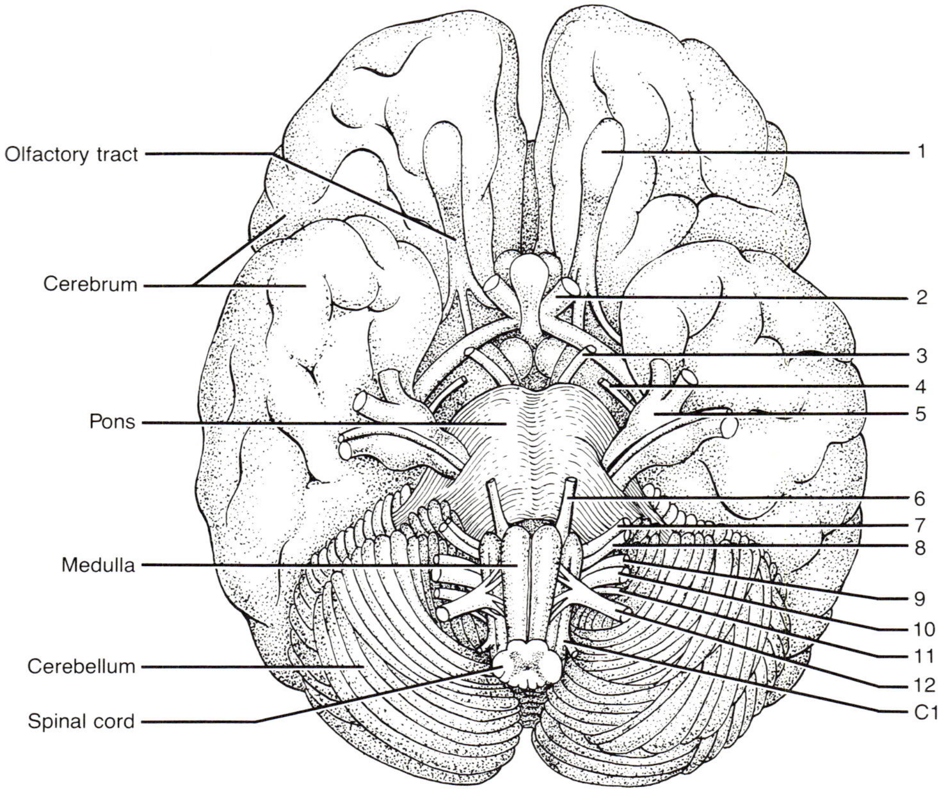

___ Abducens (VI) nerve
___ Accessory (XI) nerve
___ Facial (VII) nerve
___ Glossopharyngeal (IX) nerve
___ Hypoglossal (XII) nerve
___ Oculomotor (III) nerve
___ Olfactory bulb
___ Optic (II) nerve
___ Trigeminal (V) nerve
___ Trochlear (IV) nerve
___ Vagus (X) nerve
___ Vestibulocochlear (VIII) nerve

FIGURE 8.2 Cranial nerves of the human brain in ventral view.

ous nerves function. Use your laboratory partner as the subject in each of these tests and record your observations in the LABORATORY REPORT RESULTS at the end of the chapter. To obtain information to answer the questions, consult your textbook.

MATERIALS

Odiferous substances
Snellen eye chart
Penlight
Cotton
Ice water
Cotton applicators
Sugar solution
Swivel stool
Ticking watch
Quinine solution
Tongue depressors
Two medicine droppers

PROCEDURE

1. ***Olfactory (I) nerve***—a sensory nerve that carries nerve impulses related to smell. To test for sensory function, have the subject smell several familiar substances such as spices, first using one nostril, then the other. Odors should

be able to be distinguished equally well by each nostril. This test will not be effective if the subject has a cold or allergy.

What structures could be malfunctioning if the ability to smell is lost ***(anosmia)***? ______________

____

2. ***Optic (II) nerve***—a sensory nerve that carries nerve impulses related to vision. The left and right optic (II) nerves (Figure 8.3) run from each eye to the ***optic chiasma*** (kī-AZ-ma) where fibers from the medial half of each retina cross over to the opposite side. From the chiasma, fibers travel to the thalamus where they synapse with nerves going to the visual cortex of the occipital lobe of the cerebrum. To test for sensory function, have the subject read a portion of a printed page using each eye, wearing glasses if they have been prescribed. Do the same while using a Snellen eye chart at a distance of 20 ft.

What is the result of severing the left optic (II) nerve? ______________ of severing the optic chiasma? ______________

3. ***Oculomotor (III) nerve***—mainly a motor nerve, which has a small proprioceptive function. Motor fibers innervate the levator palpebrae superioris (the muscle that raises the upper eyelid), four extrinsic eye muscles, the sphincter (circular) muscle of the iris, and the ciliary muscle that controls lens shape.

To test the pupillary light reflex, move a small penlight from the side of the subject's face toward the front of the eye. CAUTION! *Do not make contact with the eye.*

Observe the pupil. Is this portion of the oculomotor (III) nerve automatic or somatic?

____

Observe the subject for signs of ***ptosis*** (drooping of the eyelids).

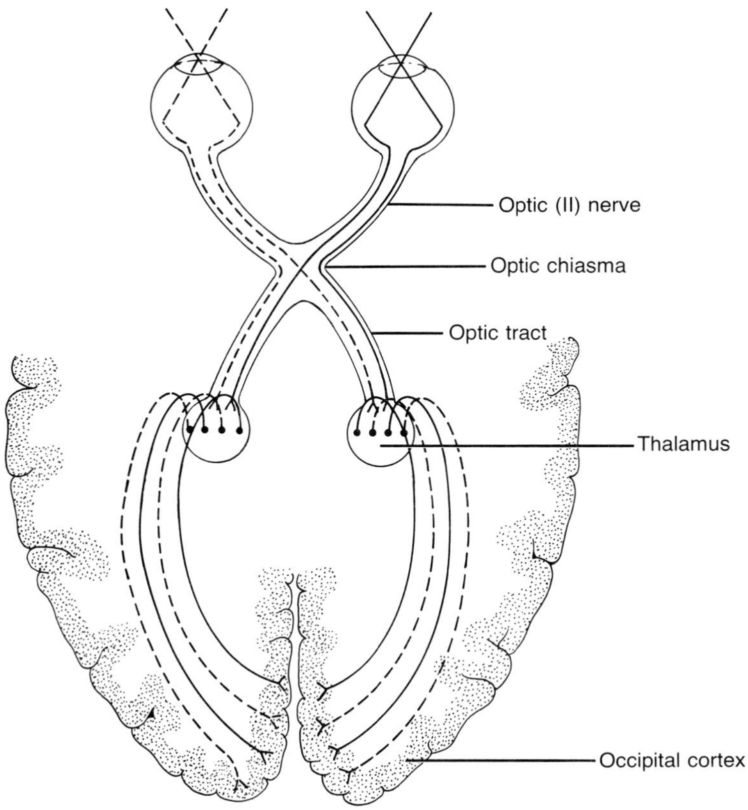

FIGURE 8.3 Transverse section through brain and eyes showing visual pathway.

What is the location of the levator palpebrae superioris muscle? ____________________

4. Innervation of the Extrinsic Eye Muscles: ***Oculomotor (III), Trochlear*** (TRŌK-lē-ar) ***(IV),*** and ***Abducens*** (ab-DOO-sens) ***(VI) nerves***—primarily motor nerves with a small proprioceptive function.

To test motor responses, have the subject hold the head still and follow your finger with the eyes. Move your finger up, down, medially, and laterally.

Indicate the innervation and movements produced by extrinsic eye muscles in the table below.

Muscle	Innervation	Action
Superior rectus		
Inferior rectus		
Lateral rectus		
Medial rectus		
Superior oblique		
Inferior oblique		

5. ***Trigeminal*** (trī-JEM-i-nal) ***(V) nerve***—a mixed nerve. Motor fibers innervate the muscles of mastication; sensory fibers arise in the structures of the eye not directly related to vision, from the nasal cavity (structures unrelated to smell), from the skin of the face and anterior scalp, and from structures in the mouth not directly related to taste.

To test for motor responses, have the subject close the jaws tightly. Now, while holding your hand under the subject's lower jaw to provide resistance, ask him/her to open their mouth.

To test sensory function, have the subject close the eyes and lightly whisk a piece of dry cotton over the mandibular, maxillary, and ophthalmic areas on each side of the face.

Are all three areas equally sensitive to stimulation? ______ Does the trigeminal (V) nerve have a larger sensory or motor distribution?

____

6. ***Facial (VII) nerve***—a mixed nerve. Motor fibers innervate muscles of facial expression and scalp muscles, the lacrimal glands, and the sublingual and submandibular salivary glands. Sensory fibers arise from the taste buds on the anterior two-thirds of the tongue.

To test the motor responses of this nerve, have the subject bring the corners of the mouth straight back, smile while showing the teeth, whistle, puff the cheeks, frown, raise and lower the eyebrows, close the eyes, and wrinkle the forehead. Check for asymmetry in the responses.

To test sensory function, touch the tip of the subject's tongue with a cotton applicator on which a sugar solution had been dropped.

Bell's palsy is inflammation of the facial (VII) nerve and/or the area around it. What would be the symptoms of this condition?

____

____

Does the facial (VII) nerve have a larger sensory or motor distribution? ____________________

7. ***Vestibulocochlear*** (ves-tib′-yoo-lō-KŌK-lē-ar) ***(VIII) nerve***—This purely sensory nerve was also known as the ***auditory*** or ***acoustic nerve.***

To test sensory function in the vestibular branch of this nerve, have the subject sit on a swivel stool and turn them 10 times. CAUTION! *Turn the stool carefully and slowly (about one turn every two seconds).* Stop the stool slowly. A normal response to experimental spinning includes

a. ***vestibular nystagmus,*** a rapid involuntary movement of the eyeballs, and

b. ***vertigo,*** or loss of equilibrium, a sense that the subject is dizzy or that the environment is moving.

Under normal conditions these symptoms indicate a disturbance of the structures responsible for the sense of balance. CAUTION! *Do not permit the subject to stand or walk until dizziness is completely gone.*

To test the sensory function of the cochlear branch of this nerve, have the subject close the eyes; test for the ability to hear a ticking watch.

What are the symptoms of damage to the vestibular branch of this nerve? ____________________

____

of damage to the cochlear branch of this nerve?

____

of damage to the entire nerve? ____________________

____

8. ***Glossopharyngeal*** (glos′-o-fa-RIN-jē-al) ***(IX) nerve***—a mixed nerve. The motor fibers inner-

vate the parotid salivary gland and, along with those of the vagus (X) nerve, innervate the muscles of swallowing. Sensory fibers arise from taste buds on the posterior third of the tongue and from the carotid sinus, a structure that is sensitive to changes in blood pressure.

To test for sensory function, drop quinine solution onto a cotton applicator and touch it *lightly* to the tip, sides, and back of the subject's tongue.

In which area of the tongue are receptors for bitter taste concentrated? ________________

9. ***Vagus (X) nerve***—a mixed nerve with a wide distribution of both motor and sensory fibers to the viscera of the thoracic and abdominal cavities.

To test for motor function of cranial nerves IX and X, touch the uvula (YOO-vū-la), a small projection from the soft palate, with a cotton-tipped applicator *slowly and very gently*. What reaction occurs? ________________

Gently hold the tongue down with a tongue depressor and have the subject say "ah." Does the uvula move? ____ Are the movements the same on both sides? ____

Have the subject swallow. Does swallowing occur easily? ____

What would be the result of severing the motor fibers of the vagus (X) nerve? ________________

____

of severing the sensory portion of the vagus (X) nerve? ________________

____

10. ***Accessory (XI) nerve***—primarily a motor nerve with a small proprioceptive function. Motor fibers innervate the muscles of swallowing and the sternocleidomastoid and trapezius muscles.

To test motor responses in the sternocleidomastoid, have the subject rotate the head against *slight* resistance that you supply by placing your hands on either side of the subject's head. To test motor response in the trapezius, have the subject shrug the shoulders while you *gently* press down on the shoulders.

Is the muscular strength equal on both sides?

____

11. ***Hypoglossal (XII) nerve***—primarily a motor nerve with a small proprioceptive function. Motor fibers innervate the muscles of the tongue.

To test for motor function, have the subject protrude the tongue. Is the protruded tongue symmetrical? ________________

Have the subject move the tongue from side to side while you *gently* resist the movements with a tongue depressor. Is there any lack of strength in the tongue muscles? ________________

Which cranial nerve(s) innervate the skeletal muscles of the tongue? ________________

the taste buds of the tongue? ________________

the receptors for touch in the tongue? ________

EXERCISE 2. Reflexes

> OBJECTIVES
>
> To describe and categorize reflexes and reflex arcs
>
> To demonstrate reflexes in the human and in the frog

Reflexes are rapid involuntary responses to changes in the environment that attempt to restore the body to homeostasis. For a reflex to occur, a nerve impulse must travel along a neural pathway called a ***reflex arc*** (see Figures 8.4, 8.5, and 8.6) which consists, in order, of the following parts:

1. ***Receptor***—the distal end of a sensory neuron that responds to a stimulus by initiating a nerve impulse in the sensory neuron.

2. ***Sensory neuron***—a nerve cell that transmits a nerve impulse from the receptor to the central nervous system (CNS).

3. ***Center***—a region within the CNS where a sensory neuron synapses with an ***association neuron*** or a ***motor neuron***. The number of synapses in the center is directly proportional to the complexity of the reflex. Reflexes are known as ***spinal reflexes*** when the reflex center is the spinal cord. These spinal reflexes occur without the involvement of higher brain centers, although the brain may alter the response by inhibiting or facilitating it.

4. ***Motor neuron***—a nerve cell that transmits a

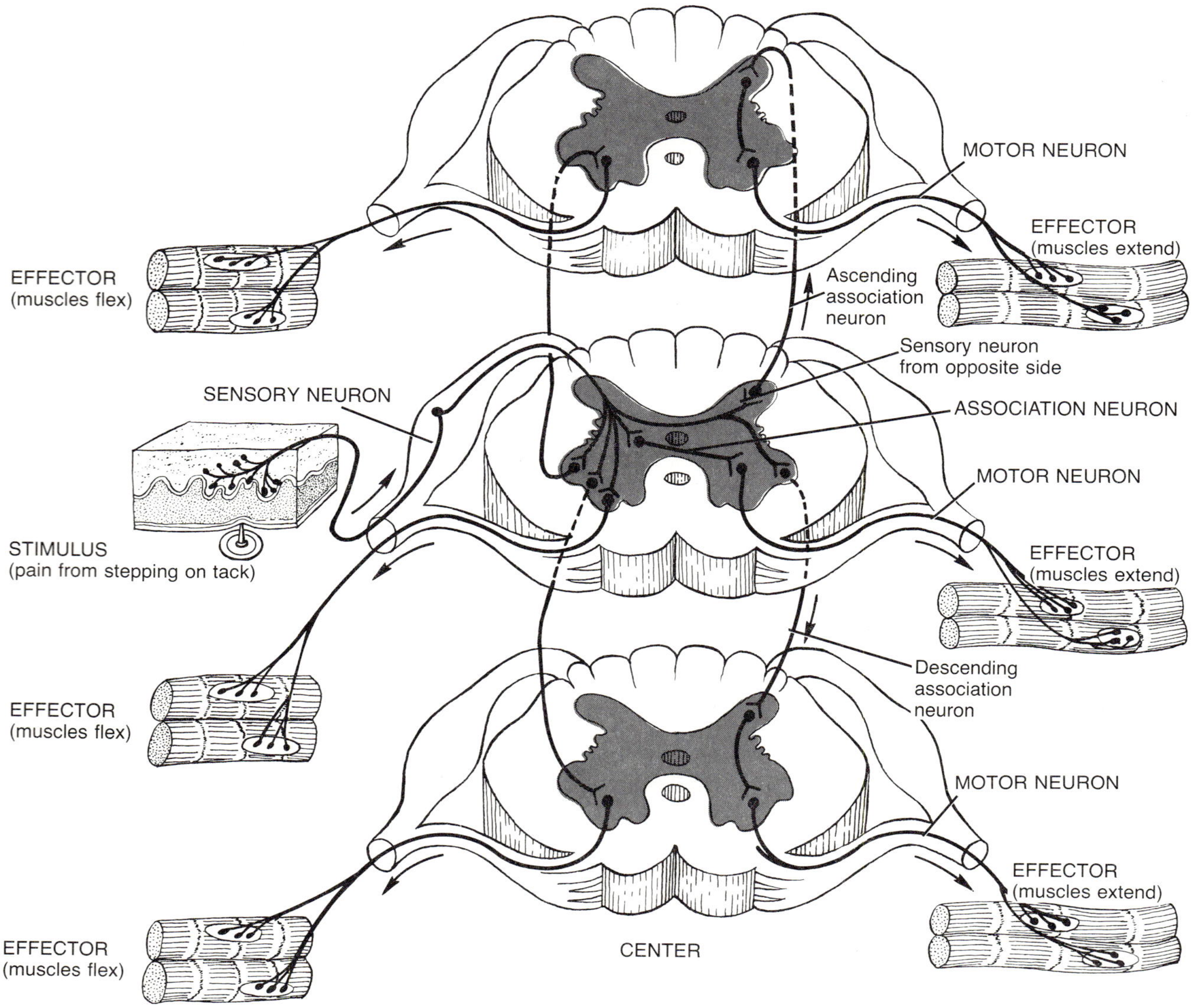

FIGURE 8.4 Withdrawal and crossed extensor reflexes. The withdrawal (flexor) reflex is shown at the left. The crossed extensor reflex is shown at the right.

nerve impulse from the CNS to the part of the body that will respond (the effector).

5. ***Effector***—the muscle or gland that responds to the motor neuron impulse. The response is a ***reflex*** or ***reflex action.***

Reflexes are categorized as ***visceral (autonomic) reflexes*** when the effector is cardiac muscle or glands. These reflexes control such involuntary processes as heart rate, salivation, and sweating. Reflexes are called ***somatic reflexes*** when the effector organ is skeletal muscle.

Monosynaptic reflexes are those that have only two neurons and hence a single synapse; ***polysynaptic reflexes*** are those in which the sensory neuron synapses with one or more association neurons which then synapse with a motor neuron.

Ipsilateral reflexes are those in which the motor impulse exits from the same side at which the sensory impulse enters. ***Contralateral reflexes*** are those in which the sensory impulse crosses over to the other side of the spinal cord from which the motor impulse exits.

The ***withdrawal reflex*** (see Figure 8.4) is an example of a polysynaptic, ipsilateral, spinal reflex. In such a reflex, a painful stimulus (like a hot stove or sharp object) triggers a sensory neuron to conduct a nerve impulse to the spinal cord where it synapses with several association neurons which then synapse with motor neurons. One of these association neurons stimulates several motor neurons that carry nerve impulses to flexor muscles and cause flexion or withdrawal of the body part from the painful stimulus. (Withdrawal reflexes are also called ***flexor reflexes.***) Other association neurons cross the spinal cord and synapse with motor neurons on the opposite side. These motor neurons carry nerve impulses to extensor muscles, which contract to maintain balance. This extension of the muscles in one limb to counterbalance the flexion of muscles in the opposite limb is called a ***crossed extensor reflex.*** It is a polysynaptic, contralateral, spinal reflex.

A. Somatic Reflexes in the Human

1. Stretch Reflexes

Stretch reflexes (see Figure 8.5) are two-neuron, monosynaptic, ipsilateral, spinal reflexes. Stretching a tendon stimulates receptors (muscle spindles) in the muscle. A nerve impulse travels along a sensory neuron through the posterior horn of the gray matter of the spinal cord to a reflex center in the cord. There the sensory neuron synapses with a motor neuron. The axon of the motor neuron exits from the anterior horn of the gray matter and travels to the effector organ: the muscle that was stretched. When the impulse reaches the muscle, the muscle contracts.

MATERIALS

Reflex hammer

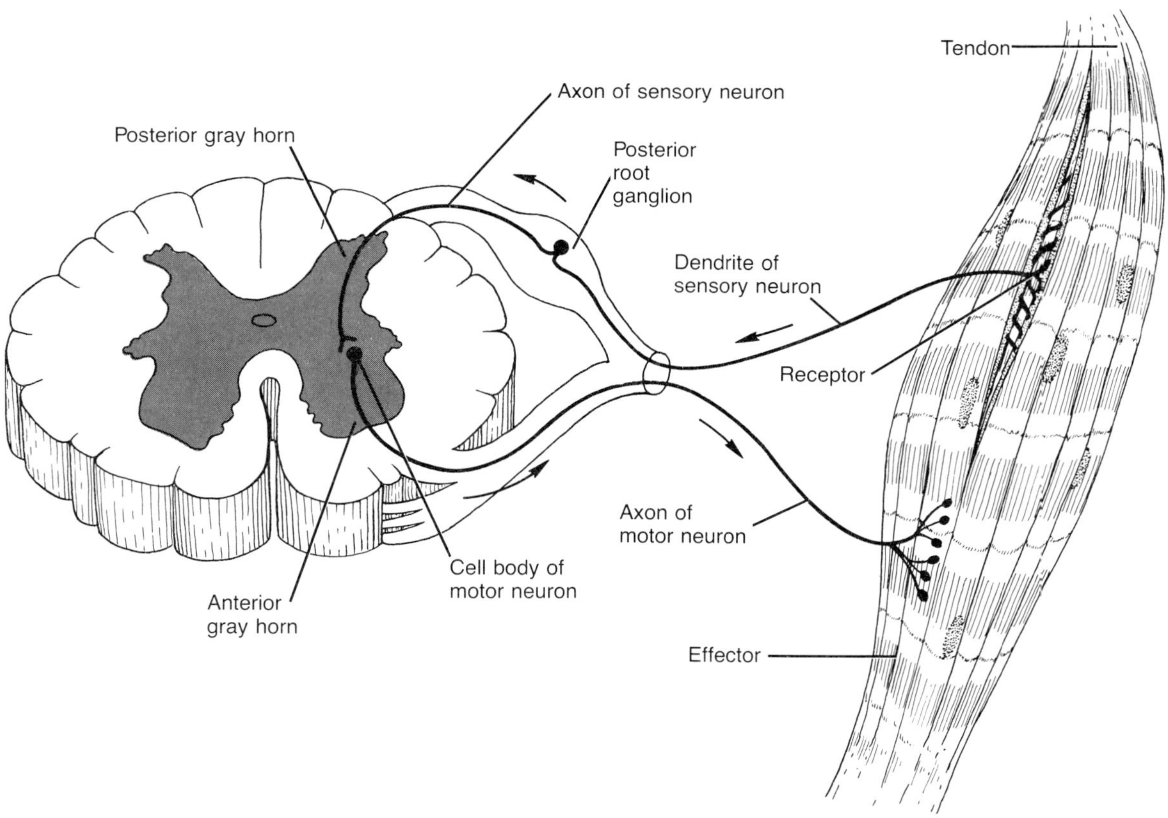

FIGURE 8.5 Components of a stretch reflex pathway.

PROCEDURE

1. Have your laboratory partner sit on the laboratory table with the legs crossed or dangling. Tap the patellar tendon with a reflex hammer.
2. Repeat step one while your partner is saying the alphabet backwards (or naming the functions of the cranial nerves).
3. CAUTION! *Assuming that your partner has no known condition that could be jeopardized by exercise,* repeat step one after your partner has engaged in vigorous physical activity (jogging, jumping in place, etc.) long enough to feel fatigued.
4. Elicit other stretch reflexes by
   a. tapping the calcaneal (Achilles) tendon. Have your partner kneel on a chair; using your left hand, dorsiflex (bend the foot in the direction of the upper surface) slightly before tapping the tendon.
   b. tapping the triceps tendon. Have your partner lean back or recline so that the arm is positioned across the abdomen. Tap the triceps brachii tendon about 5 cm (2 inches) above the elbow. (The triceps should twitch but not contract fully.)
5. Record your observations in the LABORATORY REPORT RESULTS at the end of the chapter.

2. Babinski Reflex

The ***Babinski reflex*** is used to test for the integrity of the corticospinal tract (a descending pyramidal tract leading from the cerebrum to the spinal cord). A response of plantar flexion and adduction of the toes is considered normal and is called a ***negative response.*** A ***positive Babinski response*** (dorsiflexion of the great toe and abduction of the toes) is abnormal in individuals older than 18 months or so. Infants have a positive Babinski response because the corticospinal tract is not fully developed (myelinated) until that time.

MATERIALS

Reflex hammer

PROCEDURE

1. Have your laboratory partner rest a bare foot in a relaxed position on a chair or cot, with the lateral side of the foot against the surface. Run the handle of the reflex hammer firmly up the medial side of the foot from the heel to the base of the toes.
2. Record your observations in the LABORATORY REPORT RESULTS at the end of the chapter.

B. Visceral Reflexes in the Human

Visceral reflexes (see Figure 8.6) are all polysynaptic because two motor neurons are always involved. The first motor neuron (the preganglionic neuron) leaves the reflex center and travels to a ganglion. There it synapses with the second motor neuron (the postgan-

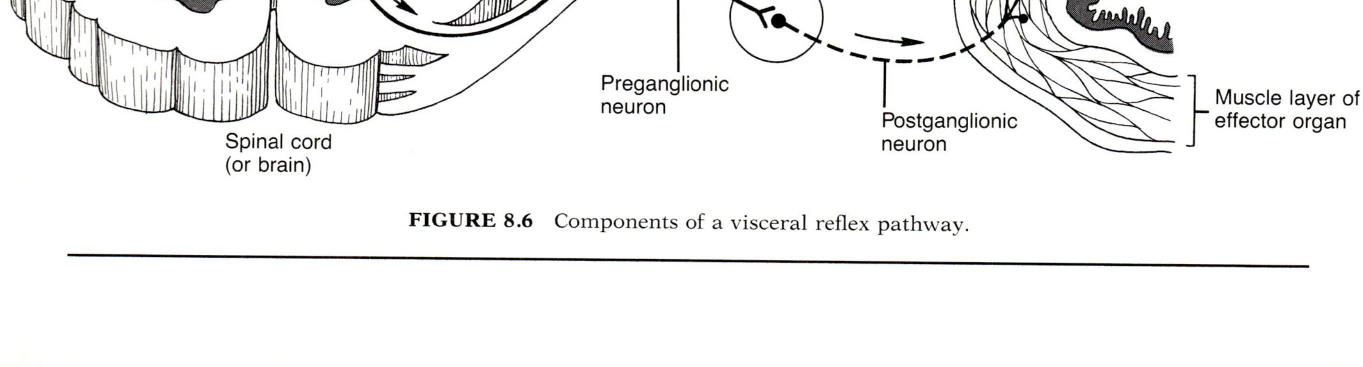

FIGURE 8.6 Components of a visceral reflex pathway.

glionic neuron) which travels to the effector organ.

Sympathetic visceral reflexes are stress responses. Sympathetic preganglionic neurons leave the spinal cord in the thoracic and lumbar areas and synapse in ganglia beside the spinal cord (paravertebral ganglia) or in the abdomen (prevertebral ganglia). Parasympathetic visceral reflexes are homeostatic responses. Parasympathetic preganglionic neurons leave the CNS from the brain or sacral region of the spinal cord and synapse in ganglia in or beside the effector organ (terminal or intramural ganglia).

1. Ciliospinal Reflex

PROCEDURE

a. Work in a team of three people. Have one person sit in *moderate* light (*not facing bright light*). Observe the size of this subject's pupils. Have one person pinch the side of the subject's neck unexpectedly.

b. Report your observations of pupillary size in the LABORATORY REPORT RESULTS at the end of the chapter.

2. Salivary Reflex

MATERIALS

Lemon juice
Sugar solution
Two medicine droppers
Small beaker and small graduated cylinder or
Graduated collection cup

PROCEDURE

a. Instruct a subject to refrain from swallowing for two minutes. At the end of that time, have them expectorate any saliva in the mouth into a small beaker. Measure the volume of saliva collected.

b. Place three drops of lemon juice on the subject's tongue and repeat step 1. (Subtract 0.15 ml from the total volume for the volume of lemon juice.)

c. Place three drops of sugar solution on the subject's tongue and repeat step 1. (Subtract 0.15 ml from the total volume for the volume of the sugar.)

d. Report your observations in the LABORATORY REPORT RESULTS at the end of the chapter.

3. Pupillary Reflexes

MATERIALS

Penlight

PROCEDURE

a. Test for the pupillary light reflex using the procedure given in Exercise 1, Section B3, on page 97.

b. Have the subject isolate the right eye by holding the hand vertically against the nose.

c. While observing the right pupil, shine a flashlight into the side of the left eye. Any change in the right pupil is called a ***consensual response,*** meaning that it is observed on one side of the body when the stimulus is applied to the opposite side.

d. Record your observations in the LABORATORY REPORT RESULTS at the end of the chapter.

Is the pupillary light response ipsilateral or contralateral? ______________________

Is the consensual response ipsilateral or contralateral? ______________________

C. Reflexes in the Frog

The following exercise will demonstrate the varying levels of complexity encountered in several common reflexes. Through the results obtained in this experiment, you should be able to determine which reflexes involve synapses within the brain and which reflexes involve synapses in the spinal cord only.

You will attempt to evoke these reflexes in an unpithed frog, a single-pithed frog, and a double-pithed frog. Single-pithing destroys the brain (and pain sensation) but leaves the spinal cord intact. Double-pithing destroys both the brain and the anterior portion of the spinal cord.

Record all observations in the LABORA-

TORY REPORT RESULTS at the end of the chapter.

MATERIALS

Frog
Pithing needle
Turtle board
String
Tissue
Wire
Ringstand and clamp
Cotton
30% acetic acid solution
Sodium hydroxide (NaOH) solution

PROCEDURE FOR UNPITHED FROG

1. Obtain a frog and observe the position of its head and legs.

2. Determine the rate of respiration by counting the number of times that the frog opens and closes its nostrils per minute.

3. Place the frog on its back and see if it rights itself (righting reflex).

4. Place the frog on a turtle board and fasten it gently around the trunk by tying it loosely with string. Slowly tilt the board and observe the animal's response (horizon reflex).

5. Pinch the toes of the hind legs and observe whether the frog withdraws its foot (withdrawal reflex).

6. Touch the frog's cornea with the twisted end of a tissue and observe the presence or absence of a corneal reflex (blinking).

7. Slap the table sharply close to the frog, and observe the animal's response to this loud noise and vibration.

PROCEDURE FOR SINGLE-PITHED FROG

1. Single-pith a frog according to the instructions in Appendix A. *NOTE. It is strongly suggested that either your instructor or a laboratory assistant perform the pithing procedure since it requires some practice and may prove difficult for inexperienced individuals.*

Before proceeding, wait 3–6 minutes until the frog has recovered from spinal shock. Spinal shock has ended when a pinch of the toes evokes a withdrawal reflex.

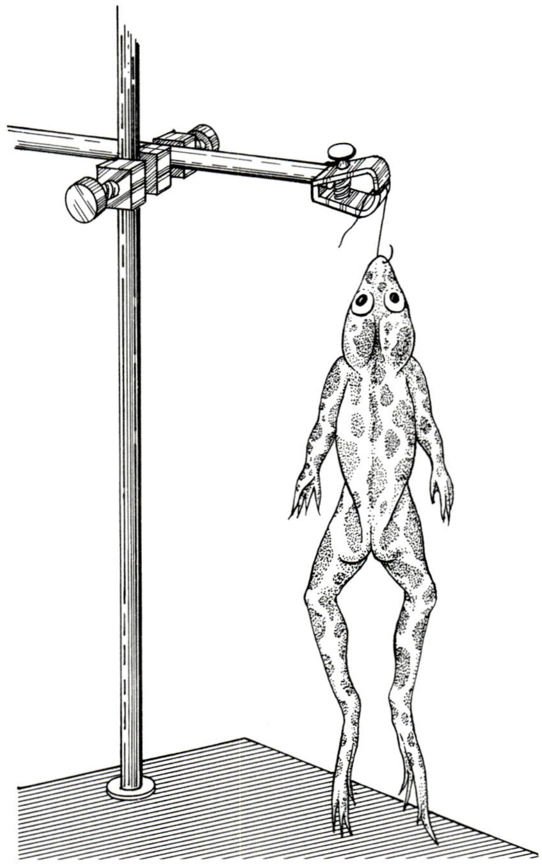

FIGURE 8.7 Pithed frog suspended from clamp.

2. Repeat the seven procedures used on the unpithed frog.

3. Insert a small wire through the anterior area of both jaws. Attach the wire so that the frog is suspended over a pan or sink with its legs hanging freely (see Figure 8.7).

4. Using a piece of cotton that has been moistened with 30% acetic acid solution, rub the lower portion of one leg. Observe the response in the stimulated leg and in the other leg.

5. Rinse the acid from the leg with a sodium hydroxide (NaOH) solution, followed by water.

6. Using a piece of cotton that has been moistened with 30% acetic acid solution, rub the skin of the anterior chest of the frog.

PROCEDURE FOR DOUBLE-PITHED FROG

1. Double-pith a frog according to the instructions in Appendix A. *NOTE. It is strongly sug-*

gested that either your instructor or a laboratory assistant perform the pithing procedure since it requires some practice and may prove difficult for inexperienced individuals.

2. Repeat the seven procedures used with the unpithed frog and the two additional procedures used with the single-pithed frog.

COMPLETE THE LABORATORY REPORT QUESTIONS AT THE END OF THE CHAPTER

LABORATORY REPORT RESULTS

PHYSIOLOGY OF THE NERVOUS SYSTEM 8

Student ____________________ Date ____________________

Laboratory Section ____________________ Score/Grade ____________________

EXERCISE 1. Brain Function

A. Tests for Cerebellar Function

Test	Successful (+)	Unsuccessful (−)
Heel to toe walk		
Balanced stand		
Heel down shin		
Finger touch		
Nose touch		
Grasp of object		

B. Cranial Nerve Function

Nerve	Test	Results
I	Identification of an odor	
II	Near vision	
	Far vision	
III	Pupillary light reflex	
	Ptosis	
III, IV, VI	Eye movement	
V	Jaw opening	
	Touch with cotton	
VII	Symmetry of facial expression	
	Sweet taste	
VIII	Response to spinning	
	Hearing	

Nerve	Test	Results
IX	Bitter taste	
IX, X	Uvular response to touch	
	Uvular response to *ah*	
	Swallowing	
XI	Sternocleidomastoid response	
	Trapezius response	
XII	Tongue protrusion	

EXERCISE 2. Reflexes

A. Somatic Reflexes in the Human

Site of tap	Result	Effector organ
Patellar tendon		
Patellar tendon with distraction		
Patellar tendon after exercise		
Calcaneal (Achilles) tendon		
Triceps brachii tendon		
Babinski reflex		

B. Visceral Reflexes in the Human

1. Result of ciliospinal reflex ______________________________
2. Salivary volume in two minutes = ____

   Salivary volume in two minutes post-lemon juice = ____

   Salivary volume in two minutes post-sugar = ____
3. Change in left pupil after light stimulus ______________________________

   Change in right pupil after light stimulus to left eye ______________________________

C. Reflexes in the Frog

Reflex activity	Unpithed frog	Single-pithed frog	Double-pithed frog
1. Head and leg position			
2. Rate of respiration			
3. Righting reflex			
4. Horizon reflex			
5. Withdrawal reflex			
6. Corneal reflex			
7. Response to noise			
	8. Acetic acid on leg		
	9. Acetic acid on chest		

What conclusions may be drawn as to the levels of complexity of the above reflexes?

What conclusions may be drawn as to the reactivity of peripheral nerves in a single- or double-pithed frog?

LABORATORY REPORT QUESTIONS

PHYSIOLOGY OF THE NERVOUS SYSTEM 8

Student ______________________ Date ______________________

Laboratory Section ______________________ Score/Grade ______________________

PART I. MULTIPLE CHOICE

_____ 1. The peripheral nervous system (PNS) (a) contains effector organs (b) consists of the brain and spinal cord (c) contains afferent and efferent neurons (d) all of the above (e) none of the above

_____ 2. Afferent neurons convey nerve impulses from (a) effector organs to the central nervous system (CNS) (b) receptors to the central nervous system (CNS) (c) the central nervous system (CNS) to the peripheral nervous system (PNS) (d) none of the above

_____ 3. The autonomic nervous system (ANS) (a) consists of afferent and efferent nerves traveling to and from the viscera (b) is under conscious control (c) has effector organs which are skeletal muscles (d) all of the above (e) none of the above

_____ 4. If vomiting and swallowing activities and the respiratory rate were depressed, the part of the brain most likely affected would be the (a) cerebrum (b) diencephalon (c) midbrain (d) pons (e) medulla oblongata

_____ 5. Which of the following is NOT a symptom of cerebellar ataxia? (a) uncoordinated movement (b) intention tremor (c) disturbances of gait and speech (d) loss of control of body temperature (e) inability to maintain balance

_____ 6. Regarding cranial nerves (a) there are twelve pairs (b) they exit the brain through foramina in the skull (c) they are designated by name and Roman numeral (d) all of the above (e) none of the above

_____ 7. The cranial nerves that are solely sensory in function are nerves number (a) I, II, and VIII (b) I and II (c) I, II, V, VII, VIII, IX and X (d) III, IV, and VI (e) V, VIII, and IX

_____ 8. The cranial nerves that innervate parts of the eye are (a) I (b) I and II (c) II, III, IV, and VI (d) III, IV, and VI (e) II and III

_____ 9. Association neurons (a) are always located in the central nervous system (CNS) (b) connect sensory and motor neurons (c) must be present in polysynaptic reflex arcs (d) all of the above (e) none of the above

_____ 10. The stretch reflex is (a) monosynaptic (b) contralateral (c) autonomic (d) all of the above (e) none of the above

_____ 11. Visceral reflexes (a) are all polysynaptic (b) are all stress responses (c) have effectors that are skeletal muscle (d) all of the above (e) none of the above

_____ 12. A response to a stimulus that occurs on the side of the body which is NOT stimulated is a (a) contralateral reflex (b) consensual response (c) both of the above (d) neither of the above

_____ 13. Spinal reflexes are all (a) autonomic (b) somatic (c) ipsilateral (d) monosynaptic (e) none of the above

_____ 14. The reflex response to a pain stimulus applied to a limb is (a) a withdrawal reflex (b) a crossed extensor reflex (c) a spinal reflex (d) all of the above (e) none of the above

_____ 15. Which reflex protects the eye from damage caused by bright light? (a) corneal reflex (b) ciliospinal reflex (c) pupillary reflex

PART II. COMPLETIONS

16. Neurons that convey nerve impulses from the central nervous system (CNS) to skeletal muscles, smooth muscles, and glands are called __________________ neurons.

17. The medulla oblongata, pons, and midbrain compose the __________________ .

18–20. Name three functions of the hypothalamus ____

____

____

21. The awareness of body position is called __________________ .

22–26. Name, in order, the five parts of a reflex arc.

____

____

____

____

____

27. Two neuron reflexes are called __________________ reflexes.

28. Reflexes in which the response is located on the same side of the body as the stimulus are called __________________ reflexes.

29. The reflex that is used to test the integrity of the corticospinal tract is the __________________ reflex.

30. The first motor neuron in a visceral reflex arc is the __________________ neuron.

PART III. CRANIAL NERVES

Give the number of the cranial nerve that is involved with

31. Smelling perfume _____

32. Hearing a brilliant lecture _____

33. Chewing gum during the lecture _____

34. Seeing a photograph in a textbook _____

35. Controlling the heart rate _____

36. Shrugging the shoulders _____

37. Moving the tongue _____

38. Tasting lunch _____

39. Feeling a tongue depressor _____

40. Smiling _____

Destruction of which cranial nerve would cause

41. Blindness ____
42. Inability to lick the lips ____
43. Anosmia ____
44. Deafness ____
45. Inability to move the eyeball laterally ____
46. Inability to open the eyelid ____
47. Inability to frown, smile, or furrow the brow ____
48. Loss of pupillary light reflex ____
49. Inability to taste bitter substances ____
50. Inability to rotate the head ____

DISCUSSION: Damage to which of the following areas might destroy the patellar reflex: cerebrum, cerebellum, cervical spinal cord, lumbar spinal cord, sacral spinal cord, spinal ganglion, or peripheral nerves? Discuss the reasons for your answer.

MUSCLE PHYSIOLOGY 9

EXERCISE 1. Biochemistry of Muscle Contraction
EXERCISE 2. Physiology of Muscle Contraction
- *A. Use of Recording Equipment*
- *B. Measurement of Muscle Contraction*
  1. *Threshold stimulus*
  2. *Single muscle twitch*
  3. *Effect of fatigue on a single muscle twitch*
  4. *Muscle response to variation in stimulus frequency*
  5. *Effect of resting length on contraction strength*

EXERCISE 3. Ergographic Measurement of Human Muscle Contraction

WORD ROOTS

endo- = within
epi- = upon
ergo- = work
fascic- = bundle
iso- = same
myo- = muscle
peri- = around
reticulo- = network
sarco- = flesh
treppe = staircase
tropo- = turning

Muscle tissue constitutes 40% to 50% of the total body weight and is composed of fibers (cells) which have the following characteristics: (1) ***excitability,*** the ability to receive and respond to stimuli; (2) ***contractility,*** the ability to contract (shorten and thicken); (3) ***extensibility,*** the ability to stretch (extend) when pulled; and (4) ***elasticity,*** the ability to return to the original shape after contraction or extension. Muscle contraction results in movement, maintenance of tone, and heat production.

Three kinds of muscle are differentiated on the basis of their histology and function (see Figure 9.1).

1. ***Skeletal muscle tissue***—usually attached to bones. Skeletal muscle is ***voluntary*** because it contracts under conscious control, and it is ***striated*** because microscopic examination reveals prominent banding patterns (striations). The cylindrical skeletal muscle fibers contain multiple nuclei and average about 25,000 μm in length and 1–2 μm in diameter.
2. ***Smooth muscle tissue***—located in the walls of viscera and blood vessels. Smooth muscle is ***involuntary*** and ***nonstriated***: spindle-shaped smooth muscle fibers contain a single nucleus and are about 100 μm long. Smooth muscle will be studied in various exercises in this book.
3. ***Cardiac muscle tissue***—found only in the wall of the heart. Cardiac muscle is ***involuntary*** and ***striated,*** although the striations are not as distinct as those in skeletal muscle. Branched cardiac muscle fibers, averaging 50 μm in length, contain a single nucleus and are separated by ***intercalated discs,*** junctions of low electrical resistance. Cardiac muscle will be studied in Chapter 17.

This chapter will focus on the physiology of skeletal muscle tissue. To review your knowledge of skeletal muscle anatomy, label Figures 9.2 and 9.3 with the following terms:

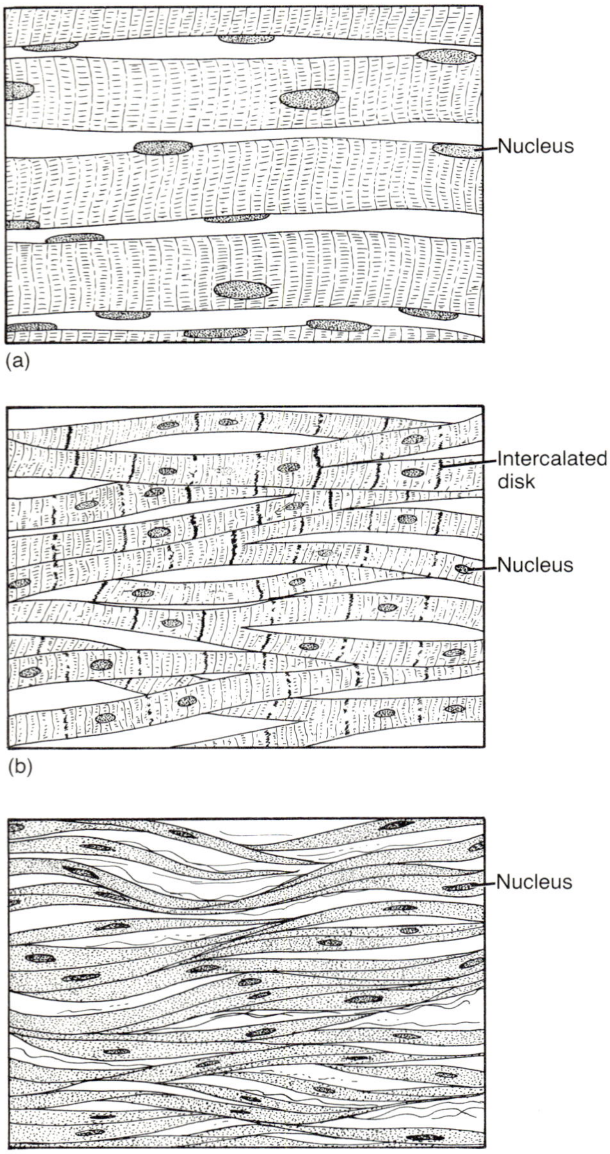

FIGURE 9.1 Types of muscle fibers (cells). (a) Skeletal muscle. (b) Cardiac muscle. (c) Smooth (visceral) muscle.

1. ***Epimysium*** (ep′-i-MĪZ-ē-um)—the connective tissue covering that surrounds the entire muscle and is continuous with the tendon or aponeurosis at the origin and insertion of the muscle.
2. ***Fascicle*** (FAS-i-kl)—a group of muscle fibers covered by a connective tissue called the perimysium.
3. ***Perimysium*** (per-i-MĪZ-ē-um)—the connective tissue covering surrounding each fascicle.
4. ***Muscle fiber (cell)***—a multinucleate cell containing myofibrils.
5. ***Endomysium*** (en′-dō-MĪZ-ē-um)—the connective tissue surrounding each muscle fiber.
6. ***Myofibril***—a group of myofilaments that run longitudinally through the muscle fiber.
7. ***Myofilaments***—thick and thin molecules that are arranged longitudinally in myofibrils. Thick myofilaments are composed of myosin; thin myofilaments of actin, troponin, and tropomyosin.
8. ***Sarcomere***—the contractile unit of a muscle fiber. It is about 2.5 μm long and extends from Z line to Z line.
9. ***I band***—the light region in a sarcomere, composed of thin myofilaments only.
10. ***Z line***—a dense region of the I band where the thin myofilaments are anchored. Z lines separate sarcomeres.
11. ***A band***—the dark region in a sarcomere represented by the length of the thick myofilaments.
12. ***H zone***—the lighter portion of the A band where there are only thick (and no thin) myofilaments.
13. ***M line***—the dense center of the H zone.
14. ***Sarcolemma***—the plasma membrane of the muscle fiber.
15. ***Mitochondrion***—the organelle that is the site of ATP (energy) production for the muscle fiber.
16. ***Sarcoplasmic reticulum***—a flattened closed sac surrounding each myofibril that releases and actively transports calcium ions during contraction and relaxation.
17. ***T (transverse) tubule***—an invagination of the sarcolemma which extends into the muscle fiber between the ends (terminal cisterns) of the sarcoplasmic reticula.
18. ***Triad***—The T tubule and the ends of the sarcoplasmic reticula that are adjacent to it.

The process of ***skeletal muscle contraction*** includes a series of electrical and chemical events. Muscle contraction occurs only if the muscle is properly stimulated. *In vivo* the stimulus is a nerve impulse carried by a ***motor neuron.*** The portion of the neuron that carries the impulse to the muscle fiber is the ***axon,*** and

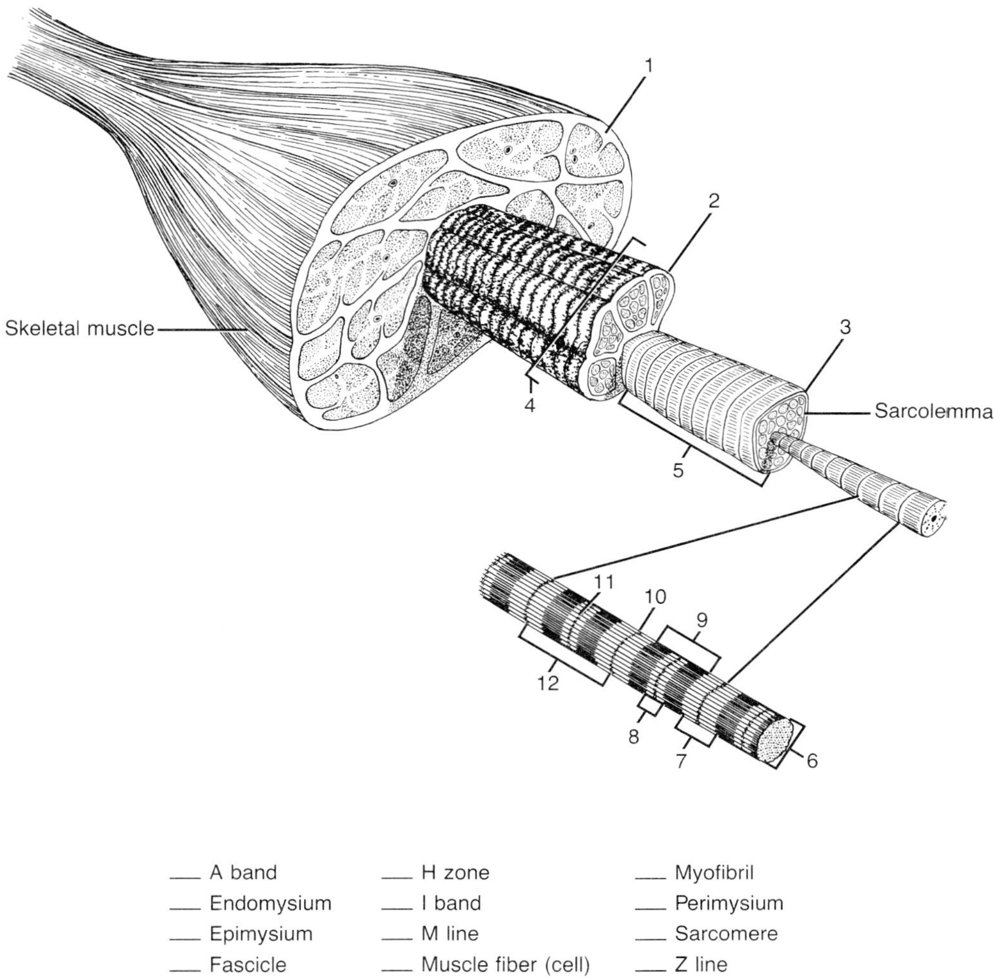

FIGURE 9.2 Diagrammatic histology of skeletal muscle tissue.

the area of contact between the axon and the muscle fiber is the ***neuromuscular (myoneural) junction.***

When the nerve impulse reaches the end of the axon in a skeletal neuromuscular junction, it causes the axon to release a ***neurotransmitter*** called ***acetylcholine (ACh)*** (a′-sēt-il-KŌ-lēn). This substance flows across the neuromuscular junction and binds to receptors on the muscle fiber membrane. The chemical stimulus of the receptors then generates a muscle action potential that travels along the sarcolemma and into the interior of the muscle fiber via the T tubules and continues through the tubules as they contact the sarcoplasmic reticulum. The action potential causes the release of calcium (Ca^{2+}) ions from the sarcoplasmic reticulum; the calcium ions flow into the spaces around the myofilaments.

The thin myofilaments are composed of actin, troponin, and tropomyosin molecules. On the actin molecules are binding sites for the heads of the myosin (thick myofilament) molecules; these sites are covered by the tropomyosin molecule. The calcium ions bind with troponin, causing a change in its molecular configuration that frees up the binding sites on the actin molecules.

As the myosin heads attach to receptors on the actin, ATP is split (hydrolyzed) into ADP and phosphate (P_i) with the release of energy. This energy causes the thin myofilaments to slide inward toward the H zone and thereby shorten the muscle fiber (see Figure 9.4). This

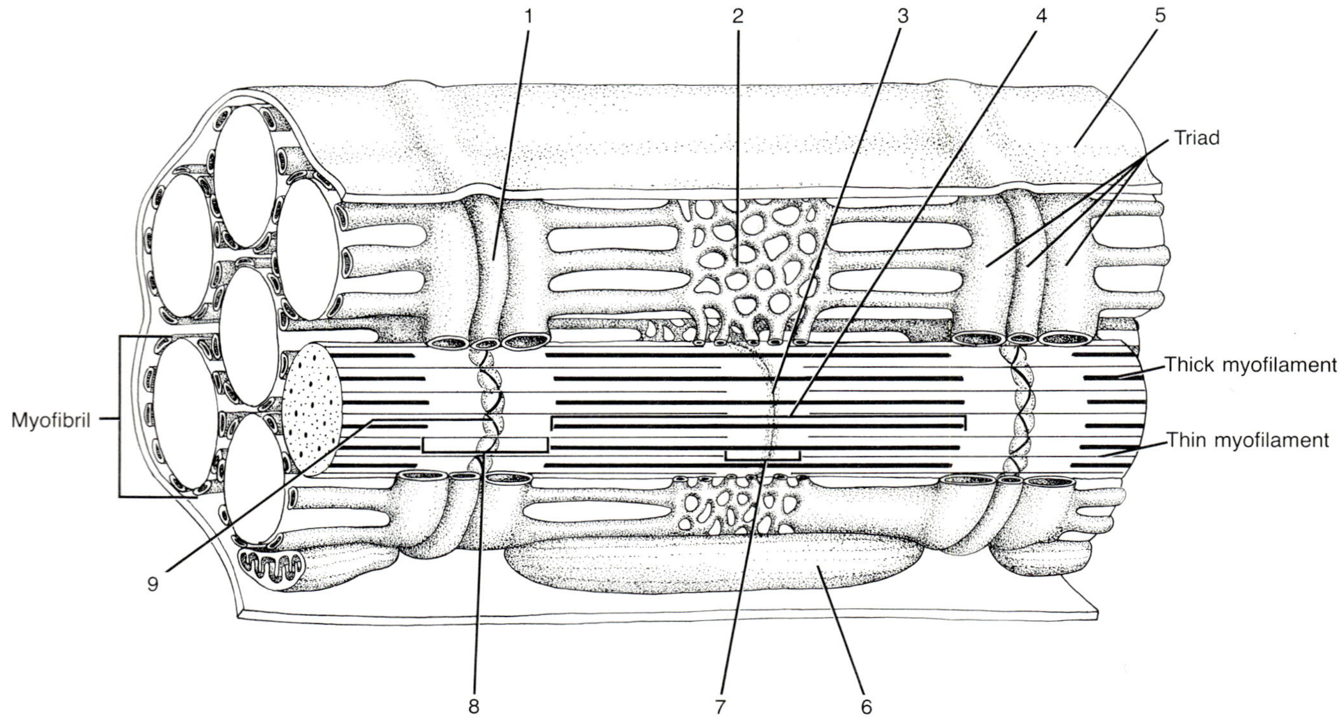

___ A band
___ H zone
___ I band
___ Mitochondrion
___ M line
___ Sarcolemma
___ Sarcoplasmic reticulum
___ T (transverse) tubule
___ Z line

FIGURE 9.3 Enlarged aspect of several skeletal muscle myofibrils, based on an electron micrograph.

action is referred to as the ***sliding filament theory*** of muscle contraction.

After the replacement of ATP on the thick myofilaments and the pumping of calcium ions back into the sarcoplasmic reticulum, the bonds between actin and myosin are broken and relaxation occurs. Relaxation requires significant energy expenditure, about half as much as contraction.

A contracting muscle fiber follows the ***all-or-none principle,*** which states that properly stimulated skeletal muscle fibers will either contract maximally or not at all. This principle does not, however, imply that the *entire muscle* must be either fully contracted or fully relaxed, as some of its fibers will be contracted and some relaxed at any given time. Thus, the muscle as a whole can have graded contractions.

EXERCISE 1. Biochemistry of Muscle Contraction

OBJECTIVES

To observe the contraction of skeletal muscle

To determine the effect of ATP and mineral ions on muscle contraction

CAUTION! *Please reread Section A, "General Procedures and Safety Precautions," and Section C, "Precautions Related to Working With Reagents" in Chapter 1 before you begin any of the exercises in this chapter. You should also read the exercises before you perform them to be sure*

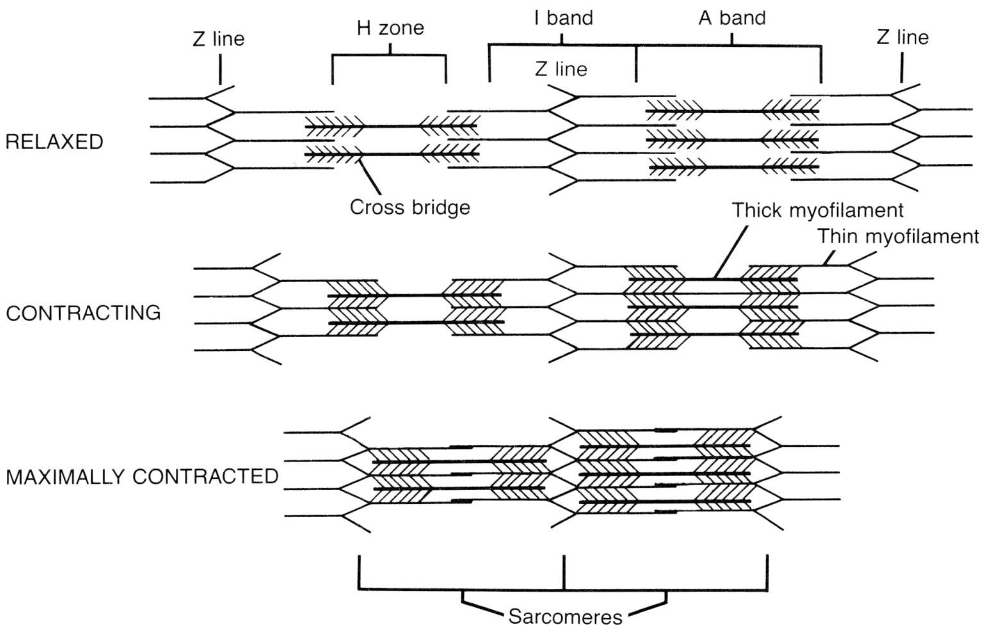

FIGURE 9.4 Sliding filament theory of muscle contraction. The positions of the various parts of two sarcomeres in relaxed, contracting, and maximally contracted states are shown. Note movement of thin myofilaments and relative size of H zone.

that you understand all of the procedures and safety precautions.

In this exercise, you will observe muscle contraction microscopically in rabbit muscle fibers which have been frozen. The muscle has been stored in buffered glycerol, which removes all water-soluble chemicals, including ATP, from the muscle. Adding ATP to the muscle will induce its contraction.

In addition, you will examine the effect of a mineral ion solution on contraction. This solution contains magnesium chloride ($MgCl_2$) and potassium chloride (KCl). Magnesium ions (Mg^{2+}) are required for the proper function of actin molecules; potassium ions (K^+) are also necessary for muscle contraction.

MATERIALS

Glycerinated skeletal muscle in 50% glycerol

Solution of 0.25% ATP in distilled water

Solution of 0.05M KCl and 0.001M $MgCl_2$ in distilled water

Solution of 0.25% ATP and 0.05M KCl and 0.001M $MgCl_2$ in distilled water

Stainless steel scissors or scalpel

Stainless steel teasing needles and fine-point forceps OR glass teasing needles

Pasteur pipette or medicine dropper

Petri dish

Microscope slides and cover slips

Millimeter scale

Compound light microscope and dissecting microscope

Safety goggles

Laboratory apron or coat

PROCEDURE FOR PREPARATION OF THE MUSCLE

1. A piece of rabbit psoas muscle has been tied to a stick. Remove the stick from the test tube, and pour the glycerol into a Petri dish.

2. Cut the strings and place the muscle into the Petri dish.

3. Using a clean stainless steel scalpel or scissors that has been rinsed in distilled water, cut the muscle into pieces about 2 cm in length.

PROCEDURE FOR OBSERVING CONTRACTION

1. Using a dissecting microscope, separate one 2 cm piece of the muscle into single muscle fibers. For this dissection use two glass needles or clean stainless steel forceps which have been rinsed in distilled water. Separating the fibers is difficult; single fibers or thin groups of fibers must be used because strands thicker than a silk thread (0.2 mm) curl when they contract.

2. Mount one strand in a drop of glycerol on a clean glass microscope slide and cover the preparation with a cover slip. A Pasteur pipette or dropper is best for transferring the fibers.

3. Using a compound light microscope, examine the strand under low and high power and note the striations. Also note that each fiber has several nuclei.

4. Transfer one to three of the thinnest strands to a minimal amount of glycerol on a second microscope slide. Do not add a cover slip. If the amount of glycerol on the slide is more than a very small drop, soak the excess into a piece of lens paper held at the edge of the glycerol farthest from the fibers.

5. Using a dissecting microscope and a millimeter ruler held beneath the slide, measure the length of the fiber(s). Record this measurement in the LABORATORY REPORT RESULTS at the end of the chapter.

6. Now flood the fiber(s) with the solution containing ATP only and observe their reaction. After 30 seconds, measure the length of the fiber(s). Record this measurement in the LABORATORY REPORT RESULTS at the end of the chapter.

7. *Using a clean slide, Pasteur pipette or dropper, and teasing needles or forceps,* repeat steps 4 and 5.

8. Flood the fiber(s) with the solution of mineral ions and observe their reaction. After 30 seconds, measure the length of the fiber(s). Record this measurement in the LABORATORY REPORT RESULTS at the end of the chapter.

9. Repeat step 7.

10. Flood the fiber(s) with a solution of ATP and mineral ions. After 30 seconds, measure the length of the fiber(s). Record this measurement in the LABORATORY REPORT RESULTS at the end of the chapter.

11. Using a compound light microscope, observe the contracted fiber under low and high power, and look for differences in appearance between muscle in a contracted and relaxed state. Record your observations in the LABORATORY REPORT RESULTS at the end of the chapter.

Which of the following markings can be seen on the relaxed muscle strand: A band, I band, Z line, H zone, M line? ________________

____

Which markings can be seen on the contracted muscle strand? ________________

Do you think the glycerol removed calcium ions from the muscle? Why? ____________

____

EXERCISE 2. Physiology of Muscle Contraction

> OBJECTIVES
>
> To demonstrate the use of recording equipment
>
> To measure muscle contraction under various conditions

Skeletal muscle can contract in various ways (see Figure 9.5) depending on the antagonistic force exerted against the movement of the muscle and on the strength and timing of the stimulus applied.

The minimum stimulus required to elicit contraction in a muscle fiber is called the ***threshold stimulus.*** The response of a muscle to a single threshold stimulus is called a ***twitch.***

Repeated stimuli to a muscle result in ***treppe,*** a series of twitches of increased strength reaching a plateau. Treppe is characteristic of muscles as they are being "warmed-up."

Rapid repeated stimuli to a muscle result in a smooth sustained contraction known as ***tetanus (tetany).***

If the antagonist, that is, the force (e.g., gravity, the weight of an object being moved) is greater than the force of contraction, the contracting muscle will increase in tone while its length remains constant. Supporting a

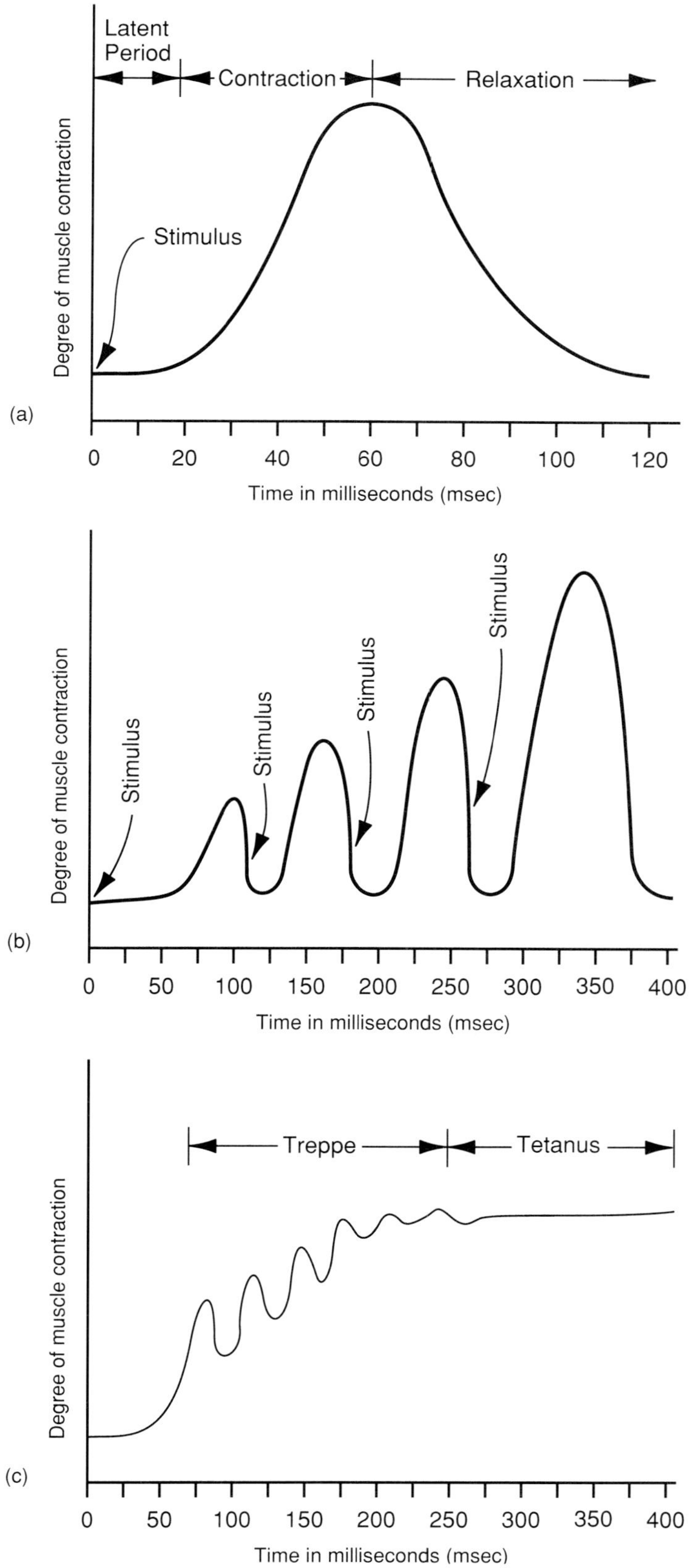

FIGURE 9.5 Myograms of various types of muscle contraction, after a stimulus is applied at time 0. (a) Twitch. (b) Treppe. (c) Tetanus.

heavy object that is fixed in position requires this ***isometric*** type of contraction.

If the strength of the contraction is sufficient to overcome the strength of the antagonistic forces, the contracting muscle shortens in length but does not increase in tone. This ***isotonic*** type of contraction is characteristic of most muscle movement.

This exercise will measure muscle contraction by measuring muscle movement; hence, we will look only at isotonic contractions. We will measure twitch, treppe, and tetanus as they are recorded on a ***myogram,*** a record of a muscle contraction.

The myograms in Figure 9.5 show a time lag between the application of a stimulus and the beginning of the contractile response. During this ***latent period*** the muscle action potential spreads across the sarcolemma and the various molecules undergo reactions which allow the myofilaments to slide. The sliding of the myofilaments causes the muscle to shorten during the ***contraction period;*** subsequently, the muscle fibers lengthen during the ***relaxation period.***

Read the following sections on the use of recording equipment *before* you do the exercise.

A. Use of Recording Equipment

There are two basic types of recording equipment used to measure muscle contraction. The ***kymograph*** (see Figure 9.6) employs a writing lever that is moved when the muscle contracts. The ***physiograph*** employs a sensing device which converts a mechanical (movement) or electrical force into a written record. Follow the procedure below if the physiograph is used in your laboratory. Follow your instructor's directions if the kymograph is to be used.

The Physiograph

The ***physiograph*** (see Figure 9.7) works by receiving a signal from a sensing device, amplifying it, and changing it into perceptible form. For example, a sensing device called a myograph transducer measures the force exerted by a contracting muscle and converts this

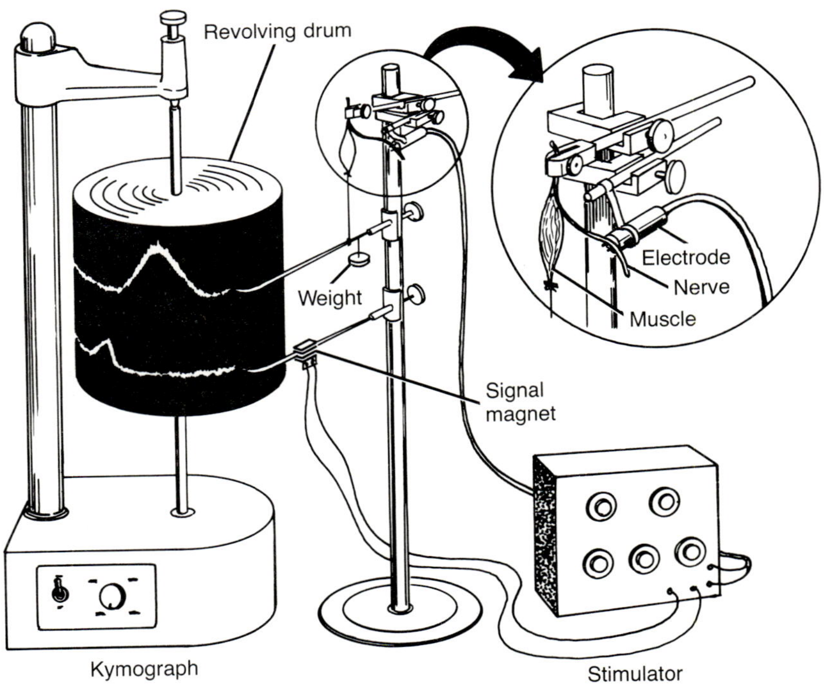

FIGURE 9.6 Kymograph and stimulator for measuring isotonic muscle contraction. (Adapted from Warren D. Dolphin, *Biology Laboratory Manual.* Dubuque, IA: Wm. C. Brown Publishers, 1983.)

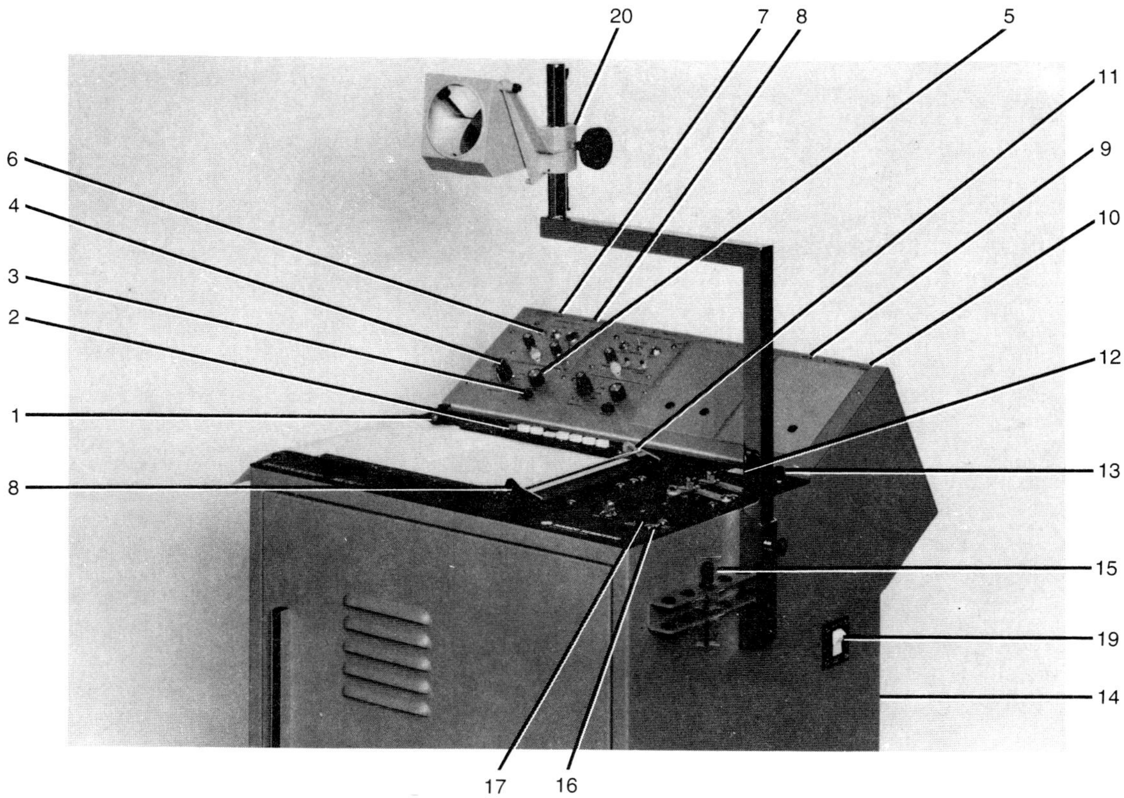

1. Chart drive tension wheel
2. Paper speed switches
3. Record
4. Sensitivity
5. Position
6. Coupler compartment
7. Auxiliary input
8. Monitor output
9. Event input
10. Event output
11. Timer switch
12. Power switch
13. Ground terminal
14. Power connector
15. Inkwell
16. External marker
17. Event marker
18. Pen lifter assembly
19. Projector power switch
20. Projector lens assembly

FIGURE 9.7 A physiograph.

mechanical force into an electrical signal. The signal is magnified by the amplifier and then changed into perceptible form by a writing pen that makes a permanent record of the contraction.

This method of recording a physiological event resembles a phonograph system in which vibrations from the record are changed into electrical signals, amplified, and changed into perceptible form by the loudspeaker.

A physiograph usually has a number of recording channels. Each is used to record a particular physiological event as it occurs. Different events may be recorded simultaneously by using different channels. Each channel consists of a sensing device to detect the event, a coupler to join the sensing device to the amplifier, an amplifier, and a writing pen. The movement of the pen is proportional to the strength of the generated current. The lowest pen on the instrument, a marker pen called TIME AND EVENTS, is used to mark the time at which stimuli are delivered.

Either electrodes or transducers can serve as the sensing device for the physiograph. ***Electrodes*** are made of sensitive metal plates or rods that can detect changes in the electrical potential of a tissue. Electrodes transmit the original unchanged electrical signal to the amplifier. ***Transducers*** convert nonelectrical signals such as movement, heat, and pressure into electrical signals.

a. ORIENTATION TO THE PHYSIOGRAPH

Plug the physiograph into an electrical outlet and turn on the master switch.

Ink Supply

The ink wells should be no more than half full. Send ink to the pens by placing a finger over the hole in the top of the ink bottle and squeezing very gently until a small drop of ink appears at the pen point. You must remove your finger before you stop squeezing the bottle or the ink will not remain in the pen assembly. When you finish using the physiograph, empty the pens by reversing the above sequence, that is, squeeze the bottle, place a finger over the hole, stop squeezing, and remove the finger from the hole when the ink has been entirely withdrawn from the tubing assembly feeding the pens. A watch glass containing water should be placed under the pen point when you empty the pens so that water will be drawn into the pen assembly as the ink is being withdrawn. Ink is gravity fed. Therefore, if the ink flow is too light, raise the ink well 3 mm.

Paper and Paper Controls

The paper drive (paper advance) control sets the paper in motion and lowers the pens. Note that the paper will move only if the leading edge of the paper is under the turning wheel. The speed of the paper is regulated by the paper speed (cm/sec) control. Activate the paper drive and observe the results of changing the speed settings.

Reuse the paper in the next steps. Open the paper storage compartment; pull the paper out of the physiograph and practice reloading. Note that the paper is fed into the physiograph printed side down. Note also that physiograph paper is ruled in metric units, usually in 5 mm or 1 mm squares.

Time and Event Marker

Activate the time marker at its lowest setting (1 sec). Observe how often the lowest pen deflects and in which direction it moves. Depress the event marker and note in which direction the lowest pen moves. This control is used to mark the time at which an event, such as the application of a stimulus, occurs. Some stimulators automatically activate the event marker when each stimulus is applied.

Amplifiers

Each amplifier unit controls one specific pen. The pens are numbered to correspond to the recording channel with which they work. Each amplifier has several controls.

1. The ***off-on switch*** must be on for the unit to be operational. A signal light indicates when the switch is on. Nonsolid-state amplifiers require about five minutes of warm-up.

2. The ***record switch*** must be on in order to record data. Turning the switch off disconnects the amplifier from the sensing device. *It must be off to make any connections to the physiograph.* On nonsolid-state physiographs, *on* is *RECORD* and *off* is *READY*. On solid-state equipment, the record state is engaged by pressing a button until it lights.

3. The ***position control*** situates the pen on the paper. Rotate this control and note the movement of the pen.

4. The ***amplitude control*** determines the amount of amplification of the incoming signal. If the amplification is low, the magnitude of the pen deflection will be small. When the amplification is increased, the magnitude of the pen deflection will also increase. This control is used to calibrate the size of the pen deflection when a known signal is presented. As you increase the sensitivity (amplitude), you also increase the susceptibility of the system to outside disturbances. If a preamplifier is used, amplification is determined by the preamplifier, not the amplifier.

5. ***Other controls*** which may or may not be present include a filter control and a polarity switch (set it to +).

b. CALIBRATION OF THE SYSTEM

Suspend a 100-g weight from the muscle transducer and adjust the sensitivity of the amplifier so that a 5 cm pen deflection is obtained. If at any time this calibration proves unsatisfactory, change the sensitivity to best fit the situation. *Record the calibration factor* for future reference during this exercise.

Calibration factor: ____________

c. USE OF THE STIMULATOR

Muscle may be stimulated by placing electrode tips directly against the muscle or by placing copper wire attached to a stimulator at both ends of the muscle. Familiarize yourself with the physiograph stimulator by noting the following features.

1. ***Off-on switch*** and the signal which lights when the switch is on.
2. ***Stimulation mode control*** which has settings for off, single stimuli, and continuous stimuli.
3. ***Frequency control*** which regulates the number of stimuli generated per second.
4. ***Duration control*** which regulates the length of each stimulus.
5. ***Voltage regulator*** which controls the strength of the stimulus.
6. Other features such as the multiplier, which may be explained by your instructor.

B. Measurement of Muscle Contraction

MATERIALS

Dissecting pan and tools
Ring stand with femur clamp
Physiograph and associated apparatus
Frog Ringer's solution
Medicine dropper

Following the instructions in Appendix A on page 365, double-pith a frog and isolate the gastrocnemius muscle. CAUTION! *It is strongly suggested that frogs be pithed by your instructor or a laboratory assistant. The procedure requires some practice and may prove difficult for inexperienced individuals.*

Place the muscle preparation in the apparatus as shown in Figure 9.8. Hold the bone firmly in a femur clamp and place the stimulating electrode in the belly of the muscle. Adjust the height of the femur clamp so that the muscle has a slight amount of tension on it. Remember that an isolated muscle has no blood supply. Therefore, moisten the muscle with frog Ringer's solution frequently. If the muscle twitches when no stimulus is being applied, moisten it immediately.

1. Threshold Stimulus

PROCEDURE

a. Set the paper speed and stimulus intensity controls at their lowest settings. Set the stimulation mode control to *single,* and the duration control, if present, to 5 milliseconds (msec).

b. Apply a single stimulus to the muscle.

c. Rinse the muscle with frog Ringer's solution at regular intervals to keep the preparation moist.

d. Increase the stimulus intensity (voltage) by one setting (0.5 V).

e. Repeat steps 2, 3, and 4 until the muscle contracts.

f. Record the threshold stimulus in the LABORATORY REPORT RESULTS at the end of the chapter.

g. Continue repeating steps 2, 3, and 4 until a maximum strength contraction has been reached. Record this voltage in the LABORATORY REPORT RESULTS at the end of the chapter.

What phenomena occur in a muscle to which subthreshold stimulus has been applied? ______

____

Does the strength of contraction increase with suprathreshold stimuli? ______________

Explain this answer with reference to the all-or-none response. ______________

____

____

____

2. Single Muscle Twitch

PROCEDURE

a. Set the physiograph paper speed at its fastest setting; leave the duration control at 5 milliseconds (msec) and the stimulation mode control at *single.*

b. Apply a single suprathreshold stimulus to the muscle.

c. Rinse the muscle with frog Ringer's solution.

d. Repeat steps 2 and 3 three times.

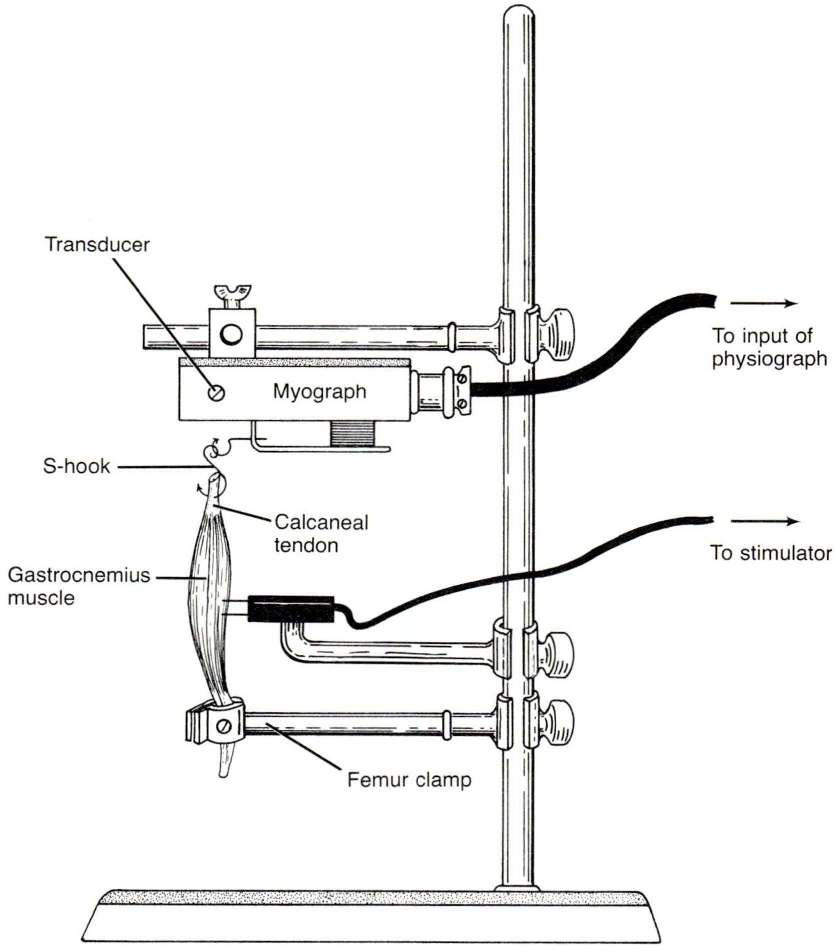

FIGURE 9.8 Frog gastrocnemius muscle preparation.

e. Turn the amplifier off and keep the muscle moist.

f. On the four tracings, measure the latent period, contraction period, and relaxation period. Record these values in the LABORATORY REPORT RESULTS at the end of the chapter. Calculate the average for each value.

What events occur during the latent period?

____

____

3. Effect of Fatigue on a Single Muscle Twitch

PROCEDURE

a. Set the physiograph paper speed at its lowest setting. Leave the duration control at 5 milliseconds (msec). Set the frequency control to 1 stimulus per second. Set the stimulation mode control to *continuous*.

b. Stimulate the muscle with a voltage just above the threshold stimulus. Continue the stimuli until the muscle fails to contract.

c. Continue the stimulation for an additional 60 seconds to determine if any recovery occurs.

d. Quickly remove the muscle and cut deep into its belly. Test the muscle with pH paper and record the pH in the LABORATORY REPORT RESULTS at the end of the chapter.

e. Record your observations on fatigue in the LABORATORY REPORT RESULTS at the end of the chapter.

Is there any change in the length of the latent period as a muscle is becoming fatigued?

Explain. ______________________________

____

____

What biochemical changes cause fatigue of a muscle? ______________________________

____

4. Muscle Response to a Variation of Stimulus Frequency

When a single threshold or suprathreshold stimulus is applied to a muscle fiber or a whole muscle, the contraction response follows the all-or-none principle. However, if two stimuli are applied in close succession, so that the second stimulus is applied before complete relaxation from the first, the second contraction is greater than the first. The extent of the increased response to the second stimulus is dependent upon the interval between the successive stimuli.

This response to increased stimulus frequency, a seeming contradiction to the all-or-none principle, is termed ***summation***. It is due to increased amounts of calcium ions accumulating within the muscle fiber. Sequestration of these ions requires time and energy expenditure, and it is not completed if a second stimulus is applied before total sequestration has occurred.

When the stimulus frequency is increased, the amount of relaxation between successive stimuli progressively decreases until further stimuli fail to increase the strength of contraction and no relaxation occurs. This pattern of response is termed ***tetanus (tetany)***. During tetanus, the contraction strength may be three or four times that seen with a single contraction.

PROCEDURE

a. Following the instructions at the beginning of Section B, make a new muscle preparation from the nondissected leg of the frog and place it in the apparatus.

b. Set the physiograph paper speed to a medium setting. Set the duration control to 5 milliseconds and the stimulus frequency to 1 stimulus per second. Set the stimulation mode control to *continuous*. Set the voltage control to a level just above threshold.

c. Progressively increase the frequency of stimulation until summation and tetany are observed.

d. Record the frequencies at which summation and tetany occur in the LABORATORY REPORT RESULTS at the end of the chapter.

e. Turn the stimulator off and rinse the muscle with frog Ringer's solution. Allow 2–3 minutes of recovery time before proceeding to the next section.

How does the strength (measured height) of contraction during tetany compare with that during twitch? Explain. ______________________________

____

____

____

5. Effect of Resting Length on Contraction Strength

PROCEDURE

a. Depending on the preparation in use, adjust either the femur clamp or muscle transducer height so that a small amount of resting tension is applied to the muscle.

b. Set the paper speed at the lowest setting, the stimulation mode control to *single*, the duration control to 5 milliseconds (msec), and the voltage control to just above threshold level.

c. Apply a single stimulus to the muscle.

d. Rinse the muscle with frog Ringer's solution.

e. Increase the resting tension very slightly.

f. Repeat steps 3, 4, and 5 until contraction strength reaches a maximum and begins to decline.

g. Graph your results in the LABORATORY REPORT RESULTS at the end of the chapter and explain your findings in the space provided.

What is the relationship between stretch and force of contraction with regard to athletic activity? ______________________________

____

____

____

NOTE: When you are through using the physiograph, follow the directions of your laboratory instructor to clean and store the equipment.

EXERCISE 3. Ergographic Measurement of Human Muscular Contraction

OBJECTIVES

To demonstrate human muscle fatigue
To demonstrate the effect of reduced blood supply on muscle fatigue

The ***ergograph*** is an apparatus that measures the amount of work done by muscles. It consists of an adjustable spring mechanism moved by muscular action which is attached to a writing device. The ergograph may be used in conjunction with a kymograph which moves recording paper at a given speed.

In this exercise the ergograph will be used to demonstrate the effect of fatigue and a compromised blood supply on skeletal muscle.

MATERIALS

Ergograph
Kymograph, paper, and writing device
Sphygmomanometer cuff

PROCEDURE

1. Work in pairs for this exercise. Set up an ergograph and a kymograph as illustrated in Figure 9.9.
2. Set the spring tension of the ergograph at its highest level.
3. Make certain that the ink supply is adequate or attach a felt tipped marker to the ergograph arm. If you are using a kymograph ink supply, place a paper towel under the ink well to prevent damage to the laboratory table.
4. Attach paper to the kymograph drum; lap the left-hand edge of the paper over the right-hand edge.
5. Raise or lower the drum until the pen tip rests about 1. 5 inches from the bottom of the paper.
6. Pull out the selector knob and set the drum speed at 9 (0.1 cm/sec).

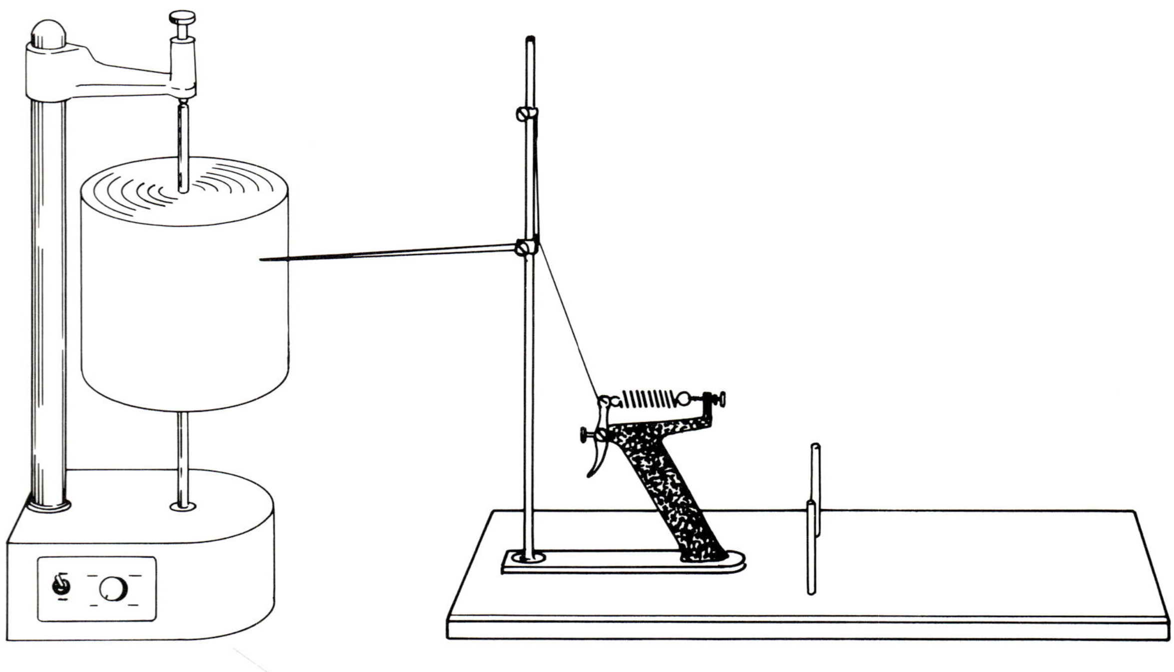

FIGURE 9.9 An ergograph and kymograph as used to measure muscle work.

7. Start the kymograph and instruct the subject to squeeze the trigger as rapidly as possible until complete fatigue develops.

8. When fatigue has developed, shut off the kymograph and have the subject rest for 5–10 minutes.

9. Place a sphygmomanometer cuff on the subject's arm and inflate the cuff until the pressure is 150 mm Hg. Repeat steps 7 and 8.

10. Calculate the amount of time required for complete fatigue under normal conditions and under conditions of compromised blood supply. Record these times in the LABORATORY REPORT RESULTS at the end of the chapter.

What condition caused the difference in the time required to generate muscle fatigue? ____

____

COMPLETE THE LABORATORY REPORT QUESTIONS AT THE END OF THE CHAPTER

MUSCLE PHYSIOLOGY 9

Student ______________________ **Date** ______________________

Laboratory Section ______________________ **Score/Grade** ______________________

EXERCISE 1. Biochemistry of Muscle Contraction

1. Initial length of muscle fiber(s) ______________________
2. Length of fiber(s) with ATP ______________________
3. Length of fiber(s) with mineral ions ______________________
4. Length of fiber(s) with ATP + ions ______________________

5. Drawing of relaxed fibers Drawing of contracted fibers

EXERCISE 2. Physiology of Muscle Contraction

1. Threshold Stimulus

a. Threshold stimulus = ____

b. Maximal strength contraction evoked by ____ volt stimulus.

2. Single Muscle Twitch

Stimulus number

	1	2	3	4	Average
Latent period					
Contraction period					
Relaxation period					

Attach a myogram of a twitch on the next page. Label the latent period, contraction period, and relaxation period.

MYOGRAM

3. Effect of Fatigue on a Single Muscle Twitch

a. Time until contraction is 50% of normal = ___________

b. Time until complete fatigue occurs = ___________

c. Number of responses during 60 seconds of stimulation after complete fatigue has occurred = ___________

d. pH of fatigued muscle = ___________

4. Muscle Response to a Variation of Stimulus Frequency

a. Frequency at which summation occurs = ___________

b. Frequency at which tetany occurs = ___________

c. Attach a myogram derived from increasing stimulus frequency below. Label phases showing summation and tetany.

MYOGRAM

5. Effect of Resting Length on Contraction Strength

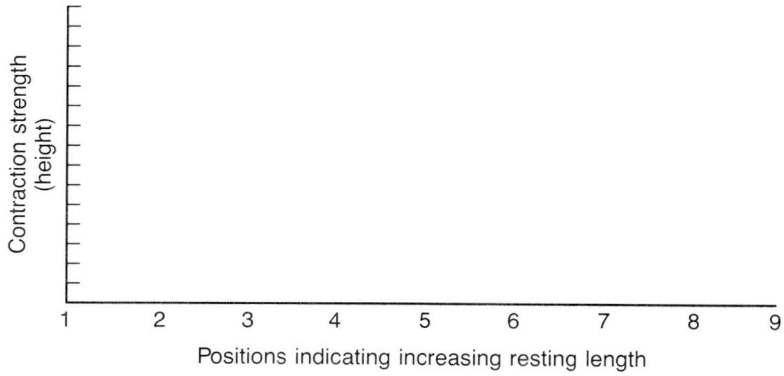

What percent increase in the strength of contraction can be obtained by increasing the resting length of muscle? ____ % Why does the strength of contraction decrease when the resting length is stretched beyond a certain limit?

EXERCISE 3. Ergographic Measurement of Muscle Contraction

a. Time for complete fatigue to develop = __________

b. Time for complete fatigue to develop with blood supply occluded = __________

c. Place kymograph tracing below. Indicate the point at which fatigue has developed.

LABORATORY REPORT QUESTIONS

MUSCLE PHYSIOLOGY 9

Student ______________________ **Date** ______________________

Laboratory Section ______________________ **Score/Grade** ______________________

PART I. MULTIPLE CHOICE

_____ 1. The ability of muscle tissue to return to its original shape after contraction or extension is called: (a) excitability (b) tetany (c) elasticity (d) extensibility (e) none of the above

_____ 2. The connective tissue that surrounds fascicles is (a) epimysium (b) perimysium (c) endomysium (d) tendon (e) aponeurosis

_____ 3. Which of the following statements is NOT true of a sarcomere? (a) there are usually more than 1,000 sarcomeres in each skeletal muscle fiber (b) sarcomeres are the contractile units of the muscle fiber (c) sarcomeres extend from M line to M line

_____ 4. The portion of a sarcomere that contains only thin myofilaments is the (a) A band (b) I band (c) H zone (d) M line

_____ 5. Thin myofilaments (a) are composed of myosin (b) have cross-bridges that rotate (c) release calcium ions upon stimulation (d) all of the above (e) none of the above

_____ 6. T tubules (a) run parallel to myofilaments (b) release calcium ions upon stimulation (c) are invaginations of the sarcolemma (d) all of the above (e) none of the above

_____ 7. The neuromuscular junction (a) lies between the dendrite of a neuron and a muscle fiber (b) lies between the axon of a neuron and a T tubule (c) is the site into which neurotransmitters are released (d) is connected to the sarcoplasmic reticulum (e) none of the above

_____ 8. During muscle contraction (a) ADP is used as the energy source (b) myosin bonds with troponin (c) calcium binds with actin (d) all of the above (e) none of the above

_____ 9. In a skeletal muscle twitch, which period occupies the least amount of time? (a) contraction period (b) relaxation period (c) latent period

PART II. MATCHING

_____ 10. Has the longest fibers

_____ 11. Striated and involuntary

_____ 12. Located in the heart

_____ 13. Has spindle-shaped fibers

_____ 14. Usually inserts on bone

_____ 15. Nonstriated

_____ 16. Cell junctions are intercalated discs

_____ 17. Striated and voluntary

_____ 18. Multinucleate

_____ 19. Composes wall of heart (myocardium)

A. Skeletal muscle
B. Smooth muscle
C. Cardiac muscle

PART III. COMPLETIONS

20. The ability of muscle to receive and respond to stimuli is called ______________ .
21. The organelle which releases and absorbs calcium ions during contraction and relaxation is the ______________ .
22. Name the three parts of the skeletal muscle triad. ______________
____
____
23. The neurotransmitter released at a neuromuscular junction is ______________ .
24. The minimum stimulus that elicits a contraction is termed a/an ______________ stimulus.
25. A contraction that causes a change in muscle tone with no decrease in length is a/an ______________ contraction.
26. A graphic diagram of a muscle contraction is a/an ______________ .

PART IV. MATCHING

____ 27. Responses to a single threshold stimulus
____ 28. Characteristic of "warm-up"
____ 29. Response to rapid repeated stimuli
____ 30. Strong, sustained contraction

A. Twitch
B. Tetany
C. Treppe

PART V. MATCHING

____ 31. Converts nonelectrical signals to electrical signals
____ 32. Controls the speed of recording
____ 33. Controls the degree of pen deflection
____ 34. Regulates the length of a stimulus
____ 35. Controls the strength of a stimulus

A. Amplifier
B. Transducer
C. Frequency control
D. Paper speed control
E. Amplitude control
F. Frequency control
G. Voltage regulator

10 SENSORY PHYSIOLOGY: GENERAL SENSES, OLFACTION, AND GUSTATION

EXERCISE 1. Cutaneous Receptors
- *A. Touch Receptors*
  - *1. Identifying touch receptors*
  - *2. Localization of the touch sensation*
  - *3. Two-point discrimination*
- *B. Pressure Receptors*
- *C. Thermoreceptors*
  - *1. Localization of heat and cold receptors*
  - *2. Adaptation of temperature receptors*
- *D. Pain Receptors*

EXERCISE 2. Proprioceptive Receptors

EXERCISE 3. Olfactory and Gustatory Receptors
- *A. Olfactory Adaptation*
- *B. Association of Smell and Taste*

WORD ROOTS

cuta-, cuti- = skin
entero- = intestinal
extero- = outside
gust- = taste
noci-, noxi- = harmful
olfact- = smell
proprio- = one's own
tact- = touch
therm- = heat
viscero- = abdominal organs

Sensation is an awareness of the conditions of the internal and external environment of the body. In order for a sensation to occur: (1) a ***stimulus*** or change in energy input, strong enough to elicit a response by the central nervous system, is necessary; (2) a ***sensory receptor*** or ***sense organ*** must act as a transducer, i.e., receive the stimulus and convert it into a nerve impulse; (3) a nerve pathway for ***conduction*** of the nerve impulse to the central nervous system is required; and (4) there must be a brain region specialized for ***translation*** of the nerve impulse into a sensation.

The nature of the sensory impulses which reach the brain is identical for sensations of heat, hearing, pain, smell, and so forth, yet the stimuli are perceived as different from one another. This characteristic of sensation is known as ***modality***, that is, the property by which sensations are distinguished from each other.

The awareness of a stimulus is not localized at the site that is stimulated but in the brain. Even though all stimuli are conducted to a small region of the brain, we can distinguish the specific location of each sensation, *i.e.*, we not only perceive pain but also whether the pain is present in the leg or the arm. This characteristic of a sensation, ***projection***, is the process by which the brain refers sensations to the learned point of stimulation.

A third characteristic of many sensations is ***adaptation***, the loss of sensation when a stimulus is still present. Bath water may feel hot upon entering it, yet the same temperature is perceived as warm even before the water has cooled; we are aware of the presence of a watch when we put it on, yet we are not aware of it touching the skin after a few moments.

Conversely, sensations often remain after the stimulus has been removed. This characteristic is that of ***afterimages.*** It can be demonstrated by focusing on a bright light and then closing the eyes; the image will persist for a measurable period of time.

Sensation may be categorized in three different ways.

Classification by Receptor Location

1. ***Exteroceptors*** (EKS-ter-ō-sep′-tors), located near the body surface, are stimulated by changes in the external environment. They transmit sensations such as hearing, sight, smell, taste, touch, pressure, temperature, and pain.

2. ***Visceroceptors*** (VIS-er-ō-sep′-tors) or ***enteroceptors***, located in blood vessels and viscera, are stimulated by changes in the internal environment. These stimuli are perceived as pain, taste, fatigue, hunger, thirst, and nausea. Two specific types of visceroceptors are ***baroreceptors (pressoreceptors)***, stimulated by changes in the hydrostatic pressure of blood, and ***osmoreceptors***, which are stimulated by changes in the solute concentration of extracellular fluid.

3. ***Proprioceptors*** (PRŌ-prē-ō-sep′-tors) or stretch receptors, located in muscles, tendons, or joints, are stimulated by stretching or movement. They provide sensations of position, movement, and muscle tension.

Classification by Type of Stimulus Received

1. ***Mechanoreceptors*** are stimulated by mechanical deformation of the receptor itself. They provide sensations of touch, pressure, vibration, proprioception (awareness of the location and movement of body parts), hearing, and equilibrium. Mechanoreceptors are also triggered by changes in blood pressure.

2. ***Thermoreceptors*** are stimulated by changes in temperature.

3. ***Nociceptors*** (nō-sē-sep′-tors) are triggered by painful stimuli.

4. ***Photoreceptors*** (electromagnetic receptors) are stimulated by light energy.

5. ***Chemoreceptors*** are stimulated by changes in the chemical environment of cells such as the presence of certain molecules on the tongue or nasal mucosa (taste and smell), and the presence of oxygen, carbon dioxide, hydrogen ions, certain other electrolytes, hormones, and glucose.

Classification by Complexity of Receptor and Neural Pathway

1. ***General senses*** involve simple receptors and neural pathways. They may be ***proprioceptive sensations*** or ***cutaneous sensations.*** The latter are subdivided into

   a. ***Tactile*** (TAK-tīl) ***sensations*** (touch, pressure, vibration)

   b. ***Thermoreceptive sensations*** (temperature)

   c. ***Pain sensations***

2. ***Special senses*** involve complex receptors and neural pathways. They are

   a. ***Olfactory*** (ol-FAK-tō-rē) ***sensations*** (smell)

   b. ***Gustatory*** (GUS-ta-tō-rē) ***sensations*** (taste)

   c. ***Visual sensations*** (sight)

   d. ***Auditory sensations*** (hearing)

   e. ***Equilibrium sensations*** (complex sensation of body orientation and balance)

EXERCISE 1. Cutaneous Receptors

A. Touch Receptors

Cutaneous receptors are not randomly distributed over the body surface; some areas contain many receptors, some areas have very few. This clustering of receptors is known as ***punctate distribution***. The following three exercises demonstrate different ways of identifying the distribution and density of touch receptors.

1. Identifying Touch Receptors

Receptors for touch are located in the dermis, just beneath the epidermis of the skin. These receptors are most numerous in the fingertips, palms, and soles of the feet; they are also abundant in the eyelids, tongue, lips, nipples, clitoris, and glans penis.

OBJECTIVE

To determine the distribution of touch receptors

MATERIALS

Light colored water-soluble felt tip pen with sharp point

Ruler

Soft bristle or Von Frey hair

PROCEDURE

1. Using a felt tip pen, mark an 8 mm square on the anterior side of a subject's forearm or back of the hand. Subdivide the square at 2 mm intervals, making 16 squares.

2. With the subject's eyes closed, press a Von Frey hair or bristle against the skin, just enough to deflect the hair, in each of the sixteen squares.

3. The subject should indicate when touch is experienced. When it is, the experimenter should record the point at which sensation was felt. For recording, use the grid in the LABORATORY REPORT RESULTS at the end of the chapter.

In how many squares was touch reported? _____ Were the areas evenly distributed or clustered? ____________

2. Localization of the Touch Sensation

OBJECTIVE

To determine the ability of different body parts to localize the point of stimulation

MATERIALS

Two water-soluble felt tip pens

Ruler

PROCEDURE

1. Have the subject close his/her eyes. Touch the skin on the thumb lightly with a pen.

2. Instruct the subject to attempt to touch the same location with a pen while keeping the eyes closed.

3. Measure the distance between the two points. Record in the LABORATORY REPORT RESULTS at the end of the chapter.

4. Repeat three times and average the distances. Record in the LABORATORY REPORT RESULTS at the end of the chapter.

5. Repeat the exercise on the palm of the hand, arm, and back of the neck and record in the LABORATORY REPORT RESULTS at the end of the chapter.

What is the relationship between the accurate localization of a stimulus and the number of tactile receptors in that area? ______________

____

____

3. Two-Point Discrimination

OBJECTIVE

To measure distances required for two-point discrimination

MATERIALS

Compass or esthesiometer

Alcohol and cotton

PROCEDURE

1. CAUTION! *Clean the points of the measuring device with alcohol or a fresh bleach solution and then rinse with water.* Place the points 2 mm apart on the tip of the subject's tongue. Ask the subject to indicate whether one or two points are perceived.

2. Apply one and two point touches randomly while decreasing the distance until only one point is perceived.

3. Open the compass to 40 mm and repeat steps 1 and 2 on back of the neck, back of the hand, side of the nose, and tip of the finger.

4. Record your measurements in the LABORATORY REPORT RESULTS at the end of the chapter.

Why is there a difference in the ability of various parts of the body to discriminate two points? ______________________________

____

B. Pressure Receptors

Pressure sensations generally result from the deformation of receptors which are deep to touch receptors. The sensations are longer lasting, have less variation in intensity, and are felt over a wider area than sensations of touch. In addition to their distribution in the skin, these receptors are found in joints and tendons, the perimysium of muscles, the mammary glands, genitals, and some viscera.

Sensations of ***vibration*** result from rapidly repetitive sensory stimuli applied to lamellated corpuscles (Pacinian receptors) and/or corpuscles of touch (Meissner's corpuscles).

> OBJECTIVE
> To determine if pressure sensitivity varies in different body regions

MATERIALS

Bristle or cardboard sliver
Laboratory manual

PROCEDURE

1. Place a large diameter bristle or a 2 × 10 mm sliver of your lab book cover beneath two pages of your lab manual.
2. Have your lab partner locate the object by running the fingers lightly over the page.
3. Continue adding pages until the object can no longer be located.
4. Repeat the search with the elbow, chin, nose, and thenar eminence at the base of the thumb.
5. Record your results in the LABORATORY REPORT RESULTS at the end of the chapter.

What is the physical effect of the object on the pressure receptors? ______________________________

C. Thermoreceptors

Cold receptors are unevenly distributed throughout the dermis and subcutaneous layer of the skin. They cluster in the mouth and genitals and are thought to be myelinated (and possibly free) nerve endings. Heat receptors are deeper and less numerous than cold receptors; they are most numerous in the soles of the feet.

Thermoreceptors are stimulated by ***relative,*** not absolute, changes in temperature; they adapt to their environment, establishing the current temperature as "physiological zero." They send few nerve impulses to the central nervous system unless a change in the stimulus occurs, that is, if temperature rises or falls.

1. Localization of Heat and Cold Receptors

> OBJECTIVE
> To localize receptors for heat and cold

MATERIALS

Water-soluble felt tip pen with sharp point
Two paper clips, metal probes, or forceps
Three beakers
Ice
Ruler
Towel
Thermometer

PROCEDURE

1. Using a felt tip pen, mark an 8 mm square on the anterior side of a subject's wrist. Subdivide the square at 2 mm intervals, making 16 squares.
2. Place an opened paper clip, metal probe, or forceps in a beaker filled with ice water. Place another in hot water (CAUTION! *Use water at about 45°C, hot enough to give a sensation of heat, but not enough to cause pain*).
3. Remove one object from the beaker, dry quickly, and touch one of the marked squares on the subject's wrist.
4. Randomize the exposures to hot and cold, but make sure to touch each square with both stimuli.
5. Have the subject report *Hot, Cold,* or *Don't know,* for each exposure.
6. Record your observations in the grid in the LABORATORY REPORT RESULTS at the end of the chapter.

Were there more receptors for heat or for cold?

____

How do you explain a perception of *Don't know*? ________________________________

____

2. Adaptation of Temperature Receptors

> OBJECTIVE
>
> To demonstrate relative versus absolute sensitivity of thermal receptors

MATERIALS

Three 1 liter beakers
Thermometer
Towel
Ice
Timer

PROCEDURE

1. Fill one 1 liter beaker with 700 ml of ice water, another with room temperature water, and a third with water at 45°C.
2. Immerse the left hand in the ice water and the right hand in the hot water for one minute.
3. Move the left hand to the room temperature water. Record the sensation in the LABORATORY REPORT RESULTS at the end of the chapter.
4. Move the right hand to the room temperature water. Record the sensation in the LABORATORY REPORT RESULTS at the end of the chapter.

How do you explain the difference in the experienced temperature of the room temperature water? ________________________________

____

D. Pain Receptors

Pain receptors are high-threshold bare nerve endings found throughout the body. Excessive stimulation of any sensory structure will cause pain. The receptors are not selective, but are stimulated by a wide variety of phenomena: excessive pressure, heat, cold, chemical stimuli, tissue ischemia, substances released from damaged cells, and so forth. Adaptation to pain stimuli occurs only rarely; this protects us from becoming used to pain and ignoring the signals of danger or disease.

Referred pain occurs when the cerebral cortex projects the sensation of pain to a body part other than the one that is receiving the painful stimulus. Examples are the pain experienced in the arm when heart muscle is damaged and the pain experienced in the forehead when ice-cold food or drink is swallowed. ***Phantom pain*** is the referred pain projected to a body part which has been amputated.

> OBJECTIVE
>
> To experience referred pain

MATERIALS

Ice water
Basin
Timer
Towel

PROCEDURE

1. Place your elbow in a large shallow pan of ice water.
2. Note the sensation in the elbow upon immersion. Is it cold, tingling, or painful?
3. Keep the elbow immersed for 2 minutes. Note the location of the sensation in 30 seconds, 1 minute, and 2 minutes.
4. Record your observations in the LABORATORY REPORT RESULTS at the end of the chapter.

EXERCISE 2. Proprioceptive Receptors

An awareness of the activities of muscles, tendons, and joints is provided by the ***proprioceptive (kinesthetic) sense.*** It informs us of the degree to which tendons are stretched and muscles are contracted. The proprioceptive sense enables us to recognize the location and rate of movement of one part of the body in relation to other parts.

It also allows us to estimate weight and to

determine the muscular work necessary to perform a task.

Proprioceptive receptors are located in skeletal muscles and tendons, in and around joints, and in the internal ear. Proprioceptors adapt only slightly. This lack of complete adaptation is beneficial because the brain must be apprised of the status of different parts of the body at all times so that adjustments can be made to ensure coordination and balance.

Proprioceptive receptors are of three types. The ***joint kinesthetic*** (kin′-es-THET-ik) ***receptors*** are located in the articular capsules and ligaments around joints. They provide feedback information on the degree and rate of angulation (change of position) of a joint. ***Muscle spindles***, most numerous in the muscles of the extremities, are the endings of sensory neurons wrapped around specialized muscle fibers. Muscle spindles provide feedback information on the degree of the muscle stretch. ***Tendon organs (Golgi tendon organs)*** are located at the junction of skeletal muscles and tendons. They function by relaying information about the degree of tension in tendons to the central nervous system.

Proprioceptors in the inner ear are the maculae and cristae that function in equilibrium. These are discussed in Chapter 11.

OBJECTIVE

To demonstrate kinesthesia

MATERIALS

Chalk

Measure

PROCEDURE

1. Face a blackboard. Position yourself close enough so that you can easily reach to mark it. Mark a small X on the board in front of you.

2. Place your chalk on the X, close your eyes, raise your arm above your head, and then attempt to make a dot on top of the X.

3. Repeat step 2 twice.

4. Record the distance between the X and the dots in the LABORATORY REPORT RESULTS at the end of the chapter.

Did repetition facilitate the accuracy of your aim? ____

EXERCISE 3. Olfactory and Gustatory Receptors

In order for ***gustatory (taste) cells*** to be stimulated, a substance must be in solution so that it can enter the taste buds where the receptors are located. These taste buds are most numerous on the tongue, but they are also found in the soft palate and pharynx. The number of taste buds decreases after age 45. Much of the experience of taste is actually an experience of smell, although texture and affective association are also involved. Adaptation to tastes occurs rapidly. The necessity of smell to the sensation of taste is amply demonstrated when the nasal mucosa is swollen from a cold or allergy.

Despite the abundance of flavors perceived, all of them are combinations of only four basic taste sensations.

1. ***Sour***. The presence of acid produces the perception of sourness; the sensation is approximately proportional to the concentration of acid.

2. ***Salty***. Most of our perception of saltiness is derived from the cations and anions of salts.

3. ***Sweet***. The sweet taste results from exposure to many different organic substances: sugars, alcohols, ketones, amino acids, esters, and so forth.

4. ***Bitter***. Bitterness is mostly caused by long chain organic substances and alkaloids like caffeine, quinine, and nicotine. We are much more sensitive to bitter tastes than to other tastes, a protective function, since many toxins are bitter.

The taste for certain substances is inherited. For example, ***phenylthiocarbamide (PTC)*** tastes sweet to some, bitter to others, and some people cannot taste it at all. As another example, artificial sweeteners produce a bitter aftertaste in individuals who have inherited the ability to taste it.

Smell is the least understood of the senses. It is thought that there are at least 50 different receptor types which are specific to certain molecules, but these types have not yet been well categorized. It is known that the ***olfactory cells*** have thresholds that vary considerably for different substances. Table 10.1 indicates the concentration of various substances required in order for them to be smelled. Note

TABLE 10.1
SELECTED OLFACTORY THRESHOLDS

Substance	mg/liter of air
Ethyl ether	5.83
Chloroform	3.3
Oil of peppermint	0.03
Artificial musk	0.0004
Methyl mercaptan (garlic)	0.0000004

that the threshold concentration of ethyl ether is 15 million (1.5×10^7) times greater than that of garlic.

Discrimination of a difference of intensity for any given odor is very poor. The concentration of an odiferous substance must be changed by about 30% before a difference can be detected. The comparable difference in our visual discrimination threshold is a 1% change in light intensity.

It is thought that we detect the direction from which an odor arises by the slight difference in the time at which it reaches each separate nostril.

In order for a substance to be smelled, three conditions must be met.

1. Its molecules must come in contact with the olfactory cells. Therefore, the substance must be partially volatile; it may have to be sniffed in to intensify the odor.
2. It must be partially water soluble, so that it can pass through the mucus to the olfactory cells.
3. It must be partially lipid soluble so that it can dissolve in the plasma membrane of the receptors.

Some olfactory stimuli such as peppers, ammonia, ether, chloroform, and sulfuric acid formed by onions cause irritation since they stimulate naked endings of the trigeminal (V) nerve in the nasal mucosa as well as the olfactory neurons.

Adaptation to odors occurs quickly. This allows unpleasant odors to be endured, and it also accounts for the failure to detect a smell which accumulates slowly. Adaptation is specific for the particular odor smelled and does not affect the perception of other odors. Olfactory adaptation is due both to fatigue of the olfactory receptors as well as action by the cerebral cortex.

A. Olfactory Adaptation

OBJECTIVE

To demonstrate olfactory adaptation

MATERIALS

A selection of substances to be smelled: oil of clove, oil of peppermint, oregano, ground coffee, vanilla or maple extract, vinegar, and so forth

Cotton

Timer

PROCEDURE

1. Instruct a subject to plug one nostril with cotton, close the eyes, and inhale through the nose and exhale through the mouth.
2. Hold a substance with a distinct odor under the nose of the subject.
3. Note the time for the odor to disappear and repeat with the other nostril.
4. As soon as olfactory adaptation has occurred, test a different substance.
5. Record your observations in the LABORATORY REPORT RESULTS at the end of the chapter.

Did the rate of adaptation seem to increase or decrease after multiple stimuli? ____________

Propose a hypothesis as to why this is so. ____

____

____

____

____

B. Association of Smell and Taste

OBJECTIVE

To demonstrate the effect of smell on taste

MATERIALS

Paper towels

Toothpicks

Cubes of potato, apple, onion, and carrot, cut into equal sizes

PROCEDURE

1. Instruct a subject to dry the tongue, close the eyes, and hold the nostrils shut.

2. Using a toothpick, place the cubes one by one on the subject's tongue.

3. Ask the subject to identify each food. Record the responses in the LABORATORY REPORT RESULTS at the end of the chapter.

4. Repeat this exercise, allowing the subject to chew the food with nostrils closed.

5. Repeat, allowing the subject to smell the food.

COMPLETE THE LABORATORY REPORT QUESTIONS AT THE END OF THE CHAPTER

LABORATORY REPORT RESULTS

10 SENSORY PHYSIOLOGY: GENERAL SENSES, OLFACTION, AND GUSTATION

Student ____________________ **Date** ____________________

Laboratory Section ____________________ **Score/Grade** ____________________

EXERCISE 1. Cutaneous Receptors

A. Touch Receptors

1. Identifying Touch Receptors

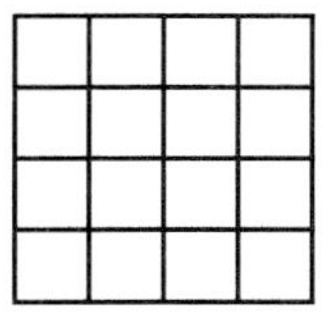

Touch Receptors on the Forearm

2. Localization of the Touch Sensation

	Distance # 1	Distance # 2	Distance # 3	Average
Thumb				
Arm				
Palm				
Nape				

3. Two-Point Discrimination

	Least Distance Between Two Points
Tongue	
Nape	
Hand	
Nose	
Finger	

B. Pressure Receptors

	Number of pages
Fingers	
Elbow	
Chin	
Nose	
Thenar eminence	

C. Thermoreceptors

1. Localization of Heat and Cold receptors

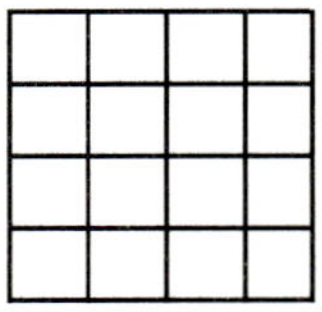

Hot stimulus

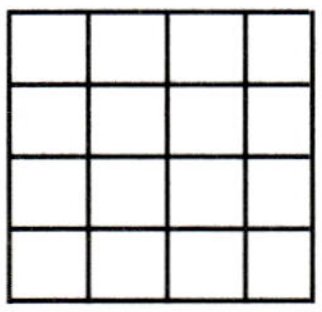

Cold stimulus

2. Adaptation of Temperature Receptors

	Reported sensation
Hand from hot water	
Hand from cold water	

D. Pain Receptors

	Reported locus of sensation
30 seconds	
1 minute	
2 minutes	

EXERCISE 2. Proprioceptive Receptors

Distance Measured

First Trial	
Second Trial	
Third Trial	

Observed movement of arms ____

____

EXERCISE 3. Olfactory and Gustatory Receptors

A. Olfactory Adaptation

Time for odor to disappear

Substance	First Nostril	Second Nostril

B. Association of Smell and Taste

Accurate Identification (+ for yes, − for no)

	On tongue	Chewed/nostrils closed	Chewed/nostrils open
Potato			
Apple			
Onion			
Carrot			

LABORATORY REPORT QUESTIONS **10**

SENSORY PHYSIOLOGY: GENERAL SENSES, OLFACTION, AND GUSTATION

Student ______________________ Date ______________________

Laboratory Section ______________________ Score/Grade ______________________

PART I. MATCHING

_____ 1. Process by which the brain refers sensations to the site of stimulus

_____ 2. The presence of sensation after a stimulus has been removed

_____ 3. The loss of sensation when a stimulus is present

_____ 4. The property by which heat and pressure are distinguished from one another

_____ 5. Transmission of a nerve impulse from a receptor to the brain

A. Adaptation
B. Afterimages
C. Conduction
D. Modality
E. Projection

_____ 6. Chemoreceptors

_____ 7. Mechanoreceptors

_____ 8. Nociceptors

_____ 9. Photoreceptors

_____ 10. Thermoreceptors

_____ 11. Proprioceptors

A. Stimulated by deformation of the receptor
B. Stimulated by light energy
C. Stimulated by temperature changes
D. Stimulated by glucose

PART II. MULTIPLE CHOICE

_____ 12. Which region of the tongue has the most receptors for bitter taste? (a) tip (b) sides (c) center (d) back

_____ 13. Which of the following is *not* a tactile sensation? (a) touch (b) pressure (c) pain (d) vibration

_____ 14. Referred pain is (a) known as phantom pain (b) a failure of projection (c) experienced by amputees (d) all of the above (e) none of the above

_____ 15. Touch receptors (a) are evenly distributed throughout the body (b) are located in the subcutaneous layer of the skin (c) are least numerous in the soles of the feet (d) all of the above (e) none of the above

_____ 16. Cold receptors (a) are less numerous than heat receptors (b) are lamellated (Pacinian) corpuscles (c) are stimulated by relative changes in temperature (d) all of the above (e) none of the above

_____ 17. In order for a substance to be smelled, it must be (a) volatile (b) partially water soluble (c) partially lipid soluble (d) all of the above (e) none of the above

_____ 18. Olfactory cells (a) are located in the superior nasal mucosa (b) adapt slowly to odors (c) are stimulated by four basic smells (d) all of the above (e) none of the above

_____ 19. Which of the following statements is *false* regarding taste? (a) the ability to taste some substances is inherited (b) a substance must be in solution in order to be tasted (c) bitter taste results from the presence of acid (hydrogen ions) (d) gustatory cells are located in the taste buds, soft palate, and pharynx

_____ 20. Taste receptors are (a) chemoreceptors (b) exteroceptors (c) special sense receptors (d) all of the above (e) none of the above

DISCUSSION: A. Is adaptation advantageous? Why or why not?

DISCUSSION: B. What is the advantage of the thermoreceptors' response to relative and not absolute temperature changes?

DISCUSSION: C. What is the advantage of the uneven distribution of tactile receptors?

SENSORY PHYSIOLOGY: VISION 11

EXERCISE 1. Ophthalmoscopy
EXERCISE 2. Errors of Refraction
A. Measurement of Visual Acuity
B. Test for Astigmatism
EXERCISE 3. The Blind Spot
EXERCISE 4. Accommodation
EXERCISE 5. Visual Reflexes
A. Photopupillary Reflex
B. Accommodation Reflex
C. Convergence Reflexes
EXERCISE 6. Binocular Vision
EXERCISE 7. Photoreceptors
A. Formation of an Afterimage
B. Test for Color Blindness
C. Color Perception

WORD ROOTS

aqua-, aque- = water
astigma-: a- = without, *stigma* = point
fundus = base
iris, irid- = colored circle
lutea = yellow
macula = spot
ophthal = eye
-opia, -opic, -ops = eye
ora = mouth
-pathy = disease
photo- = light
presby- = elder
sclera-, sclero- = hard
serrata = notched

Vision occurs when photons of light strike photoreceptors in the retina, causing a nerve impulse to arise and travel to the occipital lobe of the cerebral cortex. Label Figure 11.1 and review the following paragraph to refresh your knowledge of eye anatomy.

Six ***extrinsic eye muscles*** move the eye within its orbit to allow focus on a particular object. The exterior of the eye is covered with a ***fibrous tunic***; the posterior portion of the tunic is the white ***sclera*** (SKLE-ra), the anterior portion is the transparent ***cornea***. The ***scleral venous sinus (canal of Schlemm)*** lies at the junction of the sclera and cornea. The anterior surface of the eye is covered by the ***conjunctiva*** (kon′-junk-TĪ-va).

Just interior to the fibrous tunic is the ***vascular tunic***. Its posterior portion is the ***choroid*** (KŌ-royd); the anterior thickening of the choroid is the ***ciliary*** (SIL-ē-ar′-ē) ***body***, containing the ***ciliary muscle*** and secretory cells. The portion of the vascular tunic anterior to the ciliary body which lies beneath the cornea is the ***iris***, the colored portion of the eye. The opening in the iris is the ***pupil*** of the eye.

The most interior tunic is the ***retina*** or ***nervous tunic***. It extends anteriorly to the ***ora serrata*** (Ō-ra ser-RĀ-ta) where it meets the choroid. Along with other cell layers, the retina contains the ***photoreceptors: rods*** and ***cones***. Cones are concentrated in the central fovea within the ***macula lutea*** (MACK-yoo-la LOO-tē-a) and are stimulated by bright light of different wavelengths (colors). Rods are stimulated by dimmer light and are scattered throughout the retina except in the macula lutea. Photoreceptors synapse with ***bipolar neurons*** which synapse with ***ganglion neurons*** in the

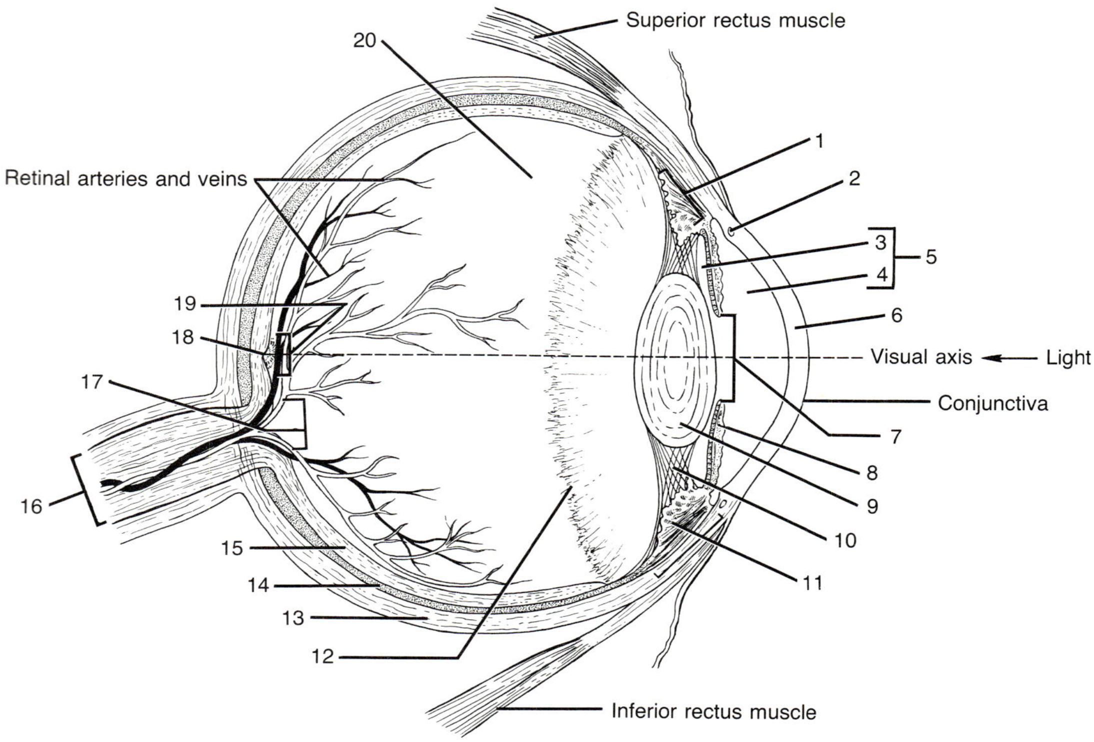

— Anterior cavity
— Anterior chamber
— Central fovea
— Choroid
— Ciliary body
— Ciliary muscle
— Cornea
— Iris
— Lens
— Macula lutea
— Optic disc
— Optic nerve
— Ora serrata
— Posterior chamber
— Posterior cavity
— Pupil
— Retina
— Sclera
— Scleral venous sinus
— Suspensory ligament

FIGURE 11.1 Diagram of midsagittal section of eye.

retina. Axons of retinal ganglion neurons leave the eye at the ***optic disc (blind spot)*** and continue to the brain as the ***optic (II) nerve***.

Suspensory ligaments extending from the ciliary body hold the lens in place. The ***posterior cavity*** of the eye is filled with ***vitreous*** (VIT-rē-us) ***humor*** and occupies the space between the retina and the posterior surface of the lens. The anterior cavity of the eye is filled with ***aqueous*** (Ā-kwē-us) ***humor*** and lies between the anterior surface of the lens and the cornea. It has two chambers: the ***posterior chamber*** between the lens and the iris and the ***anterior chamber*** between the iris and the cornea.

A review of the visual pathway: Light passes through the conjunctiva, cornea, aqueous humor, lens, and vitreous humor. Each of these structures refracts (bends) light rays as they pass from a structure of one density to a structure of another density. The cornea and lens are the most important refractive media. Light rays strike the retina and continue through the layers of ganglion and bipolar neurons to the photoreceptors. These rods and cones are excited by light energy of particular wavelengths and initiate nerve impulses which travel from photoreceptors to bipolar neurons to ganglion neurons which form the optic nerve. The optic (II) nerve transmits nerve impulses via the ***optic chiasma*** (kī-AZ-ma) and optic tract to the thalamus. These nerves synapse in the thalamus and continue to the ***occipital cortex***.

Label the structures of the eye visible in Figure 11.2.

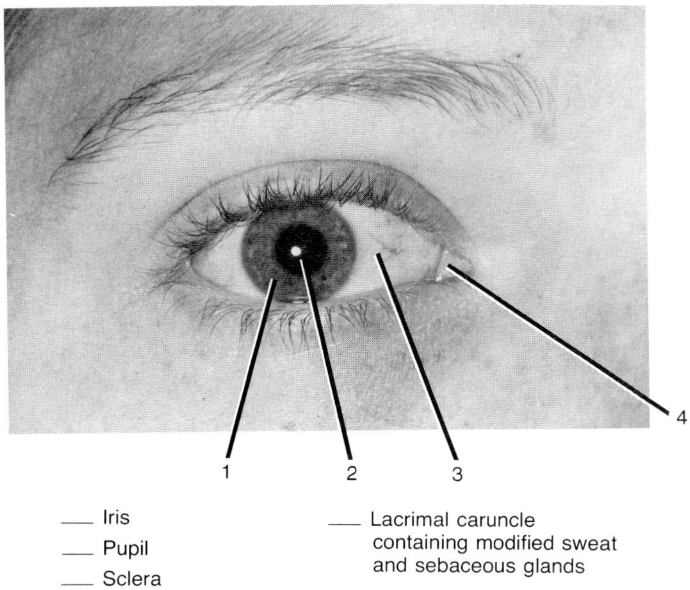

FIGURE 11.2 Anterior view of the eye.

EXERCISE 1. Ophthalmoscopy

OBJECTIVES

To demonstrate the use of the opthalmoscope

To examine the fundus of the eye

The posterior portion of the interior of the eye, known as the ***fundus***, can be examined with an ophthalmoscope (of-THAL-mō-skōp). This instrument consists of a light source to illuminate the retina, various apertures through which the light passes, a rheostat to control the intensity of light, and a series of lenses of different diopters[1] to correct for different focal distances. The use of the ophthalmoscope involves refraction of light by the examined eye and by the observer's eye. If both eyes are emmetropic (neither nearsighted nor farsighted), no lens is needed, and the lens selection setting will be 0. If there are refractive errors in either eye, the lenses of different refractive powers will provide correction for the errors.

[1]The refractive power of a lens with a focal distance of 1 meter.

An ophthalmoscope, properly held, is pictured in Figure 11.3.

If the pupil is dilated, about 50% of the retina can be seen; if undilated, about 15% is visible. The ophthalmoscope allows inspection of the retina, optic disc, macula lutea, and

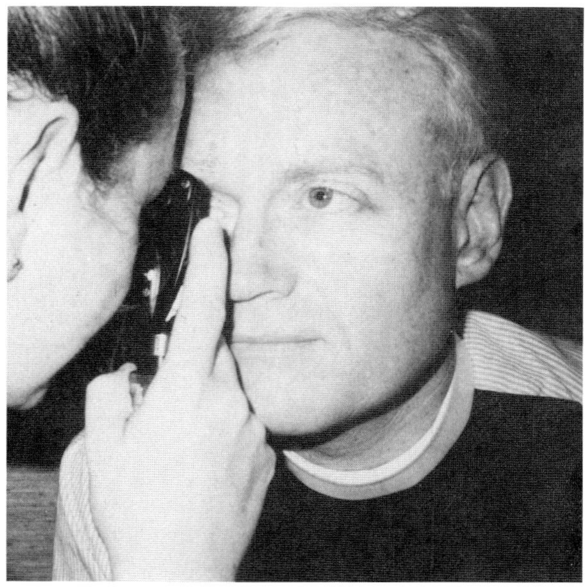

FIGURE 11.3 Use of ophthalmoscope.

central fovea plus blood vessels entering and leaving the eye. A diagram of fundal structures visible on ophthalmoscopy is shown in Figure 11.4. This examination is used for detecting and monitoring conditions such as diabetes mellitus and hypertension since these systemic diseases often cause retinopathy. It can also be used to detect the presence of foreign bodies and opacities in the lens and vitreous humor.

MATERIALS

Ophthalmoscope

PROCEDURE

1. CAUTION! *Because an ophthalmoscopic examination must be limited to one minute,* you should familiarize yourself with the use of the ophthalmoscope before you begin the examination.

a. Hold the front (the side without numbers visible through a small window) of the ophthalmoscope about 3 cm above the lab table. Using the right thumb, rotate the rheostat ring and observe the different intensities of the light beam.

b. With high light intensity, rotate the aperture selection disc and observe the five different patterns: large circle, small circle, slit, grid (for measuring and defining the location of lesions), and green field (this is a red-free field; it allows blood vessels to be seen more clearly).

c. With the large circle aperture in place, use the index finger to set the lens at +10 D (diopters) and focus on a printed letter. Continue to keep the letter in focus while rotating the lens selector down through 0 D to −10 D. Note how the focal length, the distance between the ophthalmoscope and the focused letter, must change.

2. In a darkened room, have a subject sit and look straight ahead at an object at eye level.

3. Use the green field and a lens setting of 0 D. Hold the ophthalmoscope as pictured in Figure 11.3, using your right hand and right eye to examine the subject's right eye.

4. Turn on the light source and hold the ophthalmoscope about 6 inches from the subject's eye.

CAUTION! *Direct the light beam toward the edge of the pupil rather than toward the center.* If you direct the light toward the center of the pupil, light will be refracted from the subject's

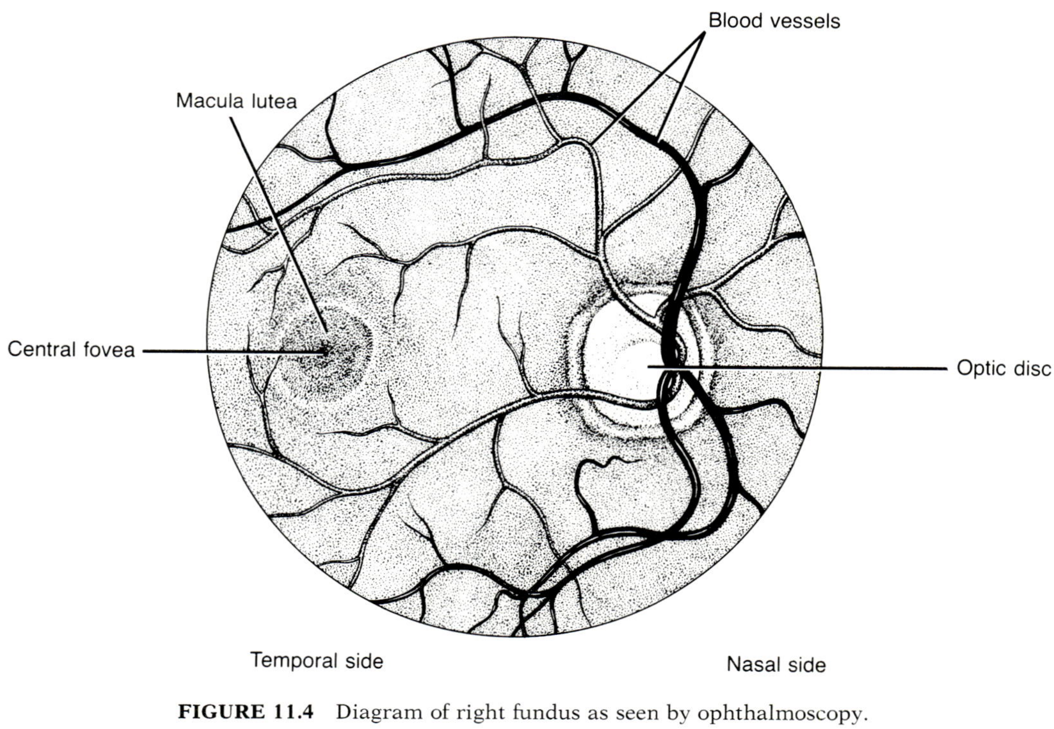

FIGURE 11.4 Diagram of right fundus as seen by ophthalmoscopy.

cornea back into your eye. You should see a red circular area in the fundus of the eye.

5. Keep this red area in view and move the ophthalmoscope *to within two inches of the subject's eye.* If the focus is not clear, rotate the lens selector until the optic disc is in sharp focus. Positive (+) settings (the numbers may be printed in black) correct for farsightedness, negative (−) settings (may be red) correct for nearsightedness. Reduce the light intensity if necessary.

6. Examine the outline of the optic disc and the blood vessels. Find the macula lutea, lateral to the optic disc; it has no blood vessels and is darker than the optic disk. Locate the central fovea in the center of the macula lutea.

CAUTION! *Remember to limit your examination time to one minute.*

How can ophthalmoscopy be used in the diagnosis of vascular disease? ____________________

____

Exercise 2. Errors of Refraction

OBJECTIVES

To describe errors of refraction
To measure visual acuity
To test for astigmatism

In order for an object to be seen clearly, its image must come to a clear focus at the central fovea. Normal vision not only depends upon the refractive power of the cornea and the lens, but also upon the distance between the lens and the retina (see Figure 11.5). An eye in which distant images (farther than 20 feet away) are refracted to focus directly on the fovea is called an ***emmetropic*** (em′-e-TRŌ-pik) ***eye***. When we focus on objects closer than 20 feet, the accommodation reflex, discussed in Exercise 5B, bulges the lens and sharpens its focus.

There are many errors of refraction. Among these are

1. ***Myopia*** (mī-Ō-pē-a) or nearsightedness in which images are focused in front of the retina. Myopia is corrected by a concave lens which causes light rays to diverge before striking the eye.

2. ***Hyperopia*** (hī′-per-Ō-pē-a), ***hypermetropia*** (hī′-per-me-TRŌ-pē-a), or farsightedness in which images strike the retina before they are focused (focused "behind" the retina). Hyperopia is corrected by a convex lens which refracts light rays before they strike the eye.

3. ***Astigmatism*** (a-STIG-ma-tizm) in which irregularities of the corneal or lens surface cause some light rays from an object to be refracted more than others; therefore, parts of an image are focused on the retina and other parts are unfocused. Astigmatism is corrected by a cylindrical lens which compensates for the irregularities in the refractive surface(s).

These errors of refraction and their correction are illustrated in Figure 11.5.

Presbyopia (prez′-bē-Ō-pē-a), the condition in which the lens loses its elasticity and cannot accommodate fully, is discussed under accommodation in Exercise 5B.

Visual acuity or sharpness of vision is tested with a Snellen eye chart. It consists of letters of various sizes which are read at a distance of 20 feet. The 20 foot distance is used so that the examination measures only refractive errors and not errors of accommodation. The numbers on the chart are the distances (in feet) at which the emmetropic eye can read the letters. Vision is said to be 20/50 if the smallest letters a subject can read at 20 feet are those in the line marked *50*, meaning that one must be 20 feet away to see a letter which could be read at 50 feet by an individual with normal refractive power. The higher the bottom number, the larger the letter must be for it to be seen at 20 feet and, of course, the weaker the refractive power.

A. Measurement of Visual Acuity

MATERIALS

Snellen eye chart
3″ × 5″ card or occluder

PROCEDURE

1. Have a subject stand 20 feet from a Snellen eye chart and cover the right eye with a 3″ × 5″ card or an occluder.

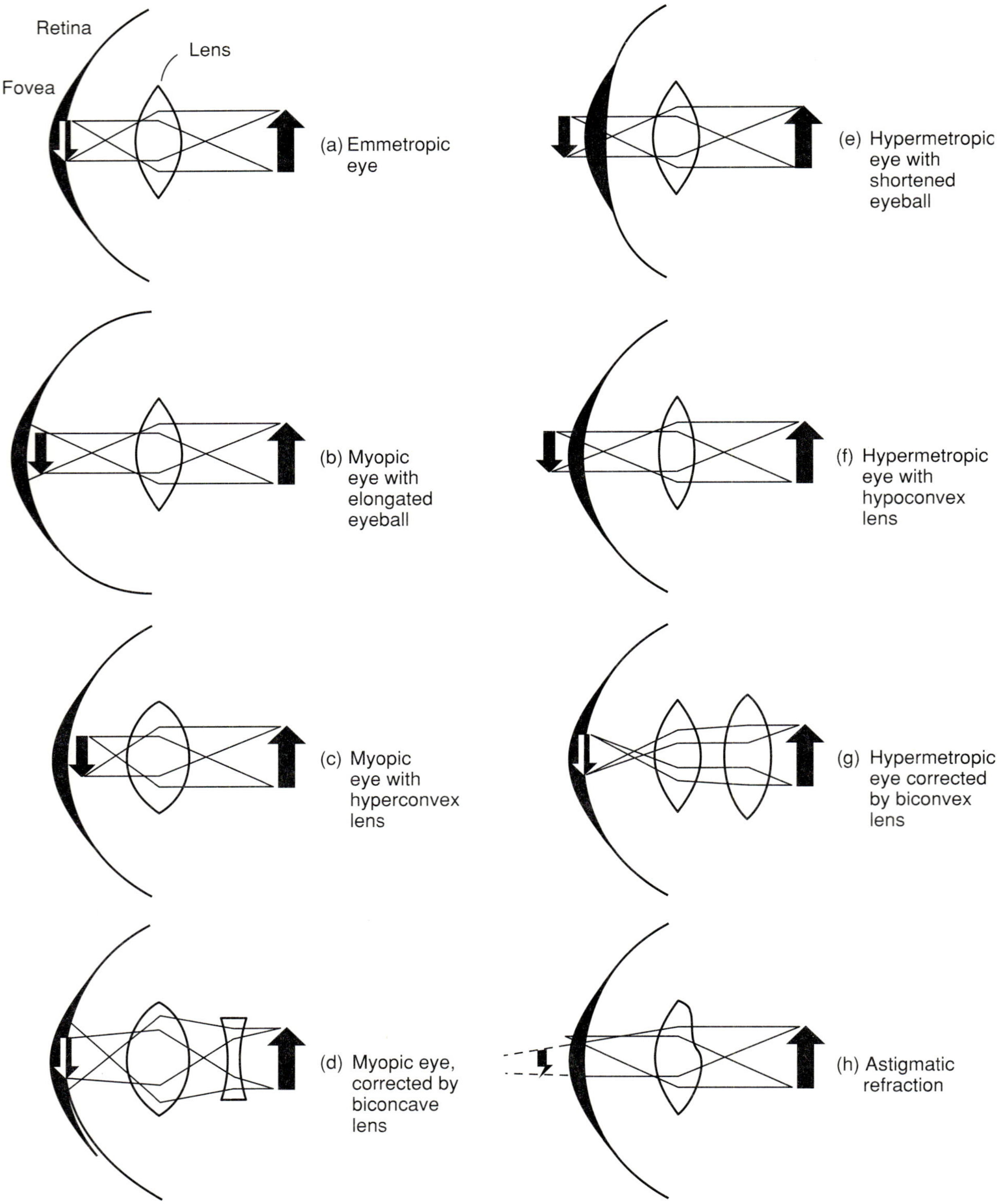

FIGURE 11.5 Normal and abnormal refraction in the eye. The lens-shaped structure represents all four refractive structures. The thick area on the retina represents the central fovea.

2. Instruct the subject to read down the chart until the letters can no longer be distinguished.

3. Record the number of the last line that can be successfully read.

4. Repeat this procedure with the left eye and repeat with both eyes open.

5. The subject shoud record the results in the LABORATORY REPORT RESULTS at the end of the chapter.

6. Examiner and subject should change places and repeat this procedure.

What does a visual acuity of 20/10 mean?

____

____

B. Test for Astigmatism

MATERIALS

Astigmatism chart or Figure 11.6

3" × 5" card or occluder

PROCEDURE

1. Remove any corrective lenses and stand close enough to an astigmatism test chart (see Figure 11.6) so that you see at least some of the radiating lines as groups of three sharp black lines.

2. Cover the left eye and stare at the *center* of the chart. If some groups of lines appear blurred or lighter in color, this indicates that astigmatism is present. Repeat with the right eye.

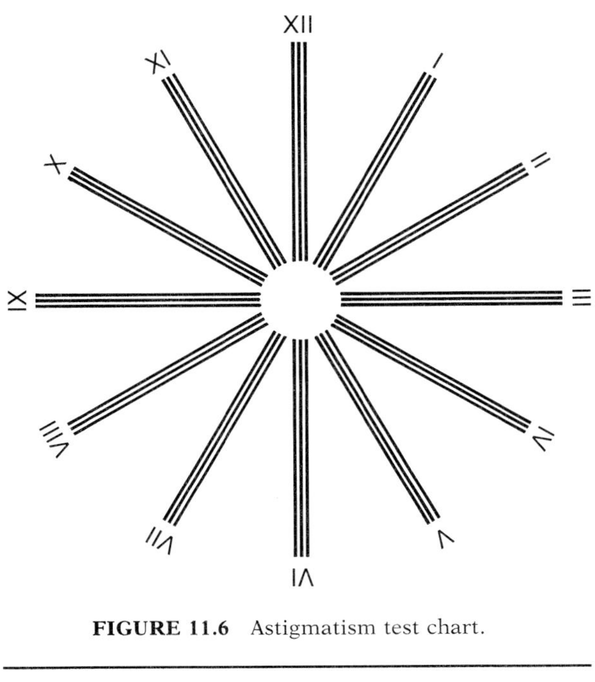

FIGURE 11.6 Astigmatism test chart.

3. Record your observations in the LABORATORY REPORT RESULTS at the end of the chapter.

4. If you wear glasses, put them on and repeat this exercise. Repeat, holding the glasses in front of you and rotating them 90 degrees.

Can an individual be both myopic and astigmatic? Explain. ______________________________

____

____

EXERCISE 3. The Blind Spot

OBJECTIVES

To demonstrate the location of the blind spot

To describe the anatomical nature of the blind spot

The ***blind spot*** of the retina is the optic disk, the point at which axons of ganglion neurons leave the eye and form the optic (II) nerve. This is also the point at which blood vessels enter and leave the eye. Since there are no photoreceptors to be excited at this site, light rays that strike it do not generate a nerve impulse.

MATERIALS

Figure 11.7

Measuring rod

PROCEDURE

1. Hold Figure 11.7 at arm's length with the cross directly in front of your right eye.

2. Close the left eye and *slowly* bring the figure closer to your face while fixing the right eye on the cross.

3. At a certain distance the circle will disappear from your vision because its image falls on the blind spot of the retina. Do not try to focus on the cross or the circle will reappear. Have your lab partner measure the distance from your eye in Figure 11.7 and record it in the LABORATORY REPORT RESULTS at the end of the chapter.

FIGURE 11.7 Test for blind spot.

Is the blind spot blind for both color vision and black and white vision? Explain. ________

____

____

EXERCISE 4. Accommodation

> OBJECTIVES
>
> To describe and demonstrate accommodation
>
> To measure the near point of accomodation

Light rays from objects farther away than 20 feet are nearly parallel when they strike the eye. Light rays from nearer objects diverge. Consequently, the eye must accommodate for this divergence; it must make the lens more convex with a stronger refracting power, in order to refract the light rays to a greater degree.

Accommodation begins with contraction of the ciliary muscle which reduces the tension on the suspensory ligaments and the lens capsule. Because the lens is elastic, the reduced tension allows it to bulge, to become more convex, and thus, to increase its refractory power. When we look at far objects, we relax the ciliary muscle. This increases the tension on the suspensory ligaments and the lens becomes flattened, less convex, less refractive, and adapted to bend the parallel light rays from distant objects.

As an object comes closer to the eye, the lens continues to accommodate until it reaches a maximum. This point is called the ***near point of accommodation***. Light rays from objects closer than this point cannot be focused on the retina so the objects appear blurry.

As with all tissues, the lens loses its elasticity with age and therefore loses its ability to accommodate. The focal distance becomes more fixed and the near point of accommodation becomes greater. This loss of the ability to accommodate is called ***presbyopia*** (old-age farsightedness). Presbyopia is corrected with bifocal or trifocal lenses which provide different refractive powers for different focal distances.

The following exercise tests for near point accommodation.

MATERIALS

Index card with a 2 mm "e" on it

Measure OR meter stick with slide

PROCEDURE

1. Close the left eye and hold the card at arm's length. Slowly move the card toward your right eye until the letter becomes blurry and out of focus.

2. Have your lab partner measure the distance between card and eye and record the measurement in the LABORATORY REPORT RESULTS at the end of the chapter. This distance is your near point accommodation. You may compare it with the population norms given in Table 11.1.

Explain why eye strain results from prolonged near vision and not from prolonged far vision.

____

EXERCISE 5. Visual Reflexes

> OBJECTIVE
>
> To describe and demonstrate the photopupillary, accommodation, and convergence reflexes

The iris contains two groups of smooth muscle fibers: ***circular (constrictor)*** and ***radial (dilator)*** fibers. The circular fibers are innervated

TABLE 11.1
CORRELATION OF AGE AND NEAR-POINT ACCOMMODATION

Age	Inches	Centimeters
10	2.95	7.5
20	3.54	9.0
30	4.53	11.5
40	6.77	17.2
50	20.67	52.5
60	32.80	83.3

by parasympathetic neurons, the radial fibers by sympathetic neurons. The muscles are stimulated by the amount of light striking the retina and by the degree of accommodation present.

The extrinsic muscles of the eye are also engaged in reflex activity when we focus on a near object. Remember that near objects have divergent light rays; these rays strike different (i.e., noncorresponding) parts of the left and right retinas. ***Convergence***, or the medial movement of the eyes, is required so that we see only one image of the object.

MATERIALS

Penlight
Occluder (optional)

PROCEDURES

A. Photopupillary Reflex

1. Seat a subject in a darkened room, or facing a dimly lit corner. Instruct the person to cover the left eye completely with one hand or an occluder.

2. Shine the beam of the light into the right eye. Observe the pupillary change and record in the LABORATORY REPORT RESULTS at the end of the chapter.

3. Remove the hand covering the subject's eye and note the size of the left pupil relative to the right one.

B. Accommodation Reflex

1. Instruct a subject to hold the hand about 12 inches from the nose and then to gaze at a distant object which is not toward a light source. Note the size of the pupils.

2. Have the subject move their point of focus to the fingers of their hand. Note any pupillary size changes and record in the LABORATORY REPORT RESULTS at the end of the chapter.

C. Convergence Reflexes

1. Hold a finger at arm's length and move it toward the nose. Note the convergence of the eyes as they focus on a near object.

2. Hold a finger about eight inches from the nose and focus on a far object. Note how many fingers are perceived when the eyes are not converged. ____________ Shift your focus to the finger. How many fingers are perceived?

____

What is the advantage of these three reflexes?

____

____

____

EXERCISE 6. Binocular Vision

OBJECTIVE

To demonstrate binocular vision, depth perception, diplopia, and eye dominance and to understand the causes of each

We are endowed with binocular vision, that is, each eye sees a different view although there is a large degree of overlap. The cerebral cortex uses the discrepancies to produce ***stereopsis*** or three-dimensional vision, an orientation of the object in space which allows us to perceive its distance from us ***(depth perception)***.

Even though there are slight differences in the views from each eye, we see a single image because the cerebral cortex integrates them into a single perception. If this integration is not present, ***diplopia*** (dip-LŌ-pē-a) or double vision results. We do not perceive an average or mean of both left and right views, rather the view from one of our eyes is dominant, i.e., it is the view we always perceive with both eyes open.

The following exercise evaluates binocular vision, depth perception, diplopia, and dominance.

MATERIALS

Book

Pencil and paper

Depth perception tester

PROCEDURES

1. Hold a book in front of you at arm's length. Place your right hand at your side and touch the nearest corner of the book with your right index finger. Close the left eye and repeat; close the right eye and repeat. Note the accuracy of your attempts and record the results in the LABORATORY REPORT RESULTS at the end of the chapter.

2. Use a depth perception tester with both eyes open and with each eye closed. Attempt to align the two arrows and measure monocular perception errors using the scale on the base. Record the results in the LABORATORY REPORT RESULTS at the end of the chapter.

3. Focus on a discrete object in the distance and press gently on your left eyelid. Note how many objects are visible while you move your eye from its normal orientation. ___________

4. Stab a pencil through a piece of paper and remove the scrap. Hold the paper at arm's length and focus on a small discrete object which just fills the hole. (You may want to use an X on the blackboard). *Without moving the paper*, close the left eye and note whether the object is still present. Repeat with right eye closed. Note your dominant eye in the LABORATORY REPORT RESULTS at the end of the chapter.

Right-handed marksmen who are right-eye dominant find difficulty aiming a shotgun. Bearing in mind that their stance requires focusing on the target with the left eye, can you explain this phenomenon? ________________

____

____

EXERCISE 7. Photoreceptors

OBJECTIVES

To describe and demonstrate afterimages
To test for color blindness
To demonstrate color perception

The rods and cones of the retina are ***photoreceptors***; that is, they contain light sensitive pigments which absorb light of different wavelengths (see Figure 11.8). ***Rhodopsin***, the light sensitive pigment in rods, consists of opsin and retinal. When a photon strikes a molecule of rhodopsin, the retinal changes from a curved to a straight shape and breaks away from the opsin. The resultant energy release initiates the impulse which causes us to perceive light.

In bright light, all the rhodopsin is decomposed so that the rods are nonfunctional. Cones function in bright light, in much the same way as rods, but they absorb light of a specific wavelength (red, blue, or green). The particular color perceived depends on which combinations of cones are stimulated. If all three are stimulated, we see white; if none are stimulated, we see black because only the rods are stimulated.

Color blindness is an inherited disorder in which certain cones are absent. It is a sex-linked disorder (see Chapter 14); about 0.5% of all females and 8% of all males are affected.

If photoreceptors are stimulated by staring at a bright object for a long period of time, they will continue firing briefly after the stimulus has been removed ***(positive afterimage)***. However, after prolonged firing, these photoreceptors become *bleached* or fatigued so that they can no longer fire, resulting in reversal of the image ***(negative afterimage)***.

A. Formation of an Afterimage

MATERIALS

Red cross or red marker and paper

White paper

Light source

PROCEDURE

1. *Stare at a light source*—CAUTION! *Do not use a bright light*—for 30 seconds. Close the eyes briefly and note the positive afterimage.

2. Open the eyes and focus on a piece of white paper. Note the negative afterimage. Record your observations in the LABORATORY REPORT RESULTS at the end of the chapter.

3. Draw a red cross on paper about 1 inch high, with lines ½ inch thick. Stare at the cross without moving the eyes for at least 30 seconds.

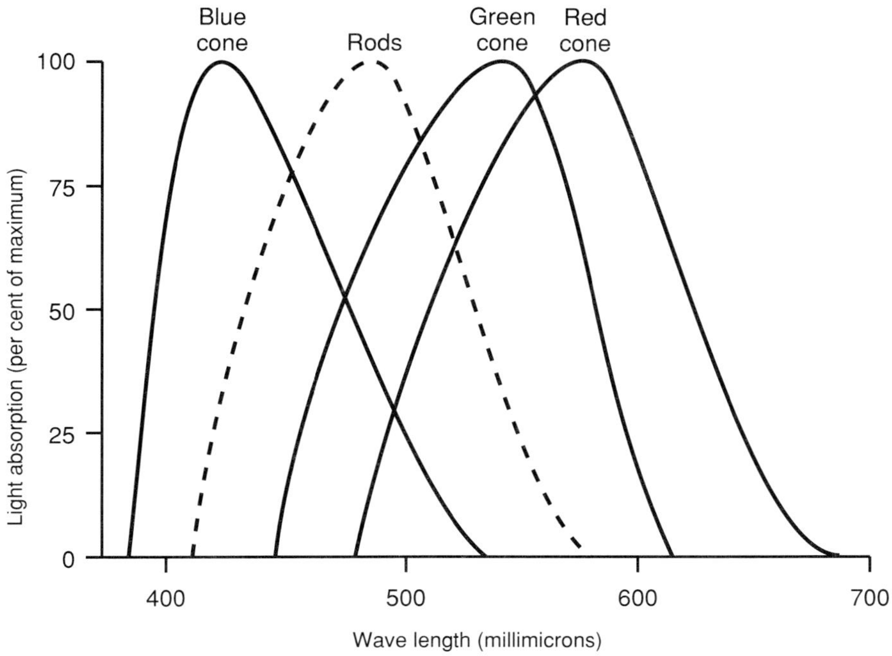

FIGURE 11.8 Light absorption by human retinal pigments. (Drawn from curves recorded by Marks, Dobelle, and MacNichol, Jr.: *Science*, 143:1181, 1964, and by Brown and Wald: *Science*, 144:45, 1964. Copyright 1964 by the American Association for the Advancement of Science.)

4. Close the eyes very briefly; open them and stare at a piece of white paper. Note the positive and negative afterimages. Record your observations in the LABORATORY REPORT RESULTS at the end of the chapter.

B. Test for Color Blindness

MATERIALS

Ishihara plates OR Holmgren test

PROCEDURE

1. View Ishihara plates in bright light and compare your responses to those in the plate book OR use Holmgren's test for matching colored threads.
2. Note the accuracy of your responses.

C. Color Perception

Chlorophyll absorbs photons of a red wavelength. Photons of all other wavelengths are refracted by it: therefore it appears green. (White minus red looks green.) When light shines through a chlorophyll solution in the dark, the green fluid absorbs and transmits only photons of a red wavelength, so red is perceived on the far side of the solution. The side of the solution adjacent to the light appears green because the photons of a red wavelength are absorbed and all others are refracted.

MATERIALS

Green leaves
Isopropyl alcohol
Two large test tubes
Water bath (hot plate and large beaker)
Test tube holder
Filter and filter paper
Ring stand
Pen light
Safety goggles
Laboratory apron or coat

PROCEDURE

1. *In a well ventilated room*, place several green leaves (tree, spinach, and so forth) with enough

alcohol to cover them in a large test tube. *Using a test tube holder* place the test tube in a water bath and heat for ten minutes. CAUTION! *Do not heat the solution directly. Do not let the alcohol boil. Keep all containers of alcohol away from flames. Be sure that the mouth of the test tube is pointing away from you and from other students.*

2. *Using a test tube holder,* filter the liquid into another test tube and observe the green color (chlorophyll) of the liquid.

3. Take the test tube into a dark room and shine a pen light through the liquid. Observe the red color.

4. Observe the color on the side of the test tube adjacent to the light source.

If an individual lacks red-sensitive cones, what colors are difficult to distinguish? ______________

____

Submariners work in a red-light environment before looking through a periscope in the dark. Rhodopsin is not broken down by red light. Explain why the red-light environment is advantageous? ______________________________

____

____

COMPLETE THE LABORATORY REPORT QUESTIONS AT THE END OF THE CHAPTER

LABORATORY REPORT RESULTS

SENSORY PHYSIOLOGY: VISION 11

Student ______________________ Date ______________________

Laboratory Section ______________________ Score/Grade ______________________

EXERCISE 2. Errors of Refraction

A. Measurement of Visual Acuity

Acuity in left eye: 20/ _____

in right eye: 20/ _____

with both eyes: 20/ _____

B. Test for Astigmatism

Planes of astigmatism, if present: ______________________

EXERCISE 3. The Blind Spot

Distance of blind spot from eye: ____________

EXERCISE 4. Accommodation

Near point accommodation distance: ____________

EXERCISE 5. Visual Reflexes

Pupillary size change in photopupillary reflex: ____________

Pupillary size change in accommodation reflex: ____________

EXERCISE 6. Binocular Vision

How accurate was your attempt to touch a point with one eye closed? ______________________

When the right eye was closed, did you have error to the left or the right? ______________________

Length of depth perception error: ______________________

Dominant eye: ______________________

EXERCISE 7. Photoreceptors

A. Formation of an Afterimage

	Positive afterimage	Negative afterimage
Light source		
Red cross		

LABORATORY REPORT QUESTIONS

SENSORY PHYSIOLOGY: VISION 11

Student ______________________ **Date** ______________________

Laboratory Section ______________________ **Score/Grade** ______________________

PART I. MULTIPLE CHOICE

_____ 1. The amount of light entering the eye is regulated by the (a) lens (b) iris (c) cornea (d) choroid (e) ciliary body

_____ 2. The part of the retina that is stimulated by colored light is the (a) ora serrata (b) optic disc (c) central fovea (d) peripheral retina (e) none of the above

_____ 3. Nearsightedness (a) is also called myopia (b) may be caused by a lens with too great refractive power (c) may be caused by too great a distance between lens and retina (d) is corrected with a biconcave lens (e) all of the above

_____ 4. Which of the following indicates the best visual acuity? (a) 20/10 (b) 20/20 (c) 20/100

_____ 5. Ophthalmoscopic examination of the fundus can reveal (a) hypermetropia (b) astigmatism (c) diplopia (d) cataract (e) none of the above

_____ 6. Presbyopia results from (a) loss of elasticity in the lens (b) loss of suspensory ligaments (c) excess aqueous humor in the anterior cavity (d) lens opacity (e) none of the above

_____ 7. The blind spot (a) is the optic disc (b) contains only rods and no cones (c) increases in size with aging (d) is the site where photoreceptor neurons leave the eye (e) none of the above

_____ 8. The circular muscles of the iris contract when (a) light becomes dim (b) we focus on a far object (c) they are stimulated by sympathetic neurons (d) all of the above (e) none of the above

_____ 9. Cones are stimulated by (a) dim light (b) light of red, blue, and yellow wavelengths (c) light of red, blue and green wavelengths

_____ 10. Accommodation (a) occurs when we focus on a far object (b) requires relaxation of the ciliary muscle (c) is less effective with increased age (d) all of the above (e) none of the above

PART II. MATCHING

_____ 11. Focus in front of the retina

_____ 12. Farsightedness

_____ 13. Corrected by a convex lens

_____ 14. Caused by reduced elasticity of the lens

_____ 15. Irregular lens curvature

_____ 16. Normal refractive power

_____ 17. Nearsightedness

A. Astigmatism
B. Emmetropia
C. Hyperopia
D. Myopia
E. Presbyopia

PART III. CIRCLE A OR B TO COMPLETE THE FOLLOWING STATEMENTS CORRECTLY

When the eye is focused on a near object, (A. sympathetic, B. parasympathetic) impulses cause the (A. radial, B. circular) muscles of the iris to contract. This contraction causes the iris to become (A. larger, B. smaller) while the pupil (A. constricts, B. dilates). The ciliary muscle (A. contracts, B. relaxes), thereby (A. increasing, B. decreasing) the tension on the suspensory ligaments. This tension change causes the lens to (A. bulge, B. flatten) and have (A. greater, B. less) refractive power. When an object is close to the eye, the extrinsic muscles cause the eyes to (A. diverge, B. converge).

DISCUSSION: What occurs when orange light is shined in front of the eyes? List all structures through which light passes and give their functions; note where and how nerve impulses arise.

SENSORY PHYSIOLOGY: HEARING

12

EXERCISE 1. Otoscopy
EXERCISE 2. Tests of Auditory Acuity
  A. Sound Localization
  B. Weber's Test
  C. Rinne's Test
  D. Audiometry
EXERCISE 3. Tests of Equilibrium
  A. Balance Test
  B. Barany Test

WORD ROOTS

ampulla = little jar
audio-, audit- = ear
deci = one-tenth
endo- = within
-lith = stone
-metry = measurement
oto- = ear
peri- = around
-scopy = examination
static, -stasis = standing still
tympano- = drum
utricle = little bag
vestibulo- = hallway

The structures of the ear are the sense organs both for hearing and equilibrium. Label Figures 12.1 and 12.2 and read the following material to refresh your knowledge of ear anatomy.

The ***external ear*** collects sound waves and directs them through the ***external auditory canal (meatus)*** to the ***tympanic*** (tim-PAN-ik) ***membrane*** or eardrum. The ***middle ear*** extends from the tympanic membrane to the ***oval*** and ***round windows***. It contains three ear ***ossicles*** (OS-si-kuls), the ***malleus*** (hammer), ***incus*** (anvil), and ***stapes*** (stirrup), two muscles, the ***tensor tympani*** and ***stapedius***, and it connects with the pharynx via the ***auditory (Eustachian) tube***.

The oval and round windows are openings in the bone which lead to the ***inner ear (labyrinth)***. The inner ear consists of a ***bony labyrinth*** which is hollowed from the temporal bone and filled with ***perilymph***. This fluid surrounds the ***membranous labyrinth***, a series of connected tubes which are filled with ***endolymph***.

The ***vestibule***, or oval central portion of the bony labyrinth, contains two sacs, the ***utricle*** (YOO-tre-k'l) and ***saccule*** (SAK-yool). The utricle opens into the ***ampullae*** (am-POOL-ē, sing. ampulla, am-POOL-a), enlargements of the three ***semicircular canals;*** the saccule opens into the cochlear duct.

The cochlear duct lies within the bony ***cochlea*** (KOK-lē-a), which twists around a bony core known as the ***modiolus*** (mō-DĪ-ō-lus). The space between the bony cochlea and the ***vestibular membrane*** (the upper surface of the cochlear duct) is the ***scala vestibuli;*** the space between the ***basilar membrane*** (the lower surface of the cochlear duct) and the bony cochlea is the ***scala tympani***. Resting on the basilar membrane is the ***spiral organ (or-***

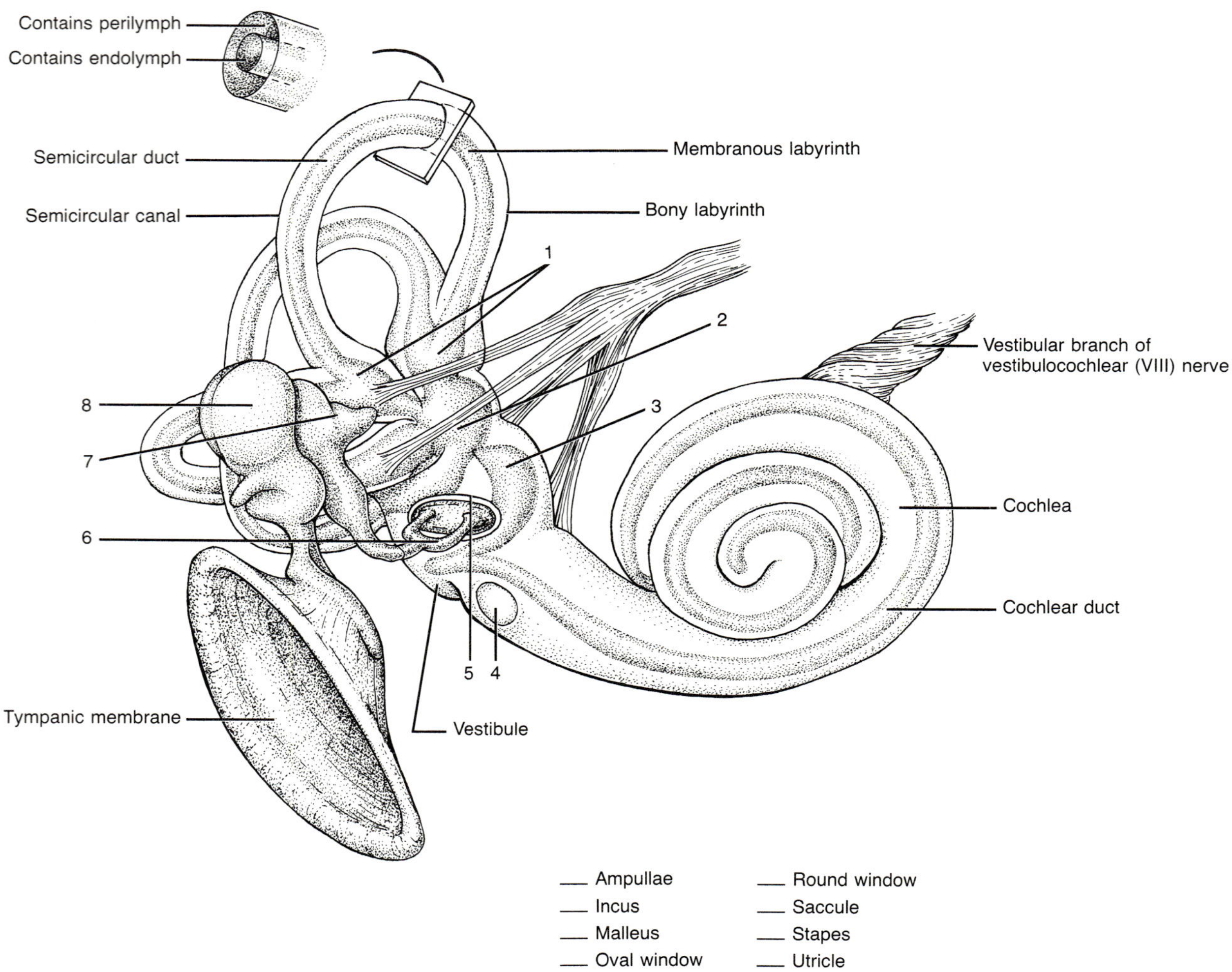

FIGURE 12.1 Schematic diagram of middle and inner ear.

gan of Corti), which includes the hair cells which are receptors for sound waves. The ***tectorial membrane*** projects over the hair cells.

A review of the auditory pathway: Sound waves deflect the tympanum, causing vibration of the malleus. This vibration is amplified as it is transmitted by the incus and the stapes. The footplate of the stapes rests on the oval window. Stapedial vibration causes movement of the perilymph in the scala vestibuli, resulting in deflection of the vestibular membrane, movement of the endolymph in the cochlear duct, and deflection of the basilar membrane. The hair cells of the spiral organ come in contact with the tectorial membrane and are bent. The mechanical stimulus initiates a nerve impulse that travels on the cochlear branch of the vestibulocochlear nerve (cranial nerve VIII) mainly to the temporal cortex (and also to the inferior colliculi).

Both the utricle and saccule also contain hair cells, which are receptors for ***static equilibrium***. These hair cells are located in a region called the ***macula*** (MAK-yoo-la), which also contains supporting cells and a gelatinous membrane in which ***otoliths*** (crystals of calcium carbonate ($CaCO_3$)) are embedded.

The semicircular canals are oriented at right angles to each other. They end in the dilated ampullae which contain receptors for ***dynamic equilibrium***. These receptor hair cells are embedded in a gelatinous ***cupula.***

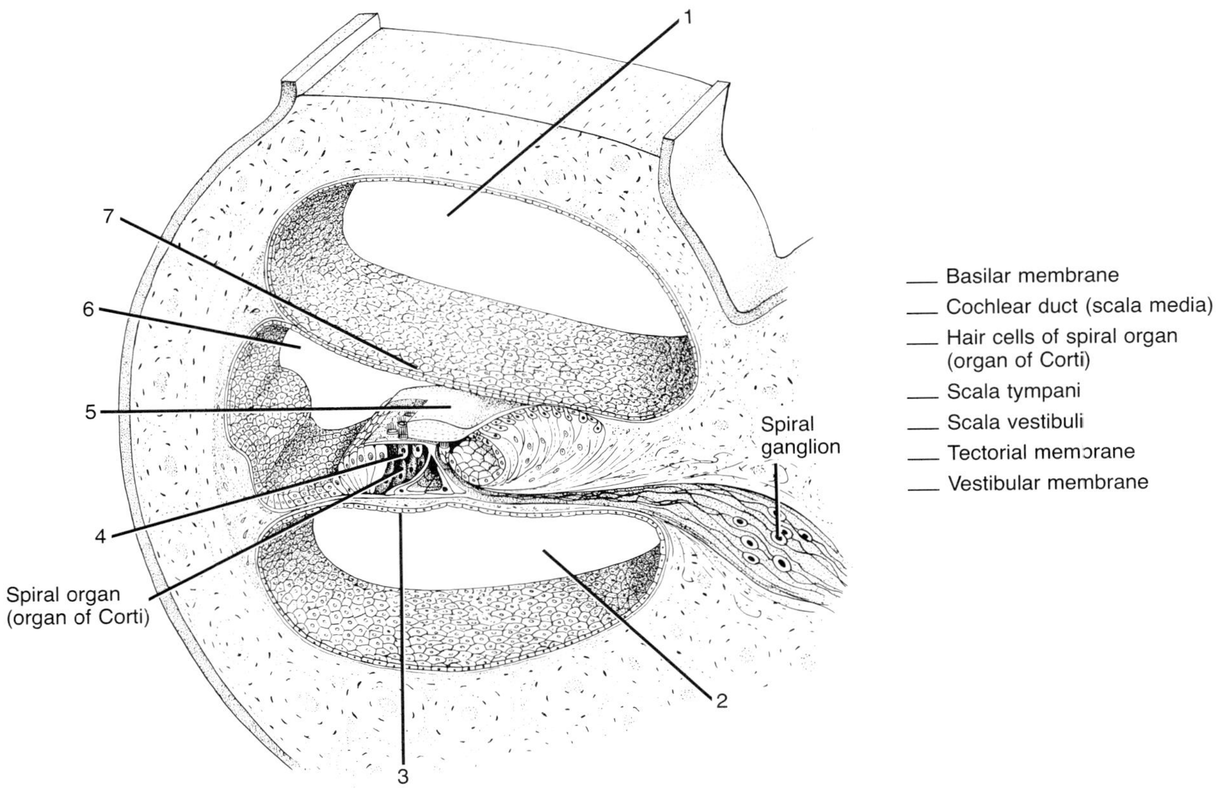

FIGURE 12.2 Cross section through the cochlea.

The function of the organs of equilibrium is discussed later in this chapter. Nerve impulses from them are carried on the ***vestibular branch*** of the ***vestibulocochlear (VIII) nerve*** to the cerebellum. The vestibulocochlear nerve transmits nerve impulses for the sensations of both hearing and equilibrium to the brain.

EXERCISE 1. Otoscopy

Otoscopic visualization of the tympanic membrane can detect infection, lesions, and the orientation of the malleus to the tympanic membrane.

OBJECTIVE

To inspect the external auditory canal (meatus) and the tympanic membrane

MATERIALS

Otoscope

Isopropyl alcohol and cotton

PROCEDURE

1. *Clean the speculum (earpiece) of the otoscope with alcohol* and turn on the light source.
2. Grasp the pinna of a subject's ear and *gently* pull it upward, backward, and a little laterally.
3. *Gently* insert the speculum of the otoscope a *short distance* into the external auditory canal (meatus). Angle the speculum downward and forward.
4. Observe the canal and the tympanic membrane. The tympanic membrane should appear pearly white; the tympanic blood vessels should be visible.
5. Clean the speculum with alcohol.
6. Record your observations in the LABORATORY REPORT RESULTS at the end of the chapter.

EXERCISE 2. Tests Of Auditory Acuity

OBJECTIVES

To describe the nature of sound
To distinguish perceptive from conductive deafness
To measure potential hearing loss

Sound waves result from the alternate compression and decompression of air. The waves have both a frequency and an amplitude. The ***frequency*** is the distance between crests of a sound wave. It is measured in ***Hertz (Hz)*** or ***cycles per second*** and is perceived as ***pitch***. The higher the frequency of a sound, the higher its pitch. Different frequencies displace different areas of the basilar membrane. The ***amplitude*** of a sound wave is perceived as ***intensity (loudness)***. Intensity is measured in ***decibels (db)***. Population norms have been calculated which measure the intensity of a sound that can just be heard, i.e., the ***threshold*** of a sound. These levels are said to have an intensity of 0 db. Each 10 db reflects a tenfold increase in intensity; thus, a sound is 10 times louder than threshold at 10 db, 100 times greater at 20 db, a million times greater at 60 db, and so on.

A. Sound Localization

The cerebral cortex localizes the source of a sound by evaluating the time lag between the entry of sound into each ear. Without turning the head, it is impossible to distinguish between the origin of sounds that arise at 30° ahead of the ear and 30° behind the ear.

MATERIALS

A ticking watch
Cotton plugs

PROCEDURE

1. In a quiet room, have a subject occlude one ear with a cotton plug and close the eyes.
2. Move a ticking watch to various points 6 inches away from the ear (side, front, top, back) and ask the subject to point to the location of the sound.
3. Note in which positions the sound was best localized. Record the results in the LABORATORY REPORT RESULTS at the end of the chapter.

B. Weber's Test

Weber's test is diagnostic of both ***conductive*** and ***perceptive deafness***. The former results from interference with sound waves reaching the inner ear (plugged external auditory canal, fusion of the ossicles, and so forth); perceptive deafness is caused by damage to the nerve pathway between the cochlea and the brain.

MATERIALS

Tuning fork
Mallet

PROCEDURE

1. In a room with a normal noise level, strike a tuning fork with a rubber mallet and place the tip of the handle on the median line of a subject's forehead.
2. Determine if the tone is equally loud in both ears.
3. Simulate conduction deafness by occluding the left ear with cotton. Repeat steps 1 and 2.
4. Analyze the results and record them in the LABORATORY REPORT RESULTS at the end of the chapter.

When the ears are unoccluded, the sound should be equally loud in both ears if hearing is normal. In conduction deafness, simulated by occluding the left ear, the sound is louder in the deaf (occluded) ear. This situation results because the normal ear is stimulated by competing background noise. If perceptive deafness were present, the sound would be louder in the normal ear because sensorineural loss produces a deficit in transmission to the cerebral cortex.

C. Rinne's Test

MATERIALS

Tuning fork of a high frequency
Mallet

PROCEDURE

1. In a quiet room, strike a tuning fork with a mallet and place the handle of the tuning fork on the right mastoid process of a subject.
2. When the sound is no longer audible to the subject, move the vibrating fork close to the external auditory canal.
3. Ask the subject to note whether sound is still heard.
4. If the subject hears the fork again when moved near the external auditory canal (by air conduction), hearing is *not* impaired.
5. Repeat the test by evaluating air conduction hearing first. Strike a tuning fork and hold it near the external auditory canal; when the sound is no longer audible, place the handle of the tuning fork on the mastoid process.
6. If the subject now hears the tuning fork again (by bone conduction), this indicates some degree of conduction deafness.
7. Repeat steps 1–6 using the left ear of the subject.
8. Assess your results and record them in the LABORATORY REPORT RESULTS at the end of the chapter.

With normal hearing ability, air conduction lasts longer than bone conduction because the sound waves are not absorbed by the tissues. In conduction deafness, bone conduction is better than air conduction because the sound waves can go to the cochlea without interference by damaged structures.

D. Audiometry

An ***audiometer*** (aw′-dē-OM-e-ter), pictured in Figure 12.3, tests auditory acuity by delivering stimuli of different frequencies at varying intensities to determine the hearing threshold for each frequency. The audiometer can use either air conduction or bone conduction. The subject reports whether or not a sound is heard. The threshold for sound detection is measured in decibels (db) of loudness. If a threshold is 30 or more decibels above the population norm for perceiving that sound, the individual is said to have a hearing loss of 30 db for that specific tone. An ***audiogram*** plots hearing loss (or normalcy) for each tested frequency in the auditory spectrum.

Children can perceive sound between 30 and 22,000 Hz. A sensorineural loss accompanies

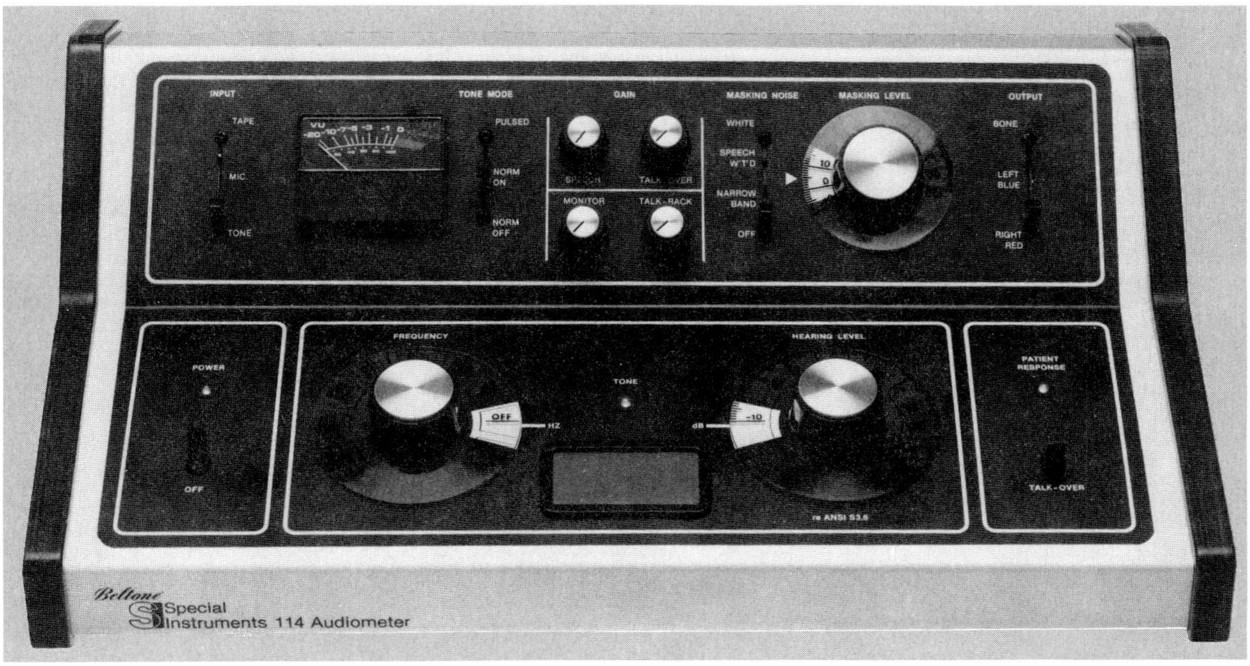

FIGURE 12.3 An audiometer.

aging. It begins after age 20, and the highest frequencies are affected first. By age 40, the upper limit is about 15,000 Hz; by age 80, it may be as low as 8,000 Hz.

MATERIALS

Audiometer

PROCEDURE

1. In a quiet room, have the subject place the earphones with the red earphone on the right ear, blue on the left.
2. With the intensity control set at audiometric zero (the tone that can just be heard by the normal ear), set the frequency control for 125 Hz.
3. Turn the output switch to red (right ear) and push the bar lever to send a continuous tone through the right earphone.
4. Instruct the subject to raise a finger when a tone is heard.
5. Increase the sound intensity *gradually* until it is heard.
6. Record the results in the LABORATORY REPORT RESULTS at the end of the chapter.
7. Repeat this procedure for 500, 1000, 2000, 4000, and 8000 Hz. Repeat for the left ear by turning the output switch to blue.
8. Plot the results in the LABORATORY REPORT RESULTS at the end of the chapter.

Why would this procedure be an inappropriate test of the hearing acuity of an older person? ______________________________

____

____

Summarize the results of the hearing tests you have performed. ____________________

____

____

____

EXERCISE 3. Tests of Equilibrium

OBJECTIVES

To describe the sense organs for equilibrium

To test for defects in the equilibrium apparatus

A sense of equilibrium is necessary to maintain balance. Proprioceptors in joints and muscles and visual input from the eyes provide some information about our spatial orientation, but the vestibular organs of the inner ear are the most important receptors.

Equilibrium is both static and dynamic. ***Static equilibrium*** is concerned with the orientation of the body (principally the head) relative to gravity and also to linear acceleration and deceleration. Through it, we are aware of whether the head is tilted and whether a car is speeding up or slowing down.

Dynamic equilibrium is concerned with changes in the rate and direction of body movement (principally the head). The receptors are sensitive to angular or dynamic acceleration and deceleration, such as occurs when spinning or turning the head.

Receptors for static equilibrium are the ***maculae*** in the walls of the ***utricle*** and ***saccule***, located on two planes perpendicular to each other. When the head is moved, the gelatinous ***otolithic membrane***, weighted by the ***otoliths***, moves at a rate slower than that of the hair cells. This is because the heavy membrane has more inertia than the hair cells. If we jump off a chair, the hair cells are pulled upward; if we accelerate, the hair cells are pulled backward (just as the body is when a car accelerates). When the head is tilted, the gelatinous membrane moves toward the gravitational force and bends the hair cells.

Receptors for dynamic equilibrium are the ***cristae*** in the ***ampullae*** of the semicircular canals. When the head spins or turns, the endolymph flows across the hair cells and bends them as water in a stream bends plants. Endolymphatic flow begins slightly after rotation begins and reverses briefly after rotation stops. Thus signals are discharged at both the beginning and end of rotation.

A. Balance Test

PROCEDURE

1. Instruct a subject to stand perfectly still with the arms at the sides and the eyes closed.
2. Observe any swaying movements. These are easier to detect if the subject stands in front of a blackboard with a light in front of the subject.
3. A mark is made at the edge of the shadow of the subject's shoulders and movement of the shadow is then observed.

If the static equilibrium system is dysfunctional the subject will sway or fall, although other proprioreceptors may compensate for the defect.

B. Barany Test

This test evaluates the function of each of the semicircular canals. A subject is rotated, and when rotation is stopped the momentum causes the endolymph in the lateral (horizontal) canal to continue spinning. The spinning bends the cupula in the direction of rotation. Other sensory input informs us that we are no longer rotating. ***Nystagmus***, the reflex movement of the eyes rapidly and then slowly, attempts to compensate for the loss of balance by visual fixation on an object. When the head is tipped toward the shoulder, the anterior semicircular canals are stimulated, so nystagmus is vertical; when the head is tipped slightly forward, the lateral canals are stimulated by the rotation, so nystagmus occurs laterally; when the head is bent onto the chest, the posterior canal receptors are stimulated, so nystagmus is rotational.

MATERIALS

Cotton swabs
Beaker of warm water
Beaker of ice water

PROCEDURE

1. Use a person who is not subject to vertigo (dizziness). Place the subject on a rotating stool, feet anchored on the stool rung and hands holding firmly to the seat. Tilt the subject's head onto one shoulder as far as possible.

CAUTION! *Watch the subject carefully and be prepared to provide support until dizziness has passed.*

2. Spin the stool 10 times in 20 seconds and then stop the spinning immediately.
3. Observe the subject's eye movements.
4. Repeat on a *different* subject (a) with the head tipped slightly forward (30°), and (b) with the chin touching the chest.
5. Record the direction of nystagmus in the LABORATORY REPORT RESULTS at the end of the chapter.

Why is rotation experienced even after spinning has ceased? ______________________

____

____

COMPLETE THE LABORATORY REPORT QUESTIONS AT THE END OF THE CHAPTER

LABORATORY REPORT RESULTS

SENSORY PHYSIOLOGY: HEARING 12

Student ______________________ **Date** ______________________

Laboratory Section ______________________ **Score/Grade** ______________________

EXERCISE 1. Otoscopy

Describe the structures viewed with the otoscope. ______________________

____

____

EXERCISE 2. Tests of Auditory Acuity

A. Sound Localization

In what regions was sound localization most accurate? ______________________

____

B. Weber's Test

Describe your results. ______________________

____

____

C. Rinne's Test

Fill in the table by answering yes or no.

	Air conduction	Bone conduction
Right ear		
Left ear		

D. Audiometry

Frequency (Hz)	Threshold: left ear	Threshold: right ear
125		
500		
1000		
2000		
4000		
8000		

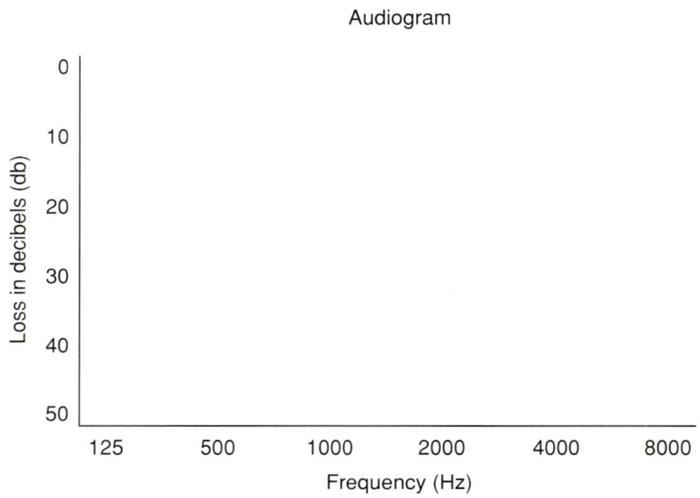

EXERCISE 3. Tests of Equilibrium
B. Barany Test

	Head to side	Head 30° toward chest	Chin on chest
Direction of nystagmus			

LABORATORY REPORT QUESTIONS

SENSORY PHYSIOLOGY: HEARING 12

Student ______________________ **Date** ______________________

Laboratory Section ______________________ **Score/Grade** ______________________

PART I. MULTIPLE CHOICE

_____ 1. The receptors for dynamic equilibrium are located in the (a) semicircular canals (b) utricle and saccule (c) cochlear duct (d) spiral organ (organ of Corti)

_____ 2. If the stapes were fused to the oval window (a) conductive deafness could result (b) perceptive deafness could result (c) vertigo could result

_____ 3. The pitch of a sound is (a) a function of the amplitude of the sound wave (b) measured in Hertz (Hz) (c) its loudness (d) all of the above (e) none of the above

_____ 4. Which of the following does *NOT* test for loss of auditory acuity? (a) audiometry (b) Weber's test (c) Rinne's test (d) Barany test

_____ 5. Which of the following is *NOT* involved in the stimulation of hair cells in the utricle? (a) endolymph (b) otoliths (c) otolithic membrane (d) cupula

PART II. MATCHING

_____ 6. Improved by a hearing aid

_____ 7. Caused by a lesion in the temporal lobe

_____ 8. Results from fusion of ear ossicles

_____ 9. Caused by damage to the cochlear branch of the vestibulocochlear (VIII) nerve

_____ 10. Bone conduction is better than air conduction of sound

A. Conductive deafness
B. Perceptive deafness

DISCUSSION: A. List all structures concerned with hearing which are affected by a sound wave. Describe their function. Note where and how nerve impulses arise.

DISCUSSION: B. Describe the function of the organs of equilibrium during linear and rotational acceleration. Note where and how nerve impulses arise.

REPRODUCTION AND DEVELOPMENT 14

EXERCISE 1. Gametogenesis
- *A. Meiosis*
- *B. Spermatogenesis*
- *C. Oogenesis*

EXERCISE 2. The Female Cycle
EXERCISE 3. Fertilization
EXERCISE 4. HCG and Pregnancy Testing
EXERCISE 5. Development

WORD ROOTS

acro- = atop
blast- = germ, sprout
diplo- = double
-gonium = generation, offspring
oo- = egg
-some = body
sperm-, spermato- = seed
troph- = nourish
zygo- = joined

The human male and female reproductive systems produce ***sex cells*** or ***gametes*** (GAM-ēts) in organs known as ***gonads*** (testes and ovaries). In addition, the male is adapted to deposit gametes within the female, and the female reproductive organs are adapted to contain the product of conception for a nine month gestation (jes-TĀ-shun) period and to deliver the fetus at the end of that period.

The female reproductive organs include the ***ovaries***, where gametes and hormones are produced: the ***uterine (Fallopian) tubes*** that conduct the ova to the ***uterus*** where the ova can implant if fertilized: the ***vagina;*** and the ***vulva***.

The male reproductive organs include the ***testes (testicles)***, where gametes and hormones are produced, a duct system through which the gametes pass, and accessory sex glands that produce the components of ***semen*** other than sperm. The ducts include the ***epididymis*** (ep′-i-DID-i-mis), ***ductus (vas) deferens***, and the ***urethra*** (yoo-RĒ-thra); the accessory sex glands are the ***prostate***, ***seminal vesicles***, and ***bulbourethral*** (bul′-bō-yoo-RĒ-thral) or ***Cowper's glands.***

Review the gross anatomy of the reproductive systems by labeling Figure 14.1 and Figure 14.2.

EXERCISE 1. Gametogenesis

In sexual reproduction, offspring are produced by the union of two gametes, one produced by each parent. The female gametes are ***ova*** (singular, ovum), and the male gametes are ***spermatozoa*** (sper′-mat-ō-ZŌ-a) or ***sperm.*** The union of the nuclei of gametes, called ***fertilization***, results in the formation of a ***zygote*** (zī-gōt).

The zygote contains 23 pairs of chromosomes. One member of each pair is derived from the egg nucleus, the other from the sperm nucleus. The zygote divides to produce two identical progeny cells, then four, then eight, and so on, by the process of mitosis (discussed in Chapter 6). Thus, the adult organism will have 23 pairs or 46 chromosomes in all somatic

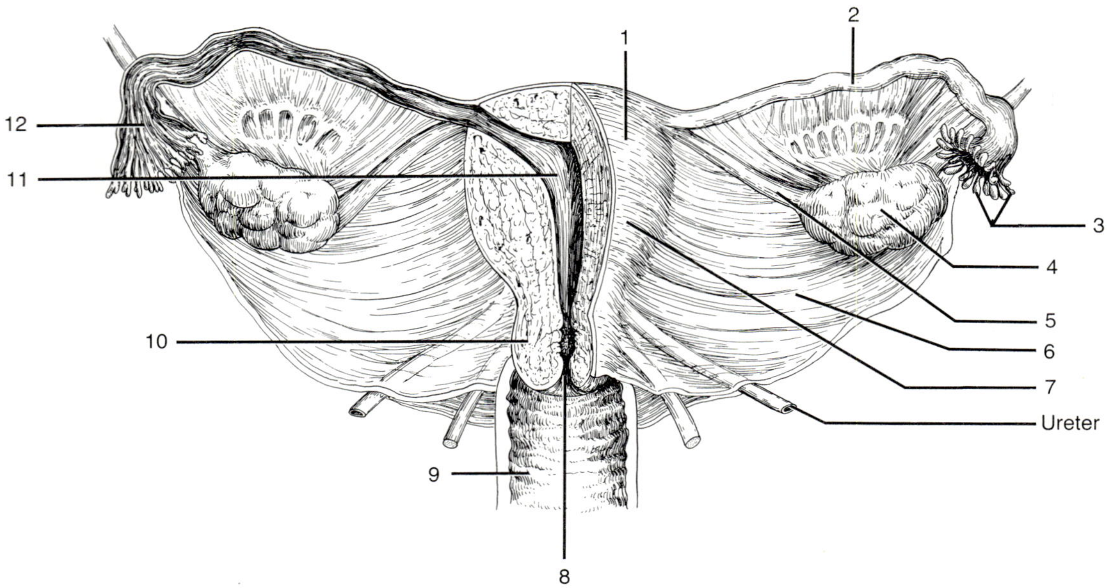

___ Body of uterus
___ Broad ligament
___ Cervical canal
___ Cervix
___ Fimbriae
___ Fundus of uterus
___ Infundibulum
___ Ovarian ligament
___ Ovary
___ Uterine cavity
___ Uterine (Fallopian) tube
___ Vagina

FIGURE 14.1 Female reproductive structures seen in posterior view. The left side of the uterus has been sectioned to show internal features.

(body) cell nuclei. The two chromosomes that belong to each pair are called ***homologous*** (hō-MOL-ō-gus) ***chromosomes.***

Because somatic cells contain both members of each chromosome pair, they are said to have $2n$ or the ***diploid number*** of chromosomes. The symbol n is used to represent the ***haploid*** (one-half) ***number,*** or the number of chromosomes in a gamete.

If the adult produced gametes with 46 chromosomes, fertilization would result in a zygote with 92 chromosomes in the first generation, and with each succeeding generation the chromosome number would double. The normative number of chromosomes is maintained from generation to generation because gametes are not formed by mitotic division but by several processes including ***meiosis*** (mī-Ō-sis) or reduction division. Meiosis produces haploid progeny cells (gametes) which have n chromosomes (23). The number of unpaired chromosomes in a gamete is also represented by n.

A. Meiosis

OBJECTIVE

To demonstrate the behavior of chromosomes in meiosis

Meiosis differs from mitosis in three important ways.

- ☐ It results in haploid (n), not diploid ($2n$) cells.
- ☐ Replication of the genetic material is followed not by one, but by two cell divisions, called ***meiosis I (reduction division)*** and ***meiosis II (equatorial division).***
- ☐ Crossing over, an exchange of genes between homologous chromosomes, may occur.

Many cell structures (the nuclear membrane, nucleolus, centrioles, and spindle) are involved

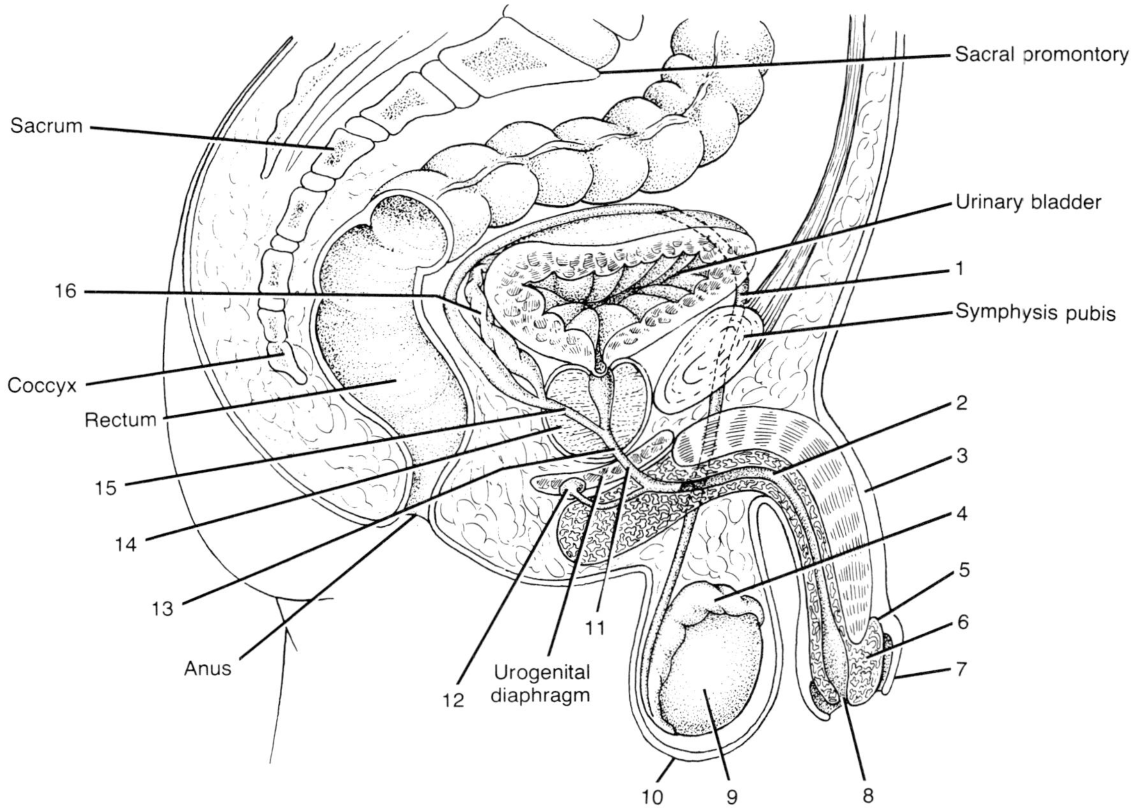

___ Bulbourethral (Cowper's) gland
___ Corona of penis
___ Ductus (vas) deferens
___ Ejaculatory duct
___ Epididymis
___ Glans penis
___ Membranous urethra
___ Penis
___ Prepuce
___ Prostate gland
___ Prostatic urethra
___ Scrotum
___ Seminal vesicle
___ Spongy (cavernous) urethra
___ Testis
___ Urethral orifice

FIGURE 14.2 Male reproductive structures seen in sagittal section.

in meiosis. In this exercise, the focus will be on the behavior of chromosomes and centromeres. We will look at a hypothetical cell in which $2n = 6$. In the process of meiosis, the genetic material replicates so that twelve chromatids are present; in meiosis I the complement is reduced to six chromatids; finally, in meiosis II four gametes, each with three chromosomes, result.

Figure 14.3 illustrates the steps in meiosis.

MATERIALS

Two long dark rods with Velcro closures

Two long light rods with Velcro closures

Two medium length dark rods with Velcro closures

Two medium length light rods with Velcro closures

Two short dark rods with Velcro closures

Two short light rods with Velcro closures

PROCEDURE

1. Obtain 12 rods as listed under Materials. The length of the rods defines them as homologous chromosomes, i.e., the long rods represent the first pair of chromosomes. The color represents their parental origin, i.e., dark rods rep-

resent chromosomes inherited from the father, light rods represent chromosomes inherited from the mother. Figure 14.3a depicts the structures represented by the rods.

2. Define a location on your laboratory table which represents the interphase nucleus of a cell about to undergo meiosis. Place rods representing three pair of homologous chromosomes in the nucleus:

One pair of long rods (light and dark)

One pair of medium length rods (light and dark)

One pair of short rods (light and dark)

These chromosomes would be invisible microscopically because, at interphase, they are uncoiled and thread-like (see Figure 14.3b).

3. Represent chromosomal replication by attaching each rod to the other rod of the same length and color at the Velcro fastener. The Velcro represents a centromere: the attached rods represent chromatid pairs (see Figure 14.3c).

4. Move both long, medium, and short chromatid pairs together into a cluster called a ***tetrad.*** During meiotic prophase, homologous pairs of chromosomes associate in this manner, called ***synapsis.*** The regions of apparent contact between chromatids are called ***chias-***

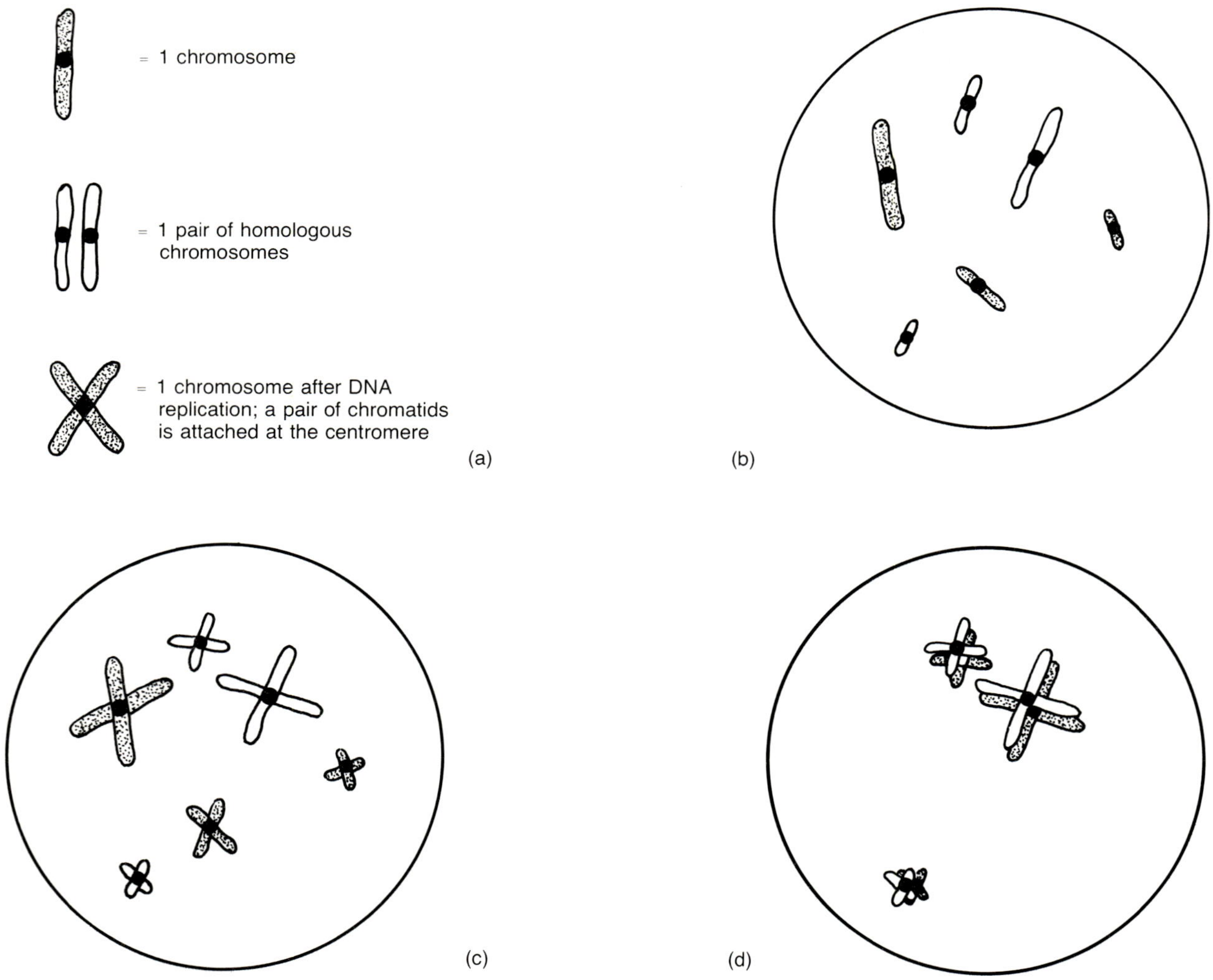

FIGURE 14.3 Meiosis. (a) Symbols. (b) Interphase I before DNA replication (G_1). (c) Interphase I after DNA replication (G_2). (d) Synapsis at Prophase I.

mata; it is here that crossing-over, or breakage of chromatids followed by exchange of genetic material, occurs. You will not be able to demonstrate crossing-over (see Figure 14.3d).

5. Mimicking metaphase, move the synapsed homologues to the equatorial plane (equator), the center of the field you have defined as the nucleus. This motion is accomplished *in vivo* by the attachment of the centromeres to spindle fibers (see Figure 14.3e).

6. Separate the members of each tetrad, so that one member of each pair of homologues moves to opposite poles. Note that the centromeres do not divide. Note that all the dark, two dark, one dark, or no dark chromosomes may move to one pole (Mendel's Law of Segregation). However, at this point, when the diploid ($2n$) number of chromosomes is reduced by one-half (chromosome number reflects a count of centromeres, not of chromatids), one member of each chromosome pair (long, medium, and short) must move to each pole (see Figure 14.3f).

7. Draw the chromosome complement of each progeny cell (see Figure 14.3g) in the LABORATORY REPORT RESULTS at the end of the chapter. Draw all other possible combinations of chromosomes.

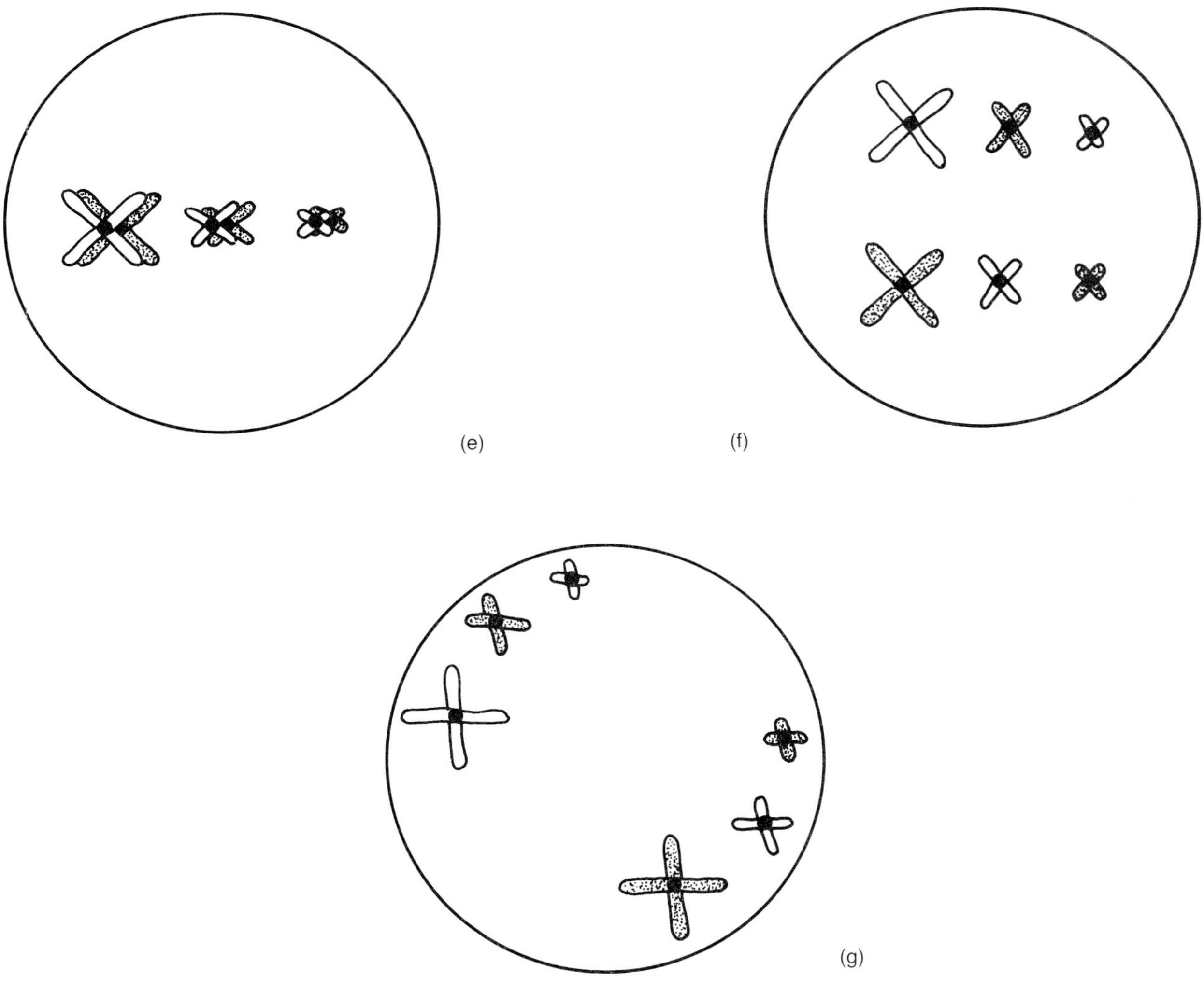

FIGURE 14.3 (*Continued*) Meiosis. (e) Metaphase I. (f) Anaphase I. (g) Telophase I.

8. Separate the two nuclei on your lab table to reflect cytokinesis. Each of the two progeny cells that have been formed will undergo meiosis II, a process that is identical to mitosis, except that interphase DNA replication does not occur (see Figure 14.3h).

9. Move the chromatid pairs to the equator of both progeny cells (see Figure 14.3i).

10. Separate the Velcro closures to mimic the splitting of the centromeres, and move the chromosomes to opposite poles (see Figure 14.3j).

11. Record the chromosome complement in each of the four haploid cells (n) that has been formed (see Figure 14.3k) in the LABORATORY REPORT RESULTS at the end of the chapter. Record all other possible combinations.

Why is there no DNA replication during meiotic interphase II? ______________________

____

____

Do you think this would be a long or a short stage? ____

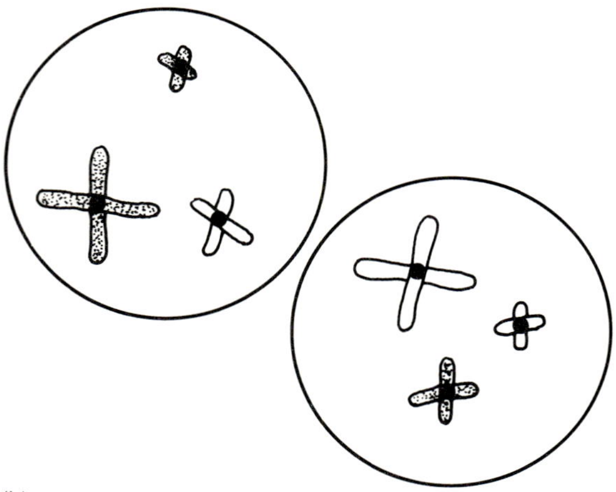

(h)

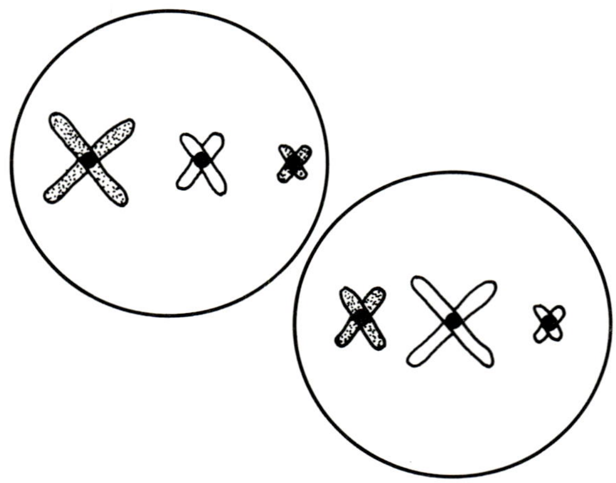

(i)

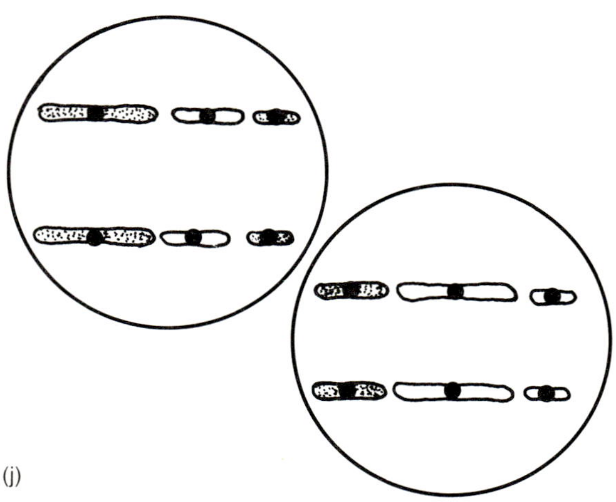

(j)

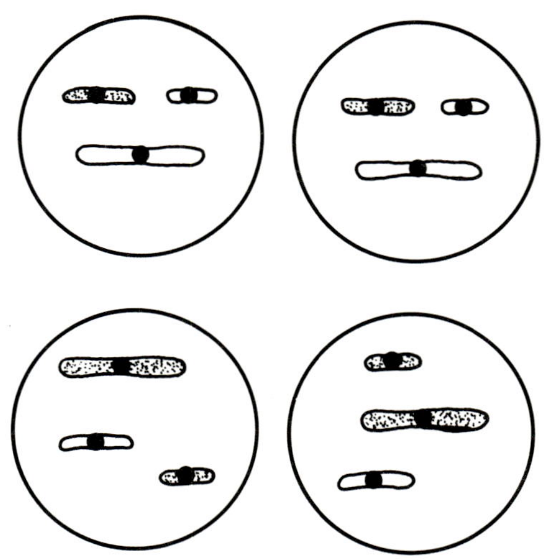

(k)

FIGURE 14.3 (*Continued*) Meiosis. (h) Interphase and Prophase II. (i) Metaphase II. (j) Anaphase II. (k) Progeny cells after Telophase II.

B. Spermatogenesis

OBJECTIVES

To describe spermatogenesis and spermiogenesis
To identify the hormonal regulation of these processes
To describe the anatomy of a spermatozoon

Coiled ***seminiferous tubules*** (Figure 14.4) within the testes are the sites of ***spermatogenesis*** (Figure 14.5). The cells in the outer border of the tubular wall are ***spermatogonia,*** diploid germinal cells which undergo mitosis throughout the reproductive life of a male, producing two progeny cells: one new spermatogonium and one cell which differentiates into a primary spermatocyte.

The diploid ***primary spermatocytes*** are pushed just inside the peripheral epithelium, toward the lumen of the tubule. They undergo meiosis, pushing their progeny cells further toward the lumen. Meiosis I results in two haploid ***secondary spermatocytes,*** and meiosis II then produces four haploid ***spermatids,*** located close to the luminal border. Because cytokinesis fails to be completed in the two meiotic divisions, these four cells remain connected by a cytoplasmic bridge. In the final stage of the process, called ***spermiogenesis*** (sper′-mē-ō-JEN-e-sis), the spermatids separate and mature into haploid ***spermatozoa (sperm).***

About 200–300 million spermatozoa (see Figure 14.6) are produced per day. Once ejaculated, they are viable for about 48 hours in the female reproductive tract. The parts of a spermatozoon are

1. Head—contains the nucleus and acrosome, which contains digestive enzymes.
2. Midpiece—contains numerous mitochondria in which the energy for locomotion is generated.
3. Tail—a typical flagellum composed of microtubules used for locomotion.

Throughout spermatogenesis and spermiogenesis, ***sustentacular*** (sus′-ten-TAK-yoo-lur) or ***nurse (Sertoli) cells*** in the seminiferous tubules play an important role. These large cells form a tight layer across the whole width of the tubule, and provide the following.

- □ Mechanical and nutritional support for the developing cells.
- □ A blood-testis barrier which isolates the developing sperm immunologically by preventing large molecules from entering the tubule.
- □ Receptor sites for follicle stimulating hormone (FSH); FSH initiates meiosis in primary spermatocytes.
- □ Inhibition of FSH (and consequent inhibition of spermatogenesis) via the release of the hormone ***inhibin;*** this feedback cycle maintains an appropriate rate of spermatogenesis.
- □ Phagocytosis of excess cytoplasm from the spermatids.

The hormonal regulation of spermatogenesis involves ***follicle stimulating hormone (FSH), luteinizing hormone (LH)*** and ***gonadotropin releasing hormone (GnRH).*** GnRH is produced in the hypothalamus and stimulates the secretion of both FSH and LH from the adenohypophysis. LH stimulates the ***interstitial endocrinocytes (cells of Leydig)*** to produce testosterone. ***Testosterone*** is necessary for the maturation of spermatids into spermatozoa.

MATERIALS

Slides of seminiferous tubule and spermatozoa
Compound microscope
Lens paper
Immersion oil

PROCEDURE

1. Examine a slide of a seminiferous tubule and label Figure 14.4b.
2. Examine a slide of human spermatozoa under oil-immersion. Since these cells are small, you will have to focus carefully. Label Figure 14.6.
3. In the LABORATORY REPORT RESULTS at the end of the chapter, draw and label a picture of a normal spermatozoon, as well as an example of any abnormalities you see.

Sperm are only viable for a few hours after ejaculation. What limitation in their structure prevents a longer life span? ________________

____

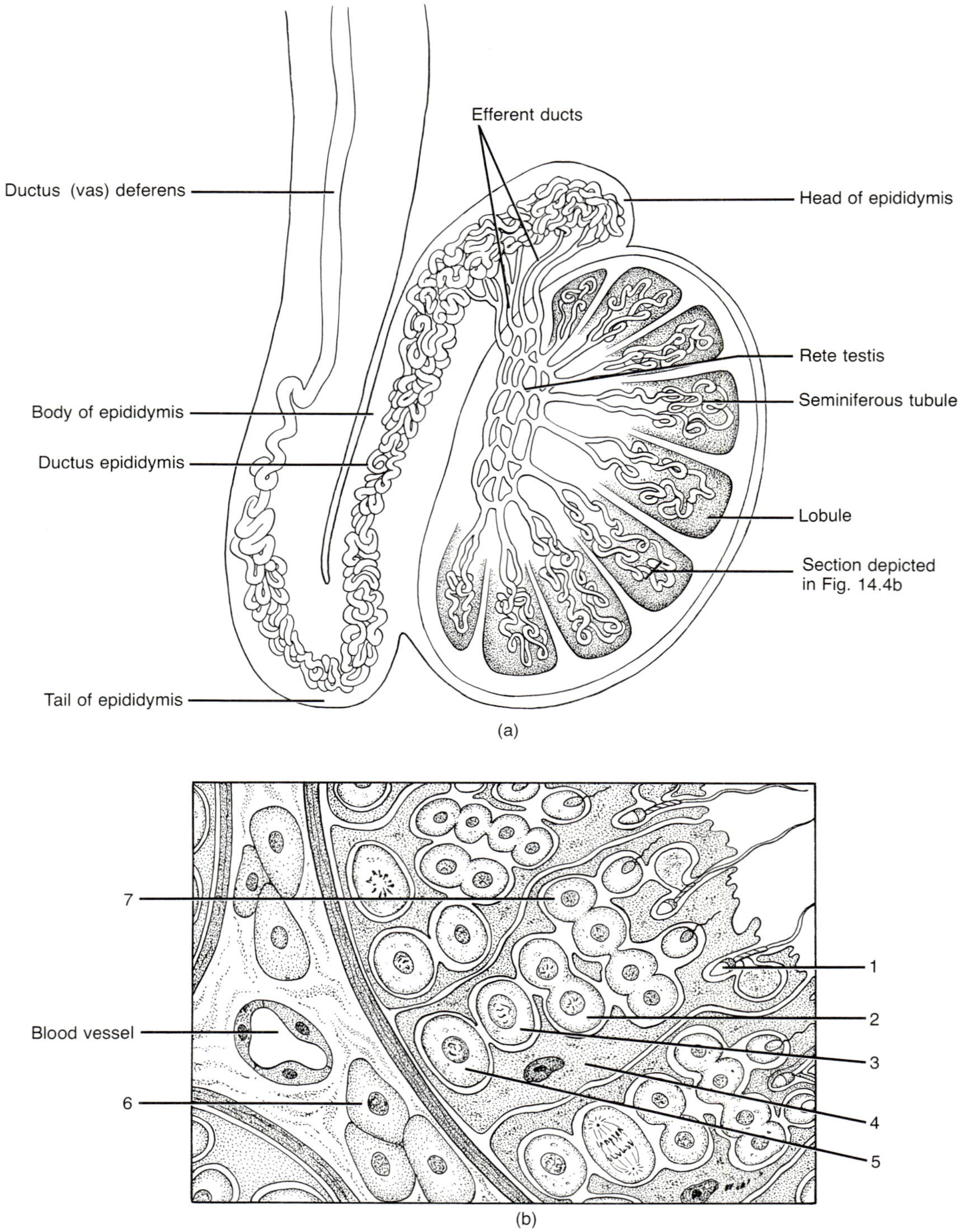

___ Interstitial endocrinocytes (cells of Leydig)
___ Primary spermatocyte
___ Secondary spermatocyte
___ Spermatid
___ Spermatogonium
___ Spermatozoon
___ Sustentacular (Sertoli) cell

FIGURE 14.4 Testes. (a) Duct system in testes of male. (b) Section of seminiferous tubule showing spermatogenesis and spermiogenesis.

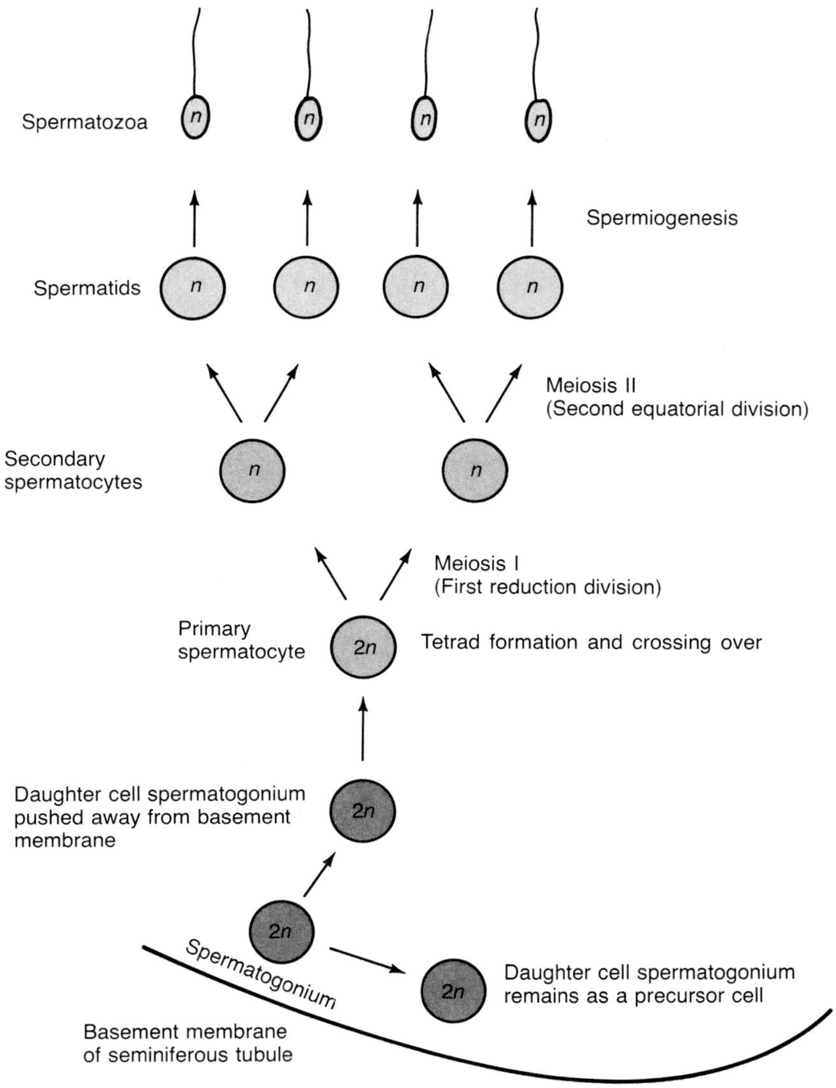

FIGURE 14.5 Spermatogenesis.

C. Oogenesis

> OBJECTIVE
> To describe oogenesis and its hormonal control

Oogenesis (Figure 14.7 and 14.8) is similar to spermatogenesis, although there are significant differences in the timing and in the number and size of the gametes produced. Oogenesis is not a continuous process like spermatogenesis. It begins during the fetal development of the female; it continues in each menstrual cycle after puberty, and it is completed only if fertilization occurs.

During fetal development, germinal cells called ***oogonia*** undergo mitosis, so that by birth, a newborn female has about 2 million ***primary oocytes***. No new oogonia are formed after birth. The primary oocytes begin meiosis

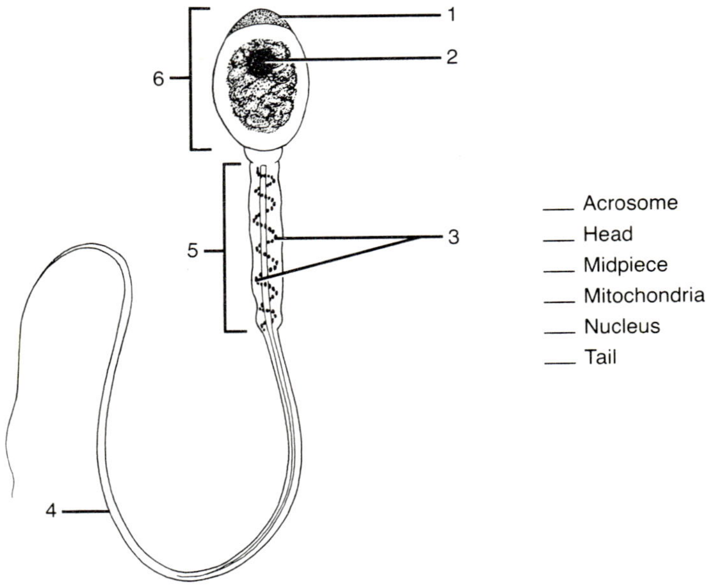

FIGURE 14.6 Parts of a spermatozoon.

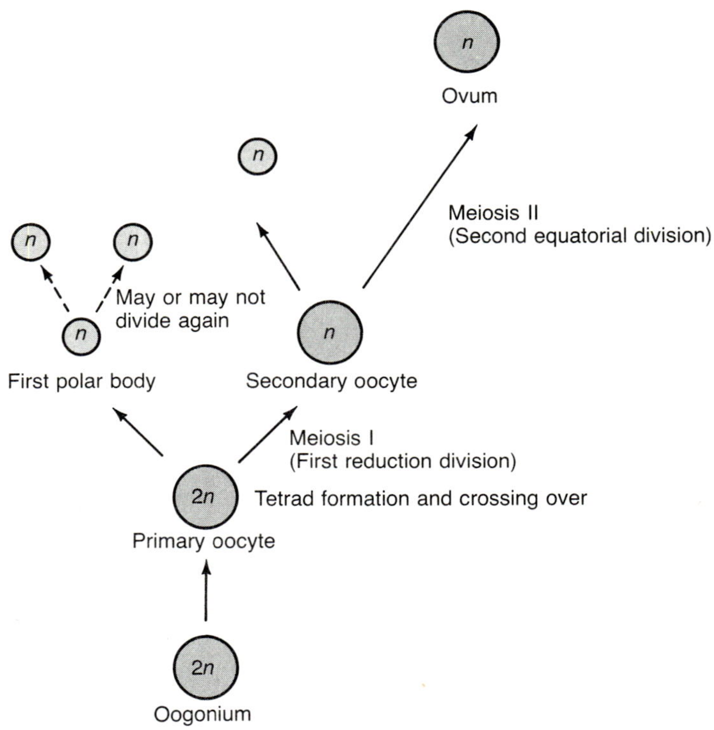

FIGURE 14.7 Oogenesis.

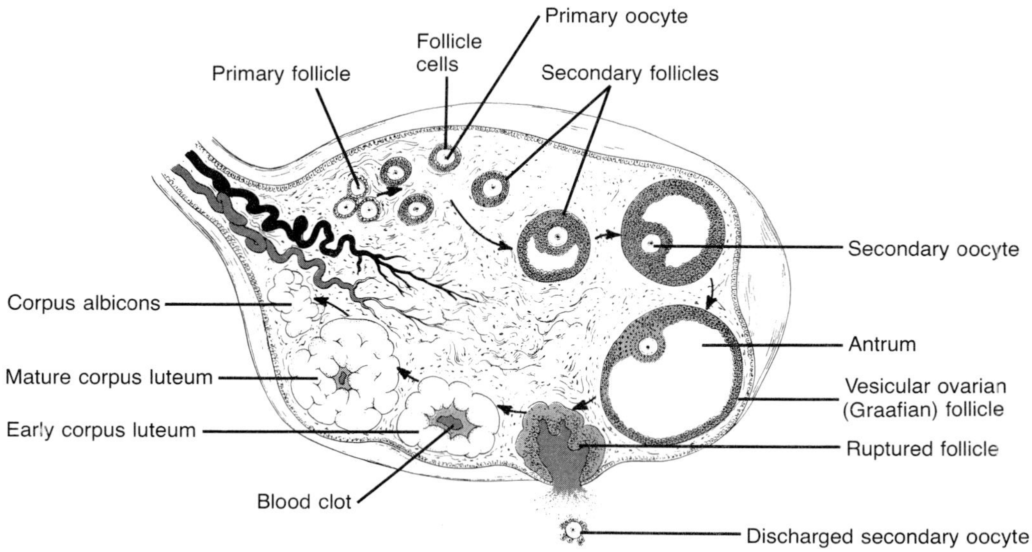

FIGURE 14.8 Sectional view of ovary during female cycle. Arrows indicate sequence of developmental stages which occur.

I, which is halted at prophase I. Many of these cells degenerate, leaving about 300,000 at ***menarche*** (the onset of menstruation).

During each monthly cycle, ***follicle stimulating hormone (FSH)*** stimulates the development of many primary oocytes: usually only one oocyte completes meiosis I. This process results in two structures: one ***secondary oocyte*** which receives all the cytoplasm and a small ***polar body,*** little more than a bare nucleus. The secondary oocyte (and occasionally the polar body) begins meiosis II, but this equatorial division halts at metaphase II unless fertilization occurs.

If this secondary oocyte is fertilized, meiosis II is completed with all the cytoplasm going to a large ***ovum*** and the production of another polar body which degenerates.

Figure 14.8 shows the development of the gamete in the ovary. The various stages depicted would not all be present at the same time. These ovarian structures are discussed in Exercise 2.

What could be the advantage of producing one large ovum and three polar bodies which degenerate? ____________________

____

____

EXERCISE 2. The Female Cycle

OBJECTIVES

To describe the cyclic changes in the ovaries and endometrium

To describe hormonal control of the cyclic changes

To define the timing of the events in the cycle

The female cycle (Figure 14.9) is a series of changes in the ovaries, endometrium, cervix, and breasts of a nonpregnant female which prepare the body for the implantation of a zygote each month. The cycle is controlled by hormones: ***β-estradiol,***[1] ***progesterone, follicle-stimulating hormone (FSH), luteinizing hormone (LH),*** and ***gonadotropin releasing hormone (GnRH),*** the hypothalamic releasing hormone for the last two hormones. The cycle lasts anywhere from 24 to 35 days; it will be described as a hypothetical (and typical) 28 day cycle which can be divided into several phases.

[1]There are at least six female hormones, collectively called ***estrogens,*** which affect the female cycle; β-estradiol is the most potent.

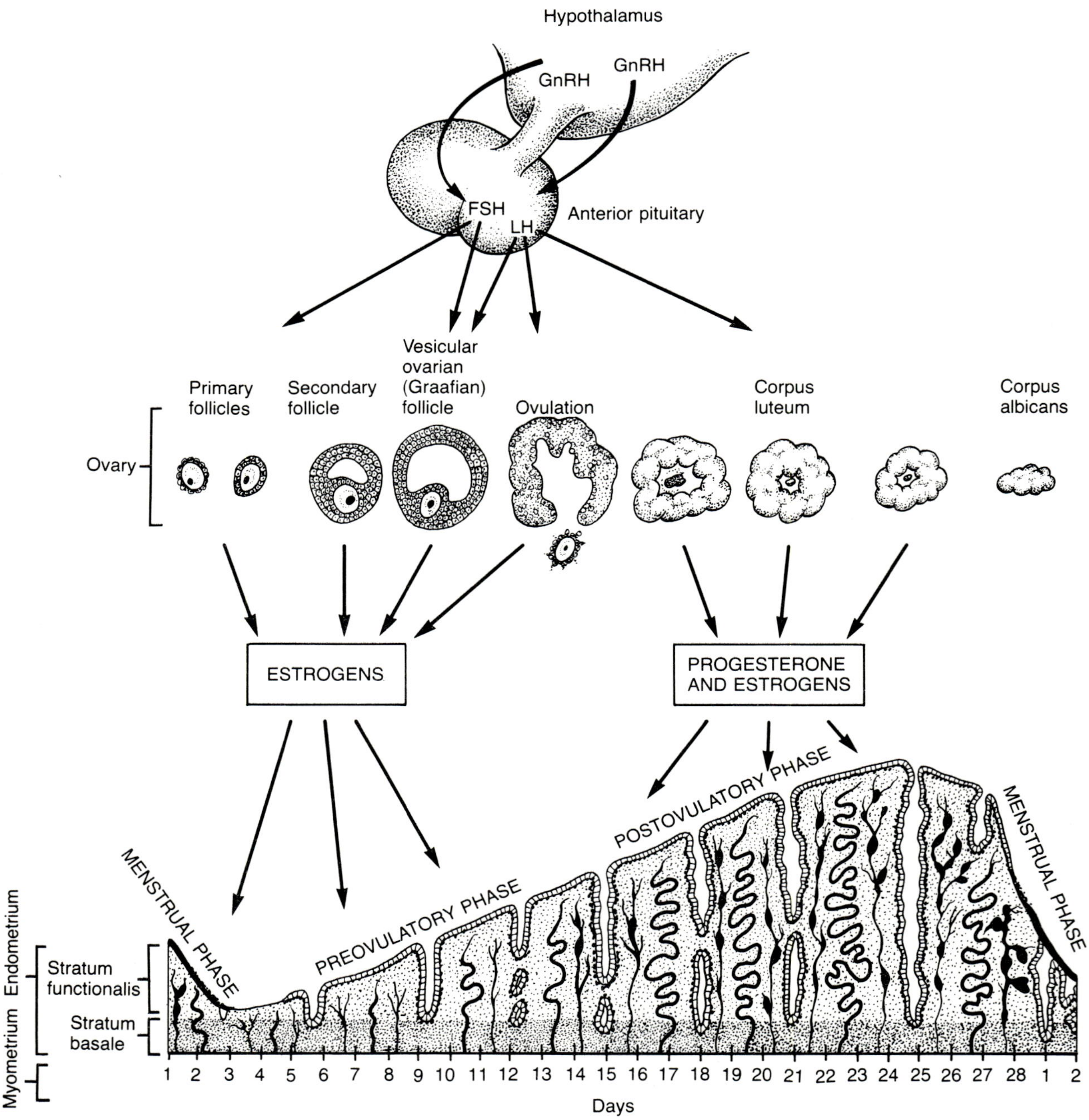

FIGURE 14.9 The female cycle.

The described length of these phases reflects the average duration in a 28 day cycle.

1. ***The Menstrual Phase (Menstruation).*** This 3–5 day phase is characterized by the discharge of blood, fluid, mucus, and epithelial cells from the endometrial lining of the uterus. It is triggered by the sudden drop in β-estradiol and progesterone levels at the end of the preceding cycle. The menstrual flow passes from the uterus through the cervix and vagina to the exterior.

2. ***The Preovulatory or Proliferative or Follicular phase.*** This phase extends from the beginning of the cycle through day 14 and includes the menstrual phase of the cycle. FSH and LH production by the anterior pituitary

gland trigger ***primary follicles*** in the ovary to develop. The follicles consist of the primary oocytes which were formed during fetal development and the follicular cells that surround them. The follicular cells secrete β-estradiol into the ***antrum*** (cavity) surrounding the primary oocyte, causing it to enlarge into a ***secondary follicle.*** The β-estradiol also stimulates the primary oocyte to complete meiosis I. When the fluid in the antrum forces the secondary oocyte to the side of the follicle, it is termed a ***mature*** or ***vesicular ovarian (Graafian) follicle.***

On day 13, a surge of luteinizing hormone (LH) and follicle-stimulating hormone (FSH) causes the rupture of the vesicular ovarian (Graafian) follicle and the release of the secondary oocyte in a process known as ***ovulation.*** The oocyte is covered with a layer of protein and polysaccharides known as the ***zona pellucida*** and a layer of granular cells, the ***corona radiata.***

During this phase, rising levels of β-estradiol promote the repair and growth of the endometrium.

3. ***The Postovulatory or Secretory or Luteal Phase.*** This phase extends from day 14 to day 28. After ovulation, the follicular cells that surrounded the secondary oocyte involute and take up fat, forming a body called the ***corpus luteum***. The corpus luteum secretes β-estradiol and progesterone in increasing quantities until day 21. These hormones increase the vascularization and glandular secretion of the endometrium and also inhibit the production of luteinizing hormone (LH). The reduced levels of LH fail to maintain the corpus luteum. Consequently, the corpus luteum shrinks into a structure known as the ***corpus albicans,*** and β-estradiol and progesterone production declines. This decline causes the inner layer (***decidua functionalis***) of the endometrium to be sloughed off in the menstrual flow.

The reduction in β-estradiol and progesterone production also releases the inhibition on FSH production, so with increased FSH, new primary follicles are stimulated to develop.

MATERIALS

Slides of ovary and endometrium
Compound microscope
Lens paper

PROCEDURE

1. Obtain slides of the ovary at various points in the female cycle. Look for primary, secondary, and vesicular ovarian (Graafian) follicles and for a corpus albicans and corpus luteum. Record drawings of your observations in the LABORATORY REPORT RESULTS at the end of the chapter.
2. Obtain slides of the endometrium at various points in the female cycle. Note any differences in thickness, distribution of blood vessels, and distribution and size of endometrial glands. Record your observations in the LABORATORY REPORT RESULTS at the end of the chapter.

EXERCISE 3. Fertilization

> OBJECTIVES
>
> To relate the time of fertilization to the events in meiosis
> To describe the formation of polar bodies in meiosis

Fertilization occurs on day 14 or 15 of the female cycle when spermatozoa meet a secondary oocyte in the distal two-thirds of the uterine (Fallopian) tube. The head of the sperm is covered by an acrosome (see Figure 14.6) containing ***hyaluronidase*** and other proteases. These enzymes, released when spermatozoa encounter the corona radiata, digest the coverings that surround the oocyte. As the sperm head penetrates the zona pellucida, a fertilization membrane is formed; this prevents the entry of more than one sperm.

As the sperm head enters the secondary oocyte, the oocyte completes meiosis II and expels a polar body. After this 12 hour process, the sperm nucleus merges with the ovum nucleus to form a ***zygote***.

MATERIALS

Slides of *Ascaris* fertilization at various stages
Compound microscope
Lens paper

PROCEDURE

1. Examine a slide of *Ascaris* showing sperm immediately prior to penetration and the entrance of the sperm head into a secondary oocyte (fertilization).

2. Examine a slide of *Ascaris* showing meiosis I and meiosis II. Find the polar bodies which have been formed.

3. Examine a slide of *Ascaris* showing female and male nuclei before and after fusion into a zygote nucleus.

4. Draw diagrams of your observations in the LABORATORY REPORT RESULTS at the end of the chapter.

EXERCISE 4. Human Chorionic Gonadotropin (HCG) and Pregnancy Testing

OBJECTIVES

To define the role of human chorionic gonadotropin (HCG)
To perform a pregnancy test and explain the mechanism of the reaction
To describe causes of false positive and false negative results in pregnancy testing

On day 21 of the menstrual cycle, the corpus luteum secretes maximal levels of β-estradiol and progesterone. If fertilization does not occur, the hormone levels decrease from day 21 to 28, causing the endometrium to be sloughed off.

If fertilization and implantation do occur, the corpus luteum is maintained for about 10 weeks, providing hormonal support for the endometrium, the site of implantation.

After only seven days of development (day 21 of the cycle) embryonic cells begin to manufacture ***human chorionic gonadotropin (HCG),*** a glycoprotein that is very similar to LH. HCG causes the corpus luteum to continue its production of β-estradiol and progesterone. After 10 weeks, the corpus luteum declines, and the placenta serves to produce the β-estradiol and progesterone necessary to maintain the endometrium.

The urine and plasma of pregnant women contain detectable levels of HCG a few days after conception. Pregnancy testing involves the measurement of HCG levels in the urine.

The hormone is detected by an immunoassay, an antigen-antibody reaction. Antibodies to HCG are added to urine, and, if HCG is present in the urine, it will form chemical bonds with the antibodies and cause their agglutination. Different antibody preparations employ various ways of visualizing this agglutination.

Prior to the development of the technique of antibody production, urine was injected into amphibians or rabbits to cause expulsion of gametes when HCG was present.

False negative results can arise if this assay is performed before HCG levels are sufficient to cause agglutination. False positives can arise in

- □ Women with tumors such as choriocarcinoma and chorioepithelioma which secrete HCG.
- □ Women with high levels of LH.
- □ Women in whom an abortion has occurred within the seven days before testing.

MATERIALS

Urine sample
Materials for pregnancy testing

PROCEDURE

1. Obtain a sample of urine from the supply table. Note the number of the sample: ______

2. Follow the directions of your instructor for performing this assay.

3. Record your results in the LABORATORY REPORT RESULTS at the end of the chapter.

What are the advantages of using this assay as opposed to injecting laboratory animals with unknown urines? ____________________

____

____

EXERCISE 5. Development

OBJECTIVE

To describe the early stages of development

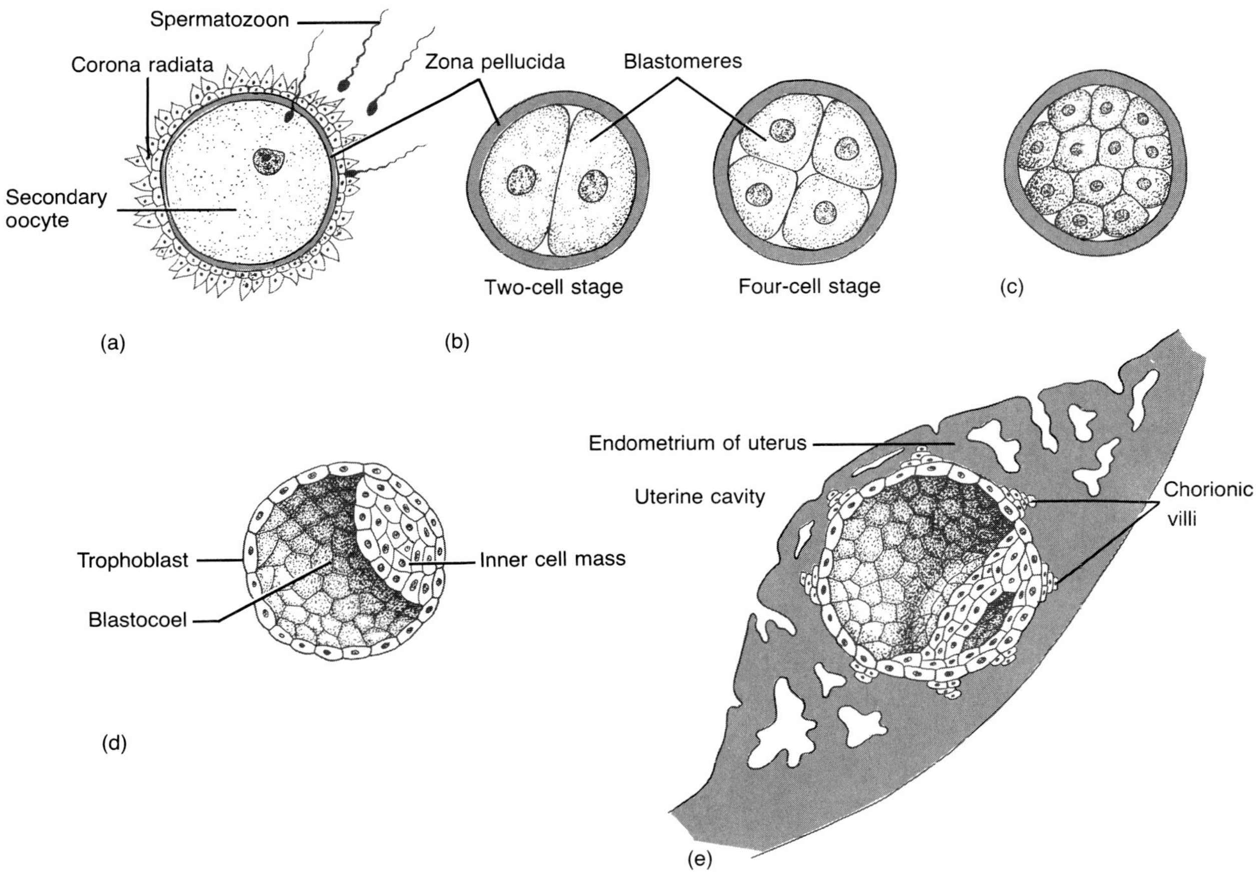

FIGURE 14.10 Fertilization and implantation. (a) Fertilization. (b) Two-cell and four-cell stages of cleavage. (c) Morula. (d) Blastocyst. (e) Implantation.

Immediately after fertilization, the zygote undergoes rapid mitotic division without cytoplasmic growth (see Figure 14.10). This early division is termed ***cleavage***. ***Blastomeres*** (BLAS-tō-mērz) are the progressively smaller and smaller cells produced by successive cleavages. After about three hours, 32 cells are present, and the structure is known as a ***morula*** (MOR-yoo-la). The morula becomes hollow and absorbs uterine fluid; mitosis continues until the morula appears like a hollow ball known as a ***blastocyst***. The outer covering of blastocyst cells is called the ***trophoblast;*** the rest of the cells are referred to as the ***inner cell mass (embryoblast);*** the cavity is known as the ***blastocoel*** (BLAS-tō-sēl).

About seven days after fertilization (day 21 in the female cycle), the trophoblast cells secrete enzymes that digest a small area in the endometrium. In the process of ***implantation*** the blastocyst attaches to the uterine wall at this spot. Extensions of the blastocyst called ***chorionic villi*** penetrate deep into the endometrial tissue.

Next, a complex invagination occurs in which the more external cells move into the blastocoel, forming a double-walled structure. Through additional movements of groups of cells, a process called ***gastrulation,*** cells differentiate into three primary germ layers. The outer layer, the ***ectoderm***, will develop into epidermal structures and the nervous system. The middle layer, the ***mesoderm,*** will form connective tissue, muscles, and the vascular and reproductive organs. The inner layer, the ***endoderm,*** will form the lining of the gut and associated glands.

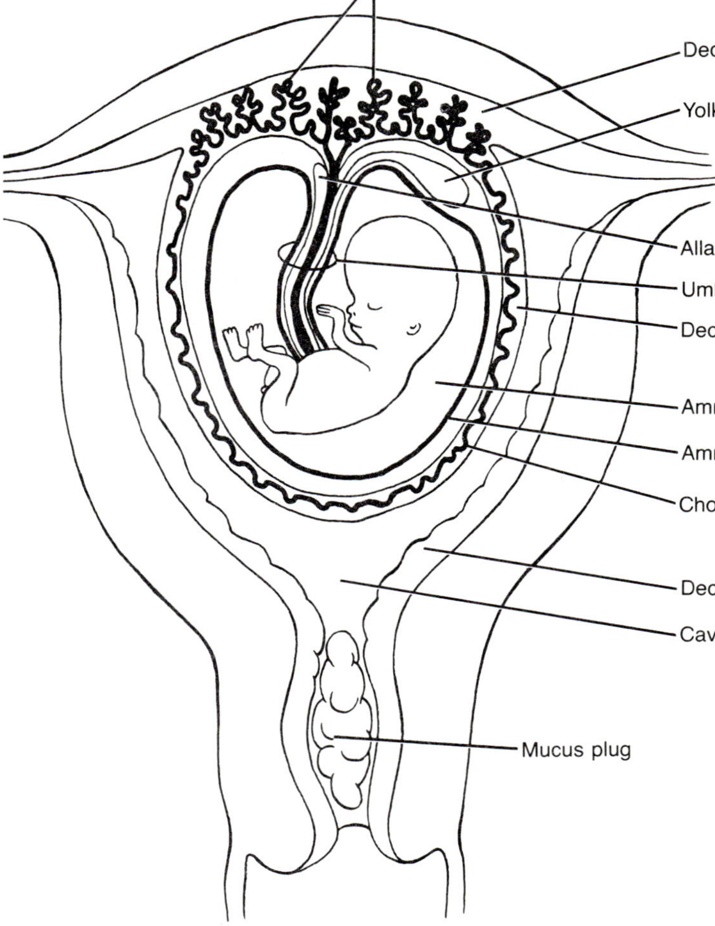

FIGURE 14.11 Embryonic membranes.

After about two weeks of development, the developing organism is known as an ***embryo.*** During the embryonic period, along with the development of the organ systems, ***embryonic membranes*** (Figure 14.11) develop as well. These membranes, the yolk sac, allantois, amnion, and chorion, protect and nourish the developing embryo.

The ***yolk sac*** serves to produce blood for the first six weeks of development until the liver forms; it also contains cells which differentiate into the primitive germ cells (spermatogonia and oogonia).

The ***allantois*** also is involved in blood cell production. It develops into the umbilical artery and vein, and it contributes to urinary bladder development.

The ***amnion*** is a sac that envelops the embryo and is filled with amniotic fluid. The fluid provides a cushion for mechanical forces on the embryo. Embryonic cells are sloughed off into this fluid; they can be examined in the procedure called ***amniocentesis*** (am′-nē-ō-sen-TĒ-sis).

The ***chorion*** participates in the formation of the ***placenta,*** a vascular organ which is also formed by the endometrial cells of the mother. It produces estrogens and progesterone and serves as the site of gas and food exchange between the mother and embryo, and later the ***fetus***.

After all major organ systems have begun to be formed at the end of week eight, the embryo is termed a fetus.

Why do you think blastomeres are progressively smaller and smaller? ______________

____

____

MATERIALS

Prepared slides of various stages in the embryonic development of the sea urchin, starfish, *Amphioxus,* or frog

PROCEDURE

1. Examine the slides of the embryonic development of one of the above species, in order from youngest to oldest. Identify a zygote, 2-, 4-, 8-, and 16-cell stage. Identify a morula and blastula (called a blastocyst in humans).

2. Draw your observations in the LABORATORY REPORT RESULTS at the end of the chapter.

COMPLETE LABORATORY REPORT QUESTIONS AT THE END OF THE CHAPTER

LABORATORY REPORT RESULTS

REPRODUCTION AND DEVELOPMENT 14

Student ______________________ Date ______________________

Laboratory Section ______________________ Score/Grade ______________________

EXERCISE 1. Gametogenesis

A. Meiosis

1. Progeny cells after Meiosis I

Other possible chromosome complements in progeny cells

2. Progeny cells after Meiosis II

Other possible chromosome complements in progeny cells

B. Spermatogenesis

Normal spermatozoon

Abnormal spermatozoon

EXERCISE 2. The Female Cycle

1. Ovarian section

2. Endometrium

	Preovulatory Phase	**Postovulatory Phase**
Thickness		
Blood vessels		
Endometrial glands		

EXERCISE 3. Fertilization

Entrance of sperm

Meiosis with Polar Bodies

Pronuclei

Fusion

EXERCISE 4. Human Chorionic Gonadotropin (HCG) and Pregnancy Testing

Results:

a. Description of reaction ______________________________

b. Test results ______________________________

EXERCISE 5. Development

2-cell stage

4-cell stage

8-cell stage

16-cell stage

morula

blastula

LABORATORY REPORT QUESTIONS

REPRODUCTION AND DEVELOPMENT 14

Student ____________________ **Date** ____________________

Laboratory Section ____________________ **Score/Grade** ____________________

PART I. MULTIPLE CHOICE

_____ 1. The cell formed by the union of the sperm nucleus and the ovum nucleus is a (a) gonad (b) gamete (c) zygote (d) pronucleus (e) polar body

_____ 2. Which of the following does NOT contain the haploid (n) number of chromosomes? (a) spermatozoon (b) oogonium (c) secondary oocyte (d) spermatid (e) primary spermatocyte

_____ 3. The symbol $2n$ represents (a) the number of chromosome pairs in a diploid nucleus (b) the number of chromosomes in a gamete (c) the number of chromosomes in a zygote (d) the number of chromatids in a dividing cell (e) none of the above

_____ 4. Meiosis (a) results in four progeny cells which have the haploid number of chromosomes (b) requires two nuclear divisions (c) is the process in which crossing-over occurs (d) all of the above (e) none of the above

_____ 5. The points where the chromatids of homologous chromosomes cross over each other are (a) synapses (b) bivalents (c) centromeres (d) tetrads (e) chiasmata

_____ 6. After meiosis I (reduction division), each progeny cell contains (a) one member of each pair of homologous chromosomes (b) the diploid number of chromosomes (c) one chromatid from each pair (d) all of the above (e) none of the above

_____ 7. Sustentacular (Sertoli) cells (a) lie in the spaces between adjacent seminiferous tubules (b) are receptor sites for testosterone (c) form a mechanical blood-testis barrier (d) phagocytize excess cytoplasm from spermatogonia (e) none of the above

_____ 8. Oogenesis (a) begins during fetal development (b) usually results in the production of one gamete during each female cycle (c) is completed only if fertilization occurs (d) all of the above (e) none of the above

_____ 9. During the preovulatory phase of the female cycle (a) β-estradiol is secreted by the primary oocyte (b) the corpus luteum increases in size (c) the endometrium increases in thickness (d) all of the above (e) none of the above

_____ 10. The ectoderm will develop into (a) nervous tissue (b) digestive organs (c) reproductive organs (d) muscles (e) none of the above

PART II. COMPLETIONS

11. Ova and spermatozoa are haploid (n) cells called ____________________ .

12. The alignment of two pairs of homologous chromatids which occurs at meiotic prophase is known as a/an ____________________ .

13. The enzyme ________________ is contained within the acrosome of a spermatozoon.

14. The function of human chorionic gonadotropin (HCG) is ________________ .

15. The first mitotic divisions of a zygote are called ________________ .

16. After eight weeks of development, the product of conception is called a(n) ________________ .

17. The attachment of the blastocyst to the uterine wall is called ________________ .

18. Women with high levels of luteinizing hormone (LH) could have a false ________________ (positive or negative) reaction in a pregnancy test.

PART III. MATCHING

____ 19. Diploid germinal cell
____ 20. Mature gamete
____ 21. Product of meiosis II
____ 22. Progeny of spermatogonial mitosis
____ 23. Produces testosterone
____ 24. Provides nutrients for developing gametes
____ 25. Product of meiosis I
____ 26. Product of spermiogenesis

A. Sustentacular (Sertoli) cell
B. Interstitial endocrinocyte (cell of Leydig)
C. Spermatozoon
D. Spermatid
E. Spermatogonium
F. Primary spermatocyte
G. Secondary spermatocyte

____ 27. Causes primary oocyte to complete meiosis I
____ 28. Along with LH, a surge of this hormone causes ovulation
____ 29. Produced by blastocyst
____ 30. Secreted into antrum
____ 31. Produced only in postovulatory phase of cycle
____ 32. Promotes growth and repair of endometrium
____ 33. Maintains corpus luteum in non-pregnant female

A. β-estradiol
B. Progesterone (PROG)
C. Luteinizing hormone (LH)
D. Follicle stimulating hormone (FSH)
E. Human chorionic gonadotropin (HCG)

____ 34. Fertilization occurs
____ 35. Ovulation occurs
____ 36. Menstruation begins
____ 37. Implantation occurs
____ 38. Progesterone level is maximal
____ 39. Primary follicle begins development
____ 40. Corpus luteum begins to develop

A. Day 1
B. Day 7
C. Day 14
D. Day 21

GENETICS 15

EXERCISE 1. The Human Karyotype
EXERCISE 2. Sex Inheritance
EXERCISE 3. Punnett Squares
EXERCISE 4. Inherited Traits
EXERCISE 5. The Hardy-Weinberg Principle
EXERCISE 6. Monohybrid and Dihybrid Crosses
EXERCISE 7. Incomplete Dominance
EXERCISE 8. Multiple Alleles
EXERCISE 9. X-Linked Inheritance
EXERCISE 10. Probability

WORD ROOTS

acro- = top
auto- = self
gameto- = to marry
hetero- = different
homo- = the same
karyo- = nucleus
meta- = middle
mono- = single
pheno- = showing
somat- = body
zygo- = tied together

Genetics is the branch of biology that studies the inheritance of anatomical and physiological traits. The traits that we possess and our ability to transmit them to our offspring are specified in large part by our genes.

Genes are specific, discrete portions of chromosomes. The nuclei in human ***somatic cells*** (all cells except sex cells) contain 23 pairs of chromosomes, the diploid number.[1] The human male has one pair of chromosomes which is not identical in appearance. These chromosomes, a larger X chromosome and a smaller Y chromosome, are called ***sex chromosomes*** to distinguish them from the 22 pairs of matching ***autosomes***. The female also has two sex chromosomes, but they are identical X chromosomes.

One member of each chromosome pair is inherited from the mother; the other member of each pair is inherited from the father. The two members of each pair are called ***homologous*** (hō-MOL-ō-gus) ***chromosomes***, and these homologues bear genes that determine the same traits. For example, both members of chromosome pair number 1 contain a gene that determines our Rh blood type, another gene that can cause an eye disease called aniridia, another that can cause a disease called phenylketonuria (PKU), and so on. The area of chromosome 1 that bears the Rh gene is the same on all number 1 chromosomes. It is called the Rh locus. A ***locus*** is the position of a gene on a chromosome. Alternative forms of genes, such as the genes for Rh positive and Rh negative blood types, always occupy the same locus.

For many traits, two or more alternative genes can occupy a given locus. These alternate forms are called ***alleles***. For example, there are three main alleles of the gene that codes for ABO blood type. Any two of these alleles occupy homologous loci on the pair of homologous chromosomes numbered 9.

[1]Diploidy and haploidy are discussed in Chapter 14.

The genes possessed by an individual constitute the ***genotype*** (JĒ-nō-tīp). Genotype may refer to a pair of alleles at a specific locus, or to the entire ***genome*** (all the genes in a cell). The physical expression of the genes is called the ***phenotype*** (FĒ-nō-tīp). The term phenotype can refer to the expression of a single trait or to the expression of all traits collectively.

Genes are not always expressed. If a gene masks the expression of its allele, it is called a ***dominant gene***, and the trait expressed is said to be a dominant trait. The homologous gene that is masked is called the ***recessive gene***. In order for a recessive trait to be expressed, both recessive genes must be present.

Genes are symbolized by letters; traditionally, the dominant gene is symbolized by an uppercase letter and a recessive gene by a lowercase letter. Individuals with two identical alleles, such as *PP* or *pp*, are said to be ***homozygous*** for the trait. When the two alleles are different, as *Pp*, they are said to be ***heterozygous***.

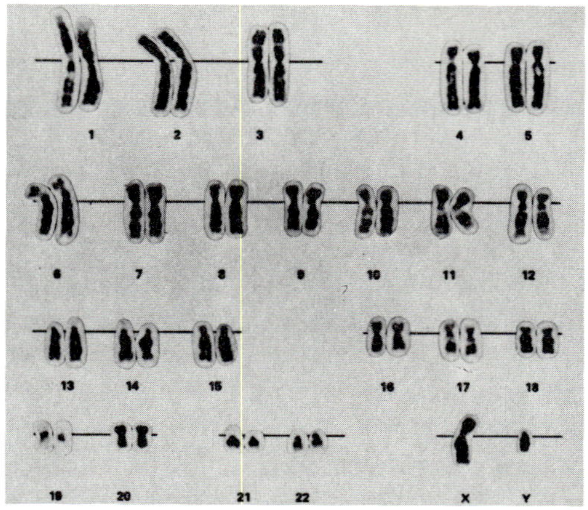

FIGURE 15.1 Karyotype of a normal human male. (Courtesy of Dr. Robert J. Sullivan.)

EXERCISE 1. The Human Karyotype

OBJECTIVES

To define and prepare a normal karyotype
To identify karyotypic sex
To recognize karyotypic anomalies

The 46 chromosomes in somatic nuclei can be arranged in homologous pairs. This pattern, shown in Figure 15.1, is known as a ***karyotype***. Karyotypes are prepared from cells that have been killed at mitotic metaphase and stained with various dyes. Giemsa stain colors chromosomal segments that are tightly coiled, revealing G bands. Q-banding involves staining with a fluorescent dye. C-banding is a modification that stains the centromeric regions of chromosomes.

Centromeres are the primary constrictions on chromosomes where chromatid pairs are held together. Chromosomes are classified as ***metacentric*** if the centromere is in the middle, ***sub-metacentric*** if the constriction is slightly off center, and ***acrocentric*** if the centromere is close to the end. Some chromosomes have a pronounced secondary constriction that pinches part of them off into a ***satellite***.

Individual chromosomes are identified by their length, location of the centromere, and banding pattern.

Abnormalities in chromosome number or size, seen in a karyotype, are termed ***cytogenetic defects***. If one chromosome is absent, the condition is termed ***monosomy***; if an extra chromosome is present, it is termed ***trisomy***. Monosomy of any chromosome other than the X chromosome is such a severe deletion that the embryo cannot develop. Trisomies of large chromosomes are also not compatible with life; however, live births of individuals with trisomy 8, 9, 13, 18, 21, and 22 have been reported. (Trisomies 8, 9, and 22 are extremely rare.) Usually, only trisomy 21 is viable beyond the first months of life. This condition, known as ***Down's syndrome***, is characterized by malformations of the face, hands, and heart, as well as mental retardation.

Abnormalities in chromosome size may be ***deletions***, in which part of a chromosome is lost. A deletion of the short arm of chromosome 5 results in ***cri du chat syndrome***, characterized by wide-set eyes, microcephaly, and a peculiar cat-like cry.

Pieces of one chromosome may be attached to another chromosome, forming a ***translocation chromosome***. Because genes are not lost or gained, there are no phenotypic effects. However, gamete formation is affected, and trisomies or monosomies may occur in the offspring.

The ***Philadelphia chromosome*** results from a translocation of a piece of the long arm of chromosome 22 to the short arm of chromosome 9. Over 95% of people with chronic myelogenous leukemia have this shortened chromosome. Even though no genetic material has been lost, there may be a position effect which can cause this cancer. It has also been suggested that a viral agent may cause the disease as well as the translocation.

An example of a translocation chromosome resulting in offspring with Down's syndrome is shown in Figure 15.2.

Figures 15.3 and 15.4 are photographs of cells that have been prepared for karyotyping. The preparation involves

1. Heparinizing a peripheral blood sample to prevent clotting and centrifuging it to separate the leucocytes.
2. Stimulating the leucocytes to grow in tissue culture by adding phytohemagglutinin, a bean extract that stimulates mitosis.
3. After 72 hours of growth, treating the culture with colchicine to arrest any mitoses at metaphase. Colchicine destroys the spin-

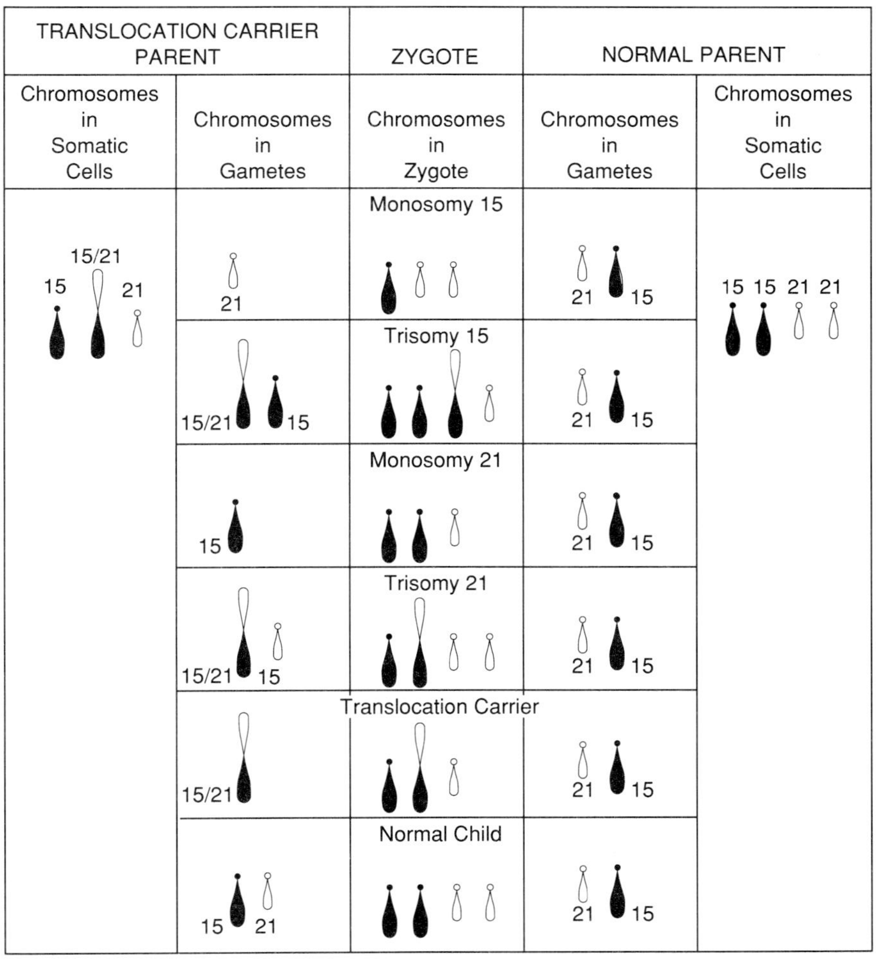

FIGURE 15.2 Inheritance of translocation Down's syndrome. The parental chromosomes on the left indicate that the parent is a translocation carrier, with chromosome 21 fused onto chromosome 15. Six different types of gametes can be formed. Of the zygotes, monosomies 15 and 21 and trisomy 15 are lethal. Of the viable offspring, one will be normal, one will be a translocation carrier, and one will have translocation Down's syndrome.

dle fibers and prevents the centromeres from dividing. Cells continue to undergo mitosis and accumulate when they are halted at metaphase.

4. Adding a hypotonic solution to cause swelling and bursting of the cells, resulting in a *metaphase spread*.

5. Fixing and staining cells on a slide, followed by microscopic examination and microphotography.

MATERIALS

Figures 15.3 and 15.4

Double-faced tape and scissors

PROCEDURE

1. Examine the metaphase spread in Figure 15.3 and count the number of chromosomes.

2. Carefully cut out the chromosomes and arrange them according to size.

3. Pair the chromosomes by matching their length, centromeric position, and G bands.

4. Place a small piece of double-faced tape on the back of each chromosome and position them on the karyotype analysis sheet provided in the LABORATORY REPORT RESULTS at the end of the chapter. Align the centromeres on the guidelines.

5. Identify the sex of the individual and any numerical or structural abnormalities that are present.

6. Record your observations in the LABORATORY REPORT RESULTS at the end of the chapter.

7. Repeat steps 1–6 with the metaphase spread in Figure 15.4.

Before 1970, no banding techniques were known. What problems do you think occurred in the preparation of karyotypes? ____________

____

____

EXERCISE 2. Sex Inheritance

OBJECTIVES

To describe the inheritance of sex
To prepare a buccal smear and identify Barr bodies

Like all traits, sex is determined by the interaction of genes and the environment. The genes that direct the development of undifferentiated embryonic genitalia are located on the X and Y chromosomes. In the absence of biochemical abnormalities, zygotes containing at least one X chromosome will develop into females, and those containing a Y and at least one X will develop into males.

Normally, all ova contain 22 autosomes and one X chromosome, and all sperm contain 22 autosomes and are either X-bearing sperm (containing an X chromosome) or Y-bearing sperm (containing a Y chromosome). Ova resulting from fertilization by X-bearing sperm will develop into females whose chromosome complement is expressed as 46,XX; ova resulting from fertilization by Y-bearing sperm will develop into 46,XY males.

Sometimes chromosomes fail to move toward opposite poles in meiotic anaphase. This is called ***nondisjunction*** and results in one sex cell having two members of a chromosome pair while the other receives none. Thus, ova can contain two X's or no X (symbolized as 0), and sperm may contain both an X and a Y chromosome, two X's or two Y's, or no sex chromosomes at all.

Because the X chromosome contains so many genes unrelated to sex and necessary for development, a zygote must contain at least one X chromosome to survive. Thus, YO and YY zygotes do not develop.

However, other zygotes with sex chromosome anomalies do develop. Several of them are listed in Table 15.1.

Extra X chromosomes (more than two in the female and more than one in the male) have a surprisingly minor effect on the individual, compared with the significant effect of other trisomies. Studies by Mary Lyon in the 1960s showed that only one X chromosome is active in any cell. Any additional X chromosomes are randomly inactivated early in development and do not express the genes contained on them. This inactivation is called ***lyonization***.

These inactivated X chromosomes remain tightly coiled and can be seen as ***Barr bodies*** (Figure 15.5). Since XY males do not have inactivated X chromosomes, no Barr bodies will be seen in normal male cells. This type of sex determination is the basis for the cytogenetic testing of athletes in order to determine their genotypic sex.

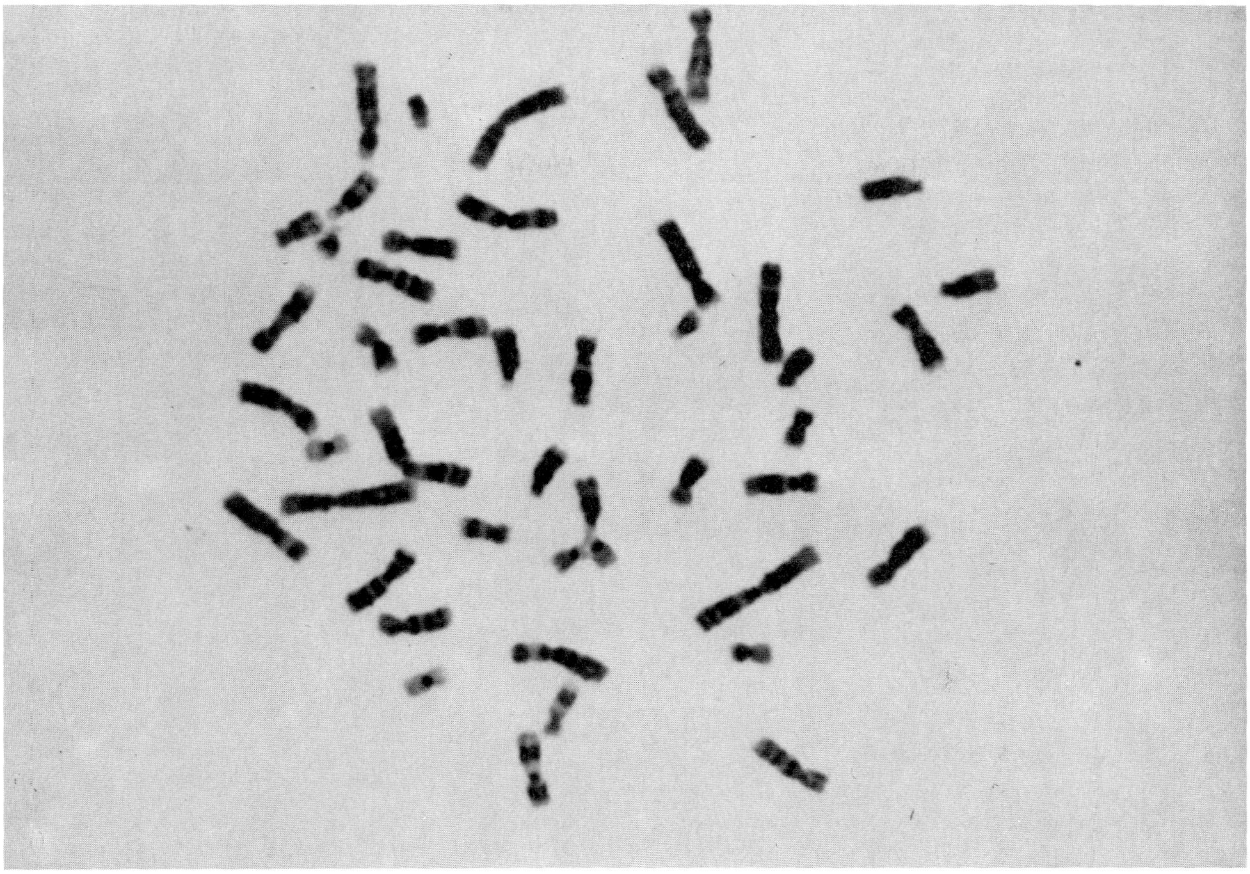

FIGURE 15.3 A metaphase spread. (Courtesy of Dr. Robert J. Sullivan.)

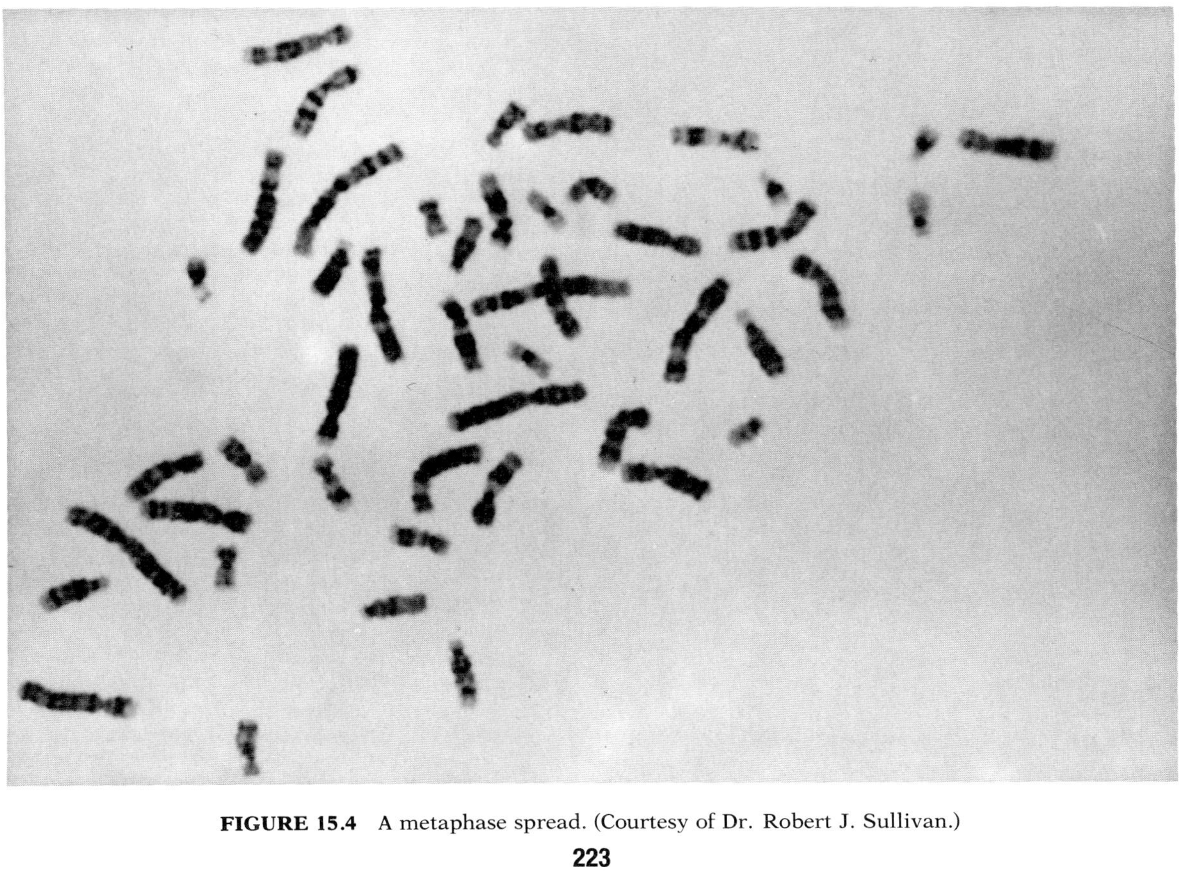

FIGURE 15.4 A metaphase spread. (Courtesy of Dr. Robert J. Sullivan.)

(This page intentionally left blank for cutting chromosomes on reverse side.)

TABLE 15.1
HUMAN SEX CHROMOSOME ANOMALIES

Sex Chromo-somes	Syndrome	Pheno-type	Frequency	Fertility	Characteristics
XO	Turner's	Female	1/300 live births	–	Short stature, sexual infantil-ism, webbed neck, cubitus valgus (lateral deviation of forearm)
XXX	Triple-X	Female	1/1400 live births	Reduced	Possible mental retardation
XXY	Kleinfelter's	Male	1/600 live births	–	Long arms, gynecomastia (male breast development), possible mental retardation
XYY	XYY	Male	1/1000 live births	+	Tall stature

MATERIALS

Toothpicks
Glass microscope slide
Two Coplin jars
Fixative
Giemsa stain
Fresh 10% bleach solution
Rubber gloves
Laboratory apron or coat

PROCEDURE

1. Make a buccal smear by *gently* scraping the inside of your cheek with the flat end of a toothpick. Discard the toothpick in a fresh 10% bleach solution and *gently* scrape the same area again. This will produce more live cells from a deeper layer of the epithelium of the mucus membrane. Discard the second toothpick in a fresh 10% bleach solution.
2. Spread the material over a clean glass slide.

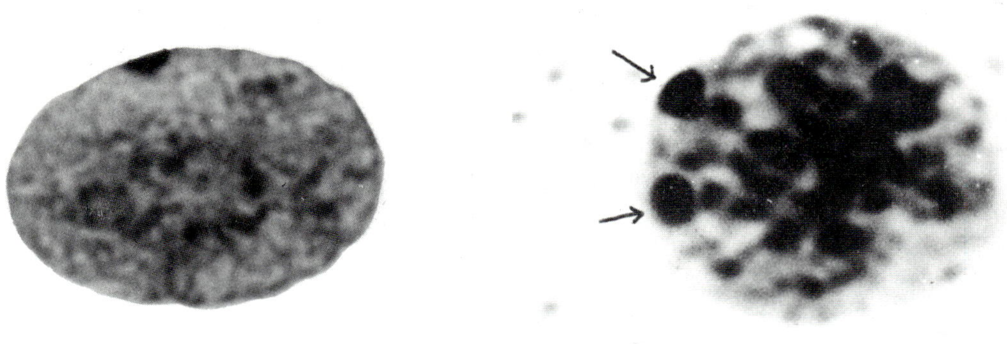

(a) (b)

FIGURE 15.5 Buccal smears. (a) Nucleus without Barr body. (b) Nucleus with Barr body.

3. Promptly place the slide in a Coplin jar filled with fixative for one minute.

4. Remove the slide and wash gently under running tap water.

5. Place the slide in a Coplin jar filled with Giemsa stain for 10–20 minutes. Fresh solutions of stain prepared within 2 hours require 10 minutes; older stains require a longer time.

6. Wash the slide gently under running water and air dry.

7. Examine the slide under high power and look for interphase nuclei. Identify Barr bodies, small disc-shaped chromatin bodies lying against the nuclear membrane. Depending on the position of the nuclei and the staining technique, Barr bodies should be seen in 30–70% of the cells of a normal female.

8. Examine a slide prepared from the buccal epithelium of a class member of the opposite sex.

9. Draw a cell containing a Barr body in the LABORATORY REPORT RESULTS at the end of the chapter.

10. Place your microscope slide in a fresh 10% bleach solution.

How many Barr bodies would you expect to be present in the cells of an individual with Turner's syndrome? _____ with Kleinfelter's syndrome? _____ with Triple-X syndrome? _____ with XYY syndrome? _____

EXERCISE 3. Punnett Squares

> OBJECTIVE
>
> To construct and use Punnett squares

To determine how the genes in gametes combine in a zygote, special charts called Punnett square are used. A ***Punnett square*** is a device that simplifies the visualization of all possible combinations of male and female gametes. To construct a Punnett square, use the following procedure.

1. Give a symbol to each trait. Use uppercase letters for dominant traits and lowercase letters for recessive traits.

2. Record the genotype of each parent. These genotypes reflect the diploid number of chromosomes, so each will have two letters representing each trait involved.

3. Determine the number of different types of gametes each parent can produce by computing it as 2^n, where n equals the number of heterozygous pairs of genes. Thus, a parent of genotype *Aa* has one heterozygous pair of genes and can make 2^1 or two types of gametes (*A* and *a*), a parent of genotype *AaBb*, with two pairs of heterozygous genes, could produce four types (2^2) of gametes (*AB*, *Ab*, *aB*, and *ab*), and a parent of genotype *AAbbCCdd*, with no pair of heterozygous genes, can produce only one (2^0) type of gamete (*AbCd*).

4. Write all possible gametes that can be produced by the mother across the top of the Punnett square. Each gamete will have only one member of each pair of genes.

5. Write the possible male gametes down the side of the Punnett square.

6. Using the model in Figure 15.6, which represents the mating of two individuals heterozygous for phenylketonuria (PKU), drop the gametes into the cells of the Punnett square. These cells will contain the genotypes of all possible zygotes.

7. Determine the genotypic ratio and phenotypic ratios of the offspring.

How many cells would be in a Punnett square representing a trihybrid cross? _____

EXERCISE 4. Inherited Traits

> OBJECTIVES
>
> To observe phenotypic variants of several traits
>
> To determine possible genotypes for these traits

The pattern of inheritance of some human traits is well known; the inheritance of other traits is complex and involves many genes. This exercise describes several phenotypic characteristics controlled by single genes. You are asked to record your phenotype and your genotype, if it can be determined. For example, if you have the phenotypically dominant trait A,

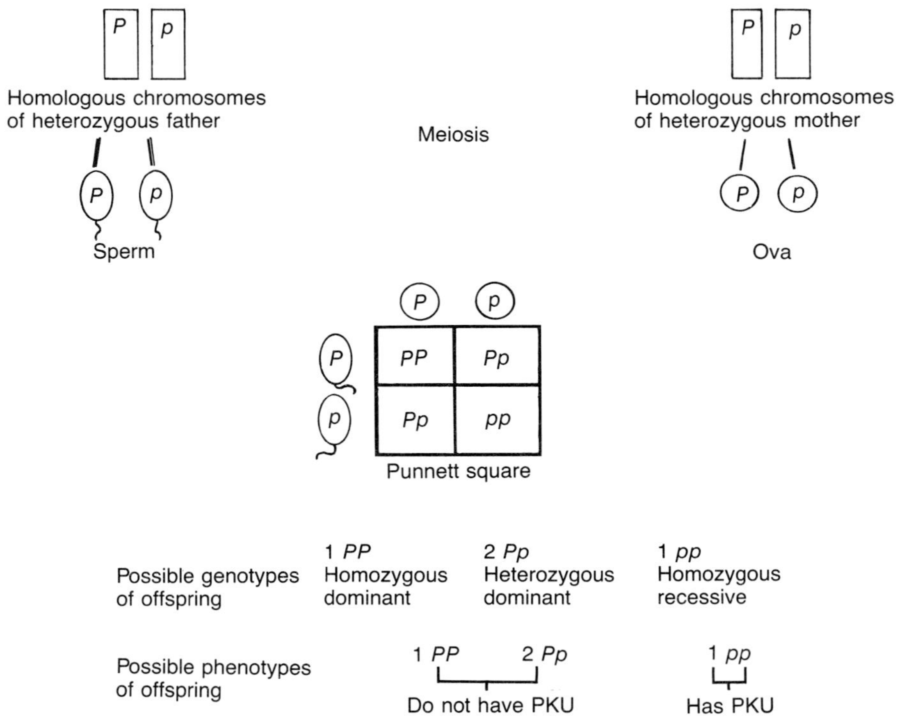

FIGURE 15.6 Inheritance of phenylketonuria (PKU).

your genotype will be *A*−, indicating that the allele symbolized as "−" is not known, since you could be homozygous dominant (*AA*) or heterozygous (*Aa*) for the trait. If you have the recessive trait *a*, your genotype will be *aa*.

PROCEDURE

Record your phenotype and genotype for the following traits in the LABORATORY REPORT RESULTS at the end of the chapter.

1. ***Attached Earlobes***. The dominant gene *E* causes earlobes that develop free from the neck; *ee* results in adherent earlobes connected to the cervical skin.
2. ***Tongue Rolling***. The dominant gene *R* causes the development of muscles that allow the tongue to be rolled into a U-shape. The *rr* genotype prohibits such rolling.
3. ***Hair Whorl Direction***. The dominant gene *W* causes the hair whorl on the cranial surface of the scalp to turn in a clockwise direction; the genotype *ww* determines a counterclockwise whorl.
4. ***Little Finger Bending***. The dominant gene *B* causes the distal segment of the little finger to bend laterally. The genotype *bb* results in a straight distal segment.
5. ***Double-jointed Thumbs***. The dominant gene *J* results in loose ligaments that allow the thumb to be bent out of the constricted orientation caused by the recessive genotype *jj*.
6. ***Widow's Peak***. The dominant gene *W* causes the hairline to extend caudally in the midline of the forehead. The recessive genotype *ww* results in a straight hairline.
7. ***Rh Factor***. A dominant gene *Rh* results in the presence of the Rh antigen on red blood cells. This antigen is not present with the recessive genotype *rhrh*. Use the results obtained in Chapter 16, Exercise 7.B to determine your phenotype.

What additional information would you need to determine your complete genotype if you have the dominant phenotype for these traits?

____

____

____

EXERCISE 5. The Hardy-Weinberg Principle

> OBJECTIVES
>
> To test for the ability to taste PTC (phenylthiocarbamide)
> To determine the population frequencies of the genes for tasting and nontasting

Looking at the dominant traits in the previous exercise, you may wonder why the whole population doesn't tend toward dominant traits and ask such questions as "Why doesn't almost everyone have a widow's peak?"

This question was answered mathematically in the early part of this century by Hardy and Weinberg in the principle named after them. It states that in a randomly breeding population, allele frequencies remain constant generation after generation. The ***Hardy-Weinberg principle*** assumes that

1. The population is large and each genotype has an equal chance to reproduce.
2. Mutation is not occurring or mutation occurs equally in two directions.
3. Individuals within the population are not migrating.

The Hardy-Weinberg principle can be expressed as $p^2 + 2pq + q^2 = 1$, where

p = the frequency of a dominant allele in the population

q = the frequency of a recessive allele in the population

$p + q = 1$, the total frequency (100%) of both dominant and recessive genes

p^2 = the percentage of the population that is homozygous dominant (AA)

q^2 = the percentage of the population that is homozygous recessive (aa), and

$2pq$ = the percentage of the population that is heterozygous (Aa).

These relations are shown in the Punnett square in Figure 15.7.

It is not possible to determine a gene frequency directly, nor is it possible to distinguish heterozygotes from homozygotes phenotypically. However, it is possible to determine (or at least to estimate from a statistically significant sample) the frequency of a recessive phenotype in a population. This percentage, q^2, can be used to calculate the other frequencies.

In this exercise you will determine the frequency of a recessive phenotype in your laboratory population. PTC (phenylthiocarbamide) is a substance that inhibits the thyroid gland from iodizing thyroid hormone. It is tasted by individuals with a dominant gene *T*; the homozygous recessive genotype *tt* is present in nontasters.

MATERIALS

PTC paper

PROCEDURE

1. Obtain a strip of paper impregnated with PTC and chew it for a few seconds.
2. Record your ability to taste PTC in the LABORATORY REPORT RESULTS at the end of the chapter and also on the chart provided in the laboratory.
3. Calculate the observed frequency of nontasters (q^2) by dividing the number of non-

	p = frequency of gene A	q = frequency of gene a
p = frequency of gene A	p^2 = homozygous dominant genotype (AA)	pq = heterozygous genotype (Aa)
q = frequency of gene a	pq = heterozygous genotype (Aa)	q^2 = homozygous recessive genotype (aa)

FIGURE 15.7 Punnett square illustrating Hardy-Weinberg Principle.

tasters in the class by the class size. Record these figures in the LABORATORY REPORT RESULTS at the end of the chapter. If the class is small, you can use the population figure of 36% as typical of American Caucasians or 9% as typical of American blacks.

4. Calculate q, the frequency of allele t, by taking the square root of q^2, the frequency of non-tasters.

5. Calculate p, the frequency of allele T, by subtracting q from 1 ($p + q = 1$).

6. Calculate $2pq$ by multiplying 2 times p times q.

7. Record these calculations in the LABORATORY REPORT RESULTS at the end of the chapter and fill in the Punnett square with the gene frequencies. Note that the frequencies do not change in the second (and subsequent) generations. What percentage of the laboratory population can be assumed to be heterozygous (Tt)?

EXERCISE 6. Monohybrid and Dihybrid Crosses

OBJECTIVE

To determine theoretical and actual genotypic and phenotypic frequencies in monohybrid and dihybrid crosses

Monohybrid crosses are those involving a mating between parents who are heterozygous for a *single pair* of alleles, such as $Aa \times Aa$. ***Dihybrid crosses*** involve a mating between parents who are heterozygous for *two pairs* of alleles, such as $AaBb \times AaBb$.

MATERIALS

Coins: quarter, dime, nickel, and penny

PROCEDURE

1. Using the blank Punnett squares in the LABORATORY REPORT RESULTS at the end of the chapter, diagram the monohybrid and dihybrid crosses of the parents listed.

2. Calculate the genotypic and phenotypic ratios of the offspring and record them in the LABORATORY REPORT RESULTS at the end of the chapter.

3. The ratios you calculated are theoretical probabilities that are possible with an infinitely large population of offspring. Mimic the crosses by using coins to represent alleles and count the frequency of offspring in the following manner.

a. Monohybrid cross. Use a nickel to represent maternal genes and a penny to represent paternal genes. Heads on either coin represent the dominant gene A; tails the recessive gene a. Flip both coins together four times (representing four offspring). Record the results in the LABORATORY REPORT RESULTS at the end of the chapter. Flip the coins eight more times and record the totals. Flip the coins 28 more times and record the totals.

b. Dihybrid cross. Use a quarter and a nickel to represent maternal genes and a dime and a penny to represent paternal genes. Dominance and recessivity are represented by

	Quarter		**Nickel**	
	Heads	Tails	Heads	Tails
Maternal Genes	A	a	B	b
	Dime		**Penny**	
Paternal Genes	A	a	B	b

Flip all four coins together 16 times and record the "genotypes" in the LABORATORY REPORT RESULTS at the end of the chapter. Flip them 32 more times and record the results.

How closely did your results approximate the theoretical ratios after a few tosses? ________

after more tosses? ________________

EXERCISE 7. Incomplete Dominance

OBJECTIVES

To describe the inheritance of sickle-cell anemia and sickle-cell trait

To explain incomplete dominance

Sickle-cell anemia is an autosomal recessive disease that affects about 1 in 400 black children born in the United States. The disease causes a change in hemoglobin structure that results in a gross abnormality in the shape of red blood cells. Heterozygotes (*Ss*) or carriers of this disease have ***sickle-cell trait***. Their red blood cells are normal unless they are exposed to low oxygen levels. Thus, the recessive gene *s* is not completely masked by the effect of the dominant gene *S*, and *S* is said to be incompletely dominant.

Complete the Punnett square that depicts the transmission of sickle-cell anemia in the LABORATORY REPORT RESULTS at the end of the chapter.

How does the expression of heterozygote *Ss* differ from that of heterozygote *Ww* (with reference to hair whorl direction)? ____________

____

EXERCISE 8. Multiple Alleles

OBJECTIVES

To understand multiple alleles and codominance

To describe the inheritance of ABO blood type

Many and possibly all genes have multiple alleles, that is, more than two allelic forms, even though the diploid cells of any individual can contain no more than two alleles.

One example of multiple alleles in humans involves the ABO blood groups discussed in Chapter 16. The four basic blood groups in the ABO system are determined by three alleles: I^A, I^B, and i. Alleles I^A and I^B are not dominant to each other (they are codominant), but either of them is dominant over allele i. These three alleles can result in six genotypes and three phenotypes as follows.

Genotype	Phenotype (blood type)
I^AI^A or I^Ai	A
I^BI^B or I^Bi	B
I^AI^B	AB
ii	O

PROCEDURE

1. Determine your ABO blood type according to the directions in Exercise 7.A in Chapter 16 or use information you have already obtained.

2. Determine all possible genotypes of yourself and of your parents and record them in the LABORATORY REPORT RESULTS at the end of the chapter.

Is it possible for a child of blood type O to have parents of blood type A and B? ____

EXERCISE 9. X-Linked Inheritance

OBJECTIVES

To distinguish between X-linked dominant and X-linked recessive inheritance

To assess color blindness and understand its mode of inheritance

Most genes borne on the X chromosome do not have alleles on the Y chromosome. Traits transmitted by these genes are said to be ***X-linked*** (or ***sex-linked***). Examples of X-linked traits are red-green color blindness, Duchenne muscular dystrophy, and hemophilia.

The inheritance of X-linked traits is different from that of autosomal traits because the male inherits only one X chromosome (from his mother), while the female inherits an X chromosome from both parents.

X-linked recessive inheritance is characterized by

1. A higher incidence of the trait in males than in females.

2. Passage of the gene (not the trait) to all daughters and no sons of an affected father; therefore, all daughters of affected fathers and normal mothers will be carriers of the trait.

3. Passage of the trait to daughters can occur only through an affected father and a carrier (or affected) mother.

X-linked dominant inheritance is characterized by

1. A higher incidence of the trait in females than males.

2. Passage of the trait to all daughters and no sons of an affected male.

3. Inheritance of the trait in mothers according to the pattern of autosomal dominant inheritance.

Red-green color blindness (there are several different types of color blindness) is an X-linked recessive trait. The ability to distinguish red from green depends entirely on genes carried on the X chromosome. A simplified explanation of red-green color blindness represents the dominant gene for normal color vision as *C* and the recessive gene that causes red-green color blindness as *c*. A single gene *c* is sufficient to cause color blindness in males, since males are ***hemizygous***, that is, they have only one X chromosome. If males have the gene *c*, there can be no dominant gene *C* to mask the effect of the recessive gene. Thus, males cannot be heterozygous carriers. In order for a female to be color blind, she must be homozygous recessive (*cc*).

Figure 15.8 demonstrates the inheritance of color blindness.

MATERIALS

Snelling, Ishihara, or Ichikawa charts or Holmgren test

PROCEDURE

1. Using the materials provided, determine your ability to distinguish red and green.

2. Record your results in the LABORATORY REPORT RESULTS at the end of the chapter.

If a mother with normal color vision has color blind sons, what is her genotype? ____

EXERCISE 10. Probability

OBJECTIVE
To learn the basic principles of probability

The ***probability*** of an event occurring is defined as

$$\frac{\text{the number of favorable outcomes}}{\text{the total number of possible outcomes}}$$

If an event is sure to occur, its probability is 1; if an event cannot happen, its probability is 0. Other probabilities are expressed as fractions. The probability of throwing heads on a coin toss is ½ (or 0.5) because there are two possibilities (heads and tails) and one favorable outcome (heads). The probability of rolling a die to get the number 5 is ⅙ because there are six possibilities and one favorable outcome.

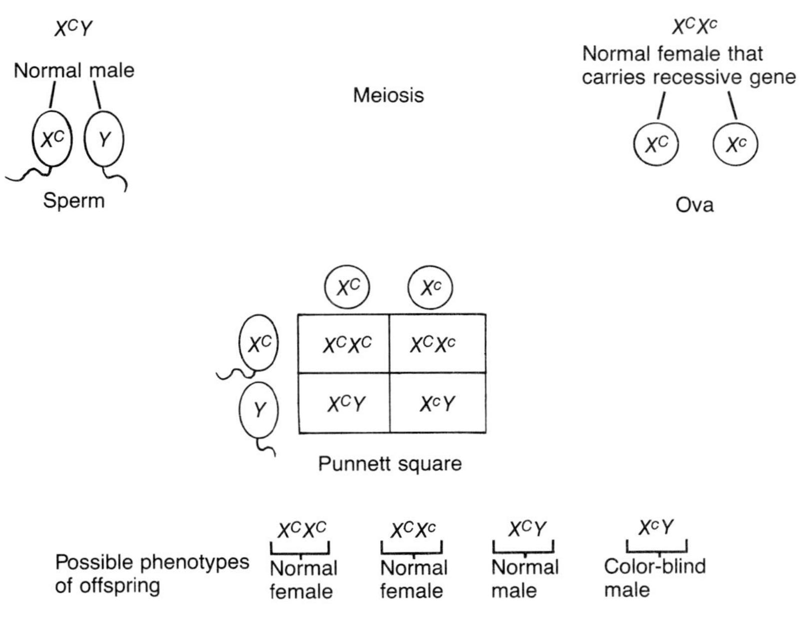

FIGURE 15.8 Inheritance of color blindness.

The probability of one OR another mutually exclusive events occurring is the sum of the separate probabilities. Thus the probability of rolling a 5 OR a 4 with a die is $1/3$ ($1/6 + 1/6$), and the probability of having a boy OR a girl is 1 ($1/2 + 1/2$).

The probability that both of two events will occur together is the product of the two separate probabilities. Thus, the probability of rolling two dice and getting two sixes is $1/36$ ($1/6 \times 1/6$). The probability of having two girls (or boys) in a row is $1/4$ ($1/2 \times 1/2$).

PROCEDURE

To practice the calculation of various probabilities, do the problems in the LABORATORY REPORT RESULTS at the end of the chapter.

COMPLETE THE LABORATORY REPORT QUESTIONS AT THE END OF THE CHAPTER

LABORATORY REPORT RESULTS

GENETICS 15

Student ______________________ Date ______________________

Laboratory Section ______________________ Score/Grade ______________________

EXERCISE 1. The Human Karyotype

A. Metaphase Spread in Figure 15.3

Number of chromosomes ____

Sex of individual ______________

Anomalies ______________

1	2	3	4	5

6	7	8	9	10	11	12

13	14	15	16	17	18

19	20	21	22	X	X or Y

B. Metaphase Spread in Figure 15.4

Number of chromosomes ____

Sex of individual ______________

Anomalies ______________

1 2 3 4 5

6 7 8 9 10 11 12

13 14 15 16 17 18

19 20 21 22 X X or Y

EXERCISE 2. Sex Inheritance

Drawing of cell with Barr body

EXERCISE 4. Inherited Traits

	Phenotype	Genotype
Attached earlobes		
Tongue rolling		
Hair whorl direction		
Little finger bending		
Double-jointed thumbs		
Widow's peak		
Rh factor		

EXERCISE 5. The Hardy-Weinberg Principle

1. Ability to taste PTC ____
2. Number of nontasters in class ____
3. Number of students in class ____
4. Frequency of nontasters (q^2) ____ %
5. $q =$ ____
6. $p =$ ____
7. $2pq =$ ____

	$p =$	$q =$
$p =$	$p^2 =$	$pq =$
$q =$	$pq =$	$q^2 =$

EXERCISE 6. Monohybrid and Dihybrid Crosses

Parents: $Aa \times Aa$

Gametes: ________

Cross:

Genotypic ratio: ________

Phenotypic ratio: ________

- -

Parents: $AaBb \times AaBb$

Gametes: ________

Cross:

Genotypic ratio: ________

Phenotypic ratio: ________

Coin Toss

	Female (nickel)	Male (penny)	Total for 4 flips	Total for 12 flips	Total for 40 flips
Dominant offspring (AA and aa)	A (heads)	A (heads)			
	A (heads)	a (tails)			
	a (tails)	A (heads)			
Recessive offspring (aa)	a (tails)	a (tails)			
	Actual ratio dominant to recessive		:	:	:
	Expected ratio dominant to recessive		3:1	9:3	30:10

Coin Toss

Female (quarter)	Male (dime)	Female (nickel)	Male (penny)	Phenotype	Total of 16 tosses	Total of 48 tosses
A	A	B	B	Double dominant (AB)		
A	A	B	b			
A	A	b	B			
A	a	B	B			
A	a	B	b			
A	a	b	B			
a	A	B	B			
a	A	B	b			
a	A	b	B			
A	A	b	b	Single dominant (Ab)		
A	a	b	b			
a	A	b	b			
a	a	B	B	Single dominant (aB)		
a	a	B	b			
a	a	b	B			
a	a	b	b	Double recessive (ab)		
Actual ratio of phenotype AB:Ab:aB:ab					: : :	
Expected ratio of phenotype AB:Ab:aB:ab					9:3:3:1	27:9:9:3

EXERCISE 7. Incomplete Dominance

Parents: Phenotype: Both have sickle cell trait.

Genotype: ____________

Gametes: ____________

Cross:

	*	**
	***	****

Phenotypes of offspring =

* = ________________________

** = ________________________

*** = ________________________

**** = ________________________

EXERCISE 8: Multiple Alleles

1. Your phenotype ____
2. Your possible genotype(s): ____
3. Possible genotypes of your parents:

____ × ____

____ × ____

____ × ____

EXERCISE 9. X-Linked Inheritance

Color blindness present ____ normal color vision ____

EXERCISE 10. Probability

1. Cystic fibrosis is an autosomal recessive disease. Two parents have an affected child. What is the probability of their having another affected child? ____

What is the probability of their having three more affected children? ____

2. If curly hair is an autosomal dominant trait, what is the probability that two curly haired parents will have a curly haired child? ____ a straight haired child? ____

3. Hemophilia is an X-linked recessive disease. The daughter of a hemophiliac marries a normal male. What is the probability that they will have a hemophiliac son? ____ a hemophiliac

daughter? ____ a normal daughter? ____ a normal son? ____ a carrier daughter? ____
What is the probability that they will have a normal son or an unaffected daughter? ____

4. If Mr. Parker is blood type AB and Mrs. Parker is blood type O, what is the probability of their having a son with blood type O? ____ a daughter of blood type AB? ____

5. Albinism is an autosomal recessive disease. What is the probability that a normal sibling of an albino brother is a carrier for the disease? ____ What is the probability that another albino will be born to this family? ____

LABORATORY REPORT QUESTIONS

GENETICS 15

Student ______________________ Date ______________________

Laboratory Section ______________________ Score/Grade ______________________

PART I. MULTIPLE CHOICE

______ 1. The structure that directs the development of a particular part of the body or biological characteristic is a (a) chromosome (b) locus (c) centromere (d) gene (e) trait

______ 2. Gametes contain (a) two sex chromosomes (b) 22 pair of autosomes (c) the diploid number of chromosomes (d) 46 chromosomes (e) none of the above

______ 3. The genotype *Aa* (a) will result in trait A being expressed (b) refers to gene loci on two chromosomes (c) is a heterozygous genotype (d) all of the above (e) none of the above

______ 4. An individual with sex chromosomes XYY (a) has Kleinfelter's syndrome (b) is a phenotypic male (c) is not likely to survive (d) has 46 chromosomes (e) all of the above

______ 5. The expression of the genes in an individual is called the (a) genotype (b) genome (c) phenotype (d) pedigree (e) locus

______ 6. Which of the following genes are located on the X chromosome? (a) hemophilia (b) sickle-cell anemia (c) Barr bodies (d) Rh blood type (e) all of the above

______ 7. Albinism is inherited as an autosomal recessive disease. What is the probability of two heterozygotes having an albino child? (a) 100% (b) 75% (c) 50% (d) 25% (e) 0%

______ 8. What is the probability of the normal sibling of an albino child being a carrier for albinism? (a) 100% (b) 67% (c) 50% (d) 25% (e) 0%

______ 9. What is the probability of the mother of an albino child being homozygous dominant for the gene for normal pigmentation? (a) 100% (b) 75% (c) 50% (d) 25% (e) 0%

______ 10. What is the blood type of a child born to a father of blood type A and a mother of blood type O? (a) A (b) O (c) AO (d) cannot be determined from the information given

______ 11. When both traits are expressed in a heterozygote, the alleles are said to be (a) hemizygous (b) codominant (c) homozygous (d) multiple alleles

______ 12. Which product of conception would be most likely to be seen in spontaneous abortions? (a) trisomy 21 (b) monosomy of an autosome (c) trisomy X (d) monosomy X

______ 13. X chromosomes above the number 1 in a cell (a) are randomly inactivated (b) appear as Barr bodies (c) are counted to determine genotypic sex (d) all of the above (e) none of the above

______ 14. The genotypic ratio of the offspring from a monohybrid cross of *Aa* × *Aa* is (a) 4:1 (b) 3:1 (c) 1:2:1 (d) 1:1 (e) 9:3:3:1

PART II. COMPLETION

1. The nucleus of each somatic cell contains ____ (number) chromosomes from each parent.
2. When one allele masks the effect of another allele it is said to be ________________ .
3. Down's syndrome is due to ________________ of chromosome 21.
4. The members of a chromosome pair are referred to as ________________ chromosomes.
5. Alternative forms of a gene are called ________________ .
6. An arrangement of the chromosomes of an individual, categorized according to number is a(n) ________________ .
7. The failure of chromosomes to separate during meiotic anaphase is called ________________ .
8. Inactive X chromosomes appear in cell nuclei as ________________ .
9. A parent of genotype *AaBbCCDDEeff* can make ____ (number) different types of gametes.
10. If freckling is caused by an autosomal dominant gene *F*, and if it occurs in 75% of a population, what is the frequency of the recessive gene *f* in the population? ____
11. Of the freckled individuals in Question 10, what percentage are homozygous? ____
12. What is the probability of two heterozygotic freckled parents having a nonfreckled son? ____
13. What is the probability of parents of three sons having a boy for their fourth child? ____
14. Albinism and nontasting of PTC are recessive traits caused by genotypes *aa* and *tt*. What proportion of the offspring of two parents heterozygous for albinism and tasting (*AaTt*) would be nontaster albinos? ________________
15. Two parents both with blood type A, Rh positive, have a child of blood type O, Rh negative. What are the genotypes of the parents? ________________
16. What proportion of the sons of a red-green color blind father and a mother with normal color vision will be red-green color blind? ________________

DISCUSSION: A. If a trait occurs in all of the sons and none of the daughters of an affected male, and if this trait is also inherited by all the grandsons and none of the granddaughters, on what chromosome is the gene most likely located?

DISCUSSION: B. Hemophilia and red-green color blindness are both inherited as X-linked recessive traits. Why do you think there are so many more color blind males than hemophiliac males?

HEMATOLOGY 16

EXERCISE 1. Blood Plasma
EXERCISE 2. Blood Cell Counts
EXERCISE 3. Hematocrit
EXERCISE 4. Hemoglobin Determination
A. Tallqvist Method
B. Use of the Hemoglobinometer
EXERCISE 5. Sedimentation Rate
EXERCISE 6. Blood Clotting
EXERCISE 7. Blood Typing
A. ABO Typing
B. Rh Typing
EXERCISE 8. Blood Pathology

WORD ROOTS

erythro- = red
-emia = blood
hemo-, hemato- = blood
leuco-, leuko- = white
-penia = lack of
phago- = eating
-poiesis = production
thrombo- = clot
vas-, vasc-, vaso- = vessel

Blood, the ***vascular fluid*** of the cardiovascular system, is required for the normal functioning of all cells in the body. Since most tissues are not in direct contact with the environment, they require blood to supply necessary substances and to remove wastes.

One function of blood is the transport of respiratory gases (O_2 and CO_2), nutrients, metabolic wastes, hormones, and enzymes. Blood is also of critical importance for the regulation of body temperature and fluid and electrolyte balance. Because of its clotting ability, blood prevents fluid loss. And its buffering action helps to regulate pH. Blood cells are also important in defense against infection.

Blood is a fluid connective tissue, consisting of two portions: (1) ***plasma***, the fluid portion which contains dissolved substances, and (2) ***formed elements***, cells and cell-like bodies suspended in the plasma. The most common classification of the formed elements in blood is

Erythrocytes (red blood cells)
Leucocytes (white blood cells)
Granular leucocytes (granulocytes)
Neutrophils
Eosinophils
Basophils
Agranular leucocytes (agranulocytes)
Lymphocytes
Monocytes
Thrombocytes (platelets)

Erythrocytes (e-RITH-rō-sīts), also called red blood cells (RBCs), are deformable, biconcave, nonnucleated discs, about 7.5 μm in diameter (see Figures 16.1a and 16.2). Because they lack nuclei, they cannot reproduce or carry on extensive metabolic activities. ***Hemoglobin***, a red pigment, occupies most of the cell volume. Erythrocytes transport oxygen and, to a much lesser extent, carbon dioxide. An RBC becomes nonfunctional and is destroyed after about 120 days.

Leucocytes (LOO-kō-sīts), also called white blood cells or WBCs, are nucleated cells that are larger than RBCs (see Figures 16.1b and 16.2). If unstained, WBCs appear pale. These

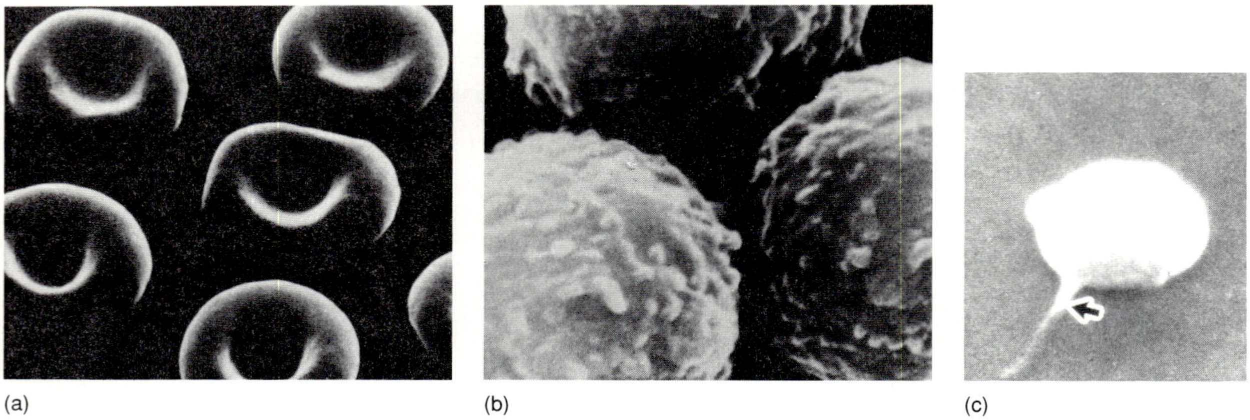

FIGURE 16.1 Scanning electron micrographs of blood cells. (a) Erythrocytes (2260×). (b) Leucocytes (7000×). (c) Thrombocycte (2260×).

cells function in phagocytosis, antibody production, and allergic reactions. In the blood, the life span of leucocytes ranges from a few hours to a few months; leucocytes that migrate into tissues may live several years.

Thrombocytes (THROM-bō-sīts) or platelets (see Figures 16.1c and Figure 16.2) are formed when small fragments pinch off from metamegakaryocytes. Thus, they are formed elements but not true cells. Platelets are non-nucleated and irregularly shaped; they prevent blood loss by initiating a chain of reactions that results in blood clotting. The life span of platelets is about one week.

NOTE: The exercises in this chapter are sufficient for laboratory demonstration, but they are not necessarily clinically accurate.

EXERCISE 1. Blood Plasma

OBJECTIVES

To know the main constituents of blood plasma

To determine the pH of blood plasma

When the formed elements are removed from blood, a straw-colored liquid called ***plasma*** remains. Over half of normal blood consists of plasma, a substance composed of about 92% water and 8% solutes. Among the solutes are proteins (albumins, globulins, and clotting factors), nonprotein nitrogen (NPN) substances (urea, uric acid, creatine, and creatinine), foods (amino acids, glucose, fatty acids, and glycerol), regulatory substances (enzymes and hormones), and electrolytes.

Plasma can be separated from whole blood by centrifugation, a process that separates heavier from lighter components. After centrifugation, the bottom of the tube will contain a red layer of erythrocytes; above these packed RBCs will be a buffy coat of leucocytes and platelets; the plasma will be in the top (lightest) layer.

MATERIALS

Latex gloves

Blood plasma from a clinical agency or from centrifugation of mammalian blood (other than human blood)

Graduated cylinder

Test tube

pH paper

Dropper bottle of 0.1N HCl

Glass stirring rod

Container of fresh 10% bleach solution

Safety goggles

Laboratory apron or coat

PROCEDURE

CAUTION! *Please reread Section A, "General Procedures and Safety Precautions," Section B, "Precautions Related to Working With Blood, Other Body Fluids or Blood Products," and Sec-*

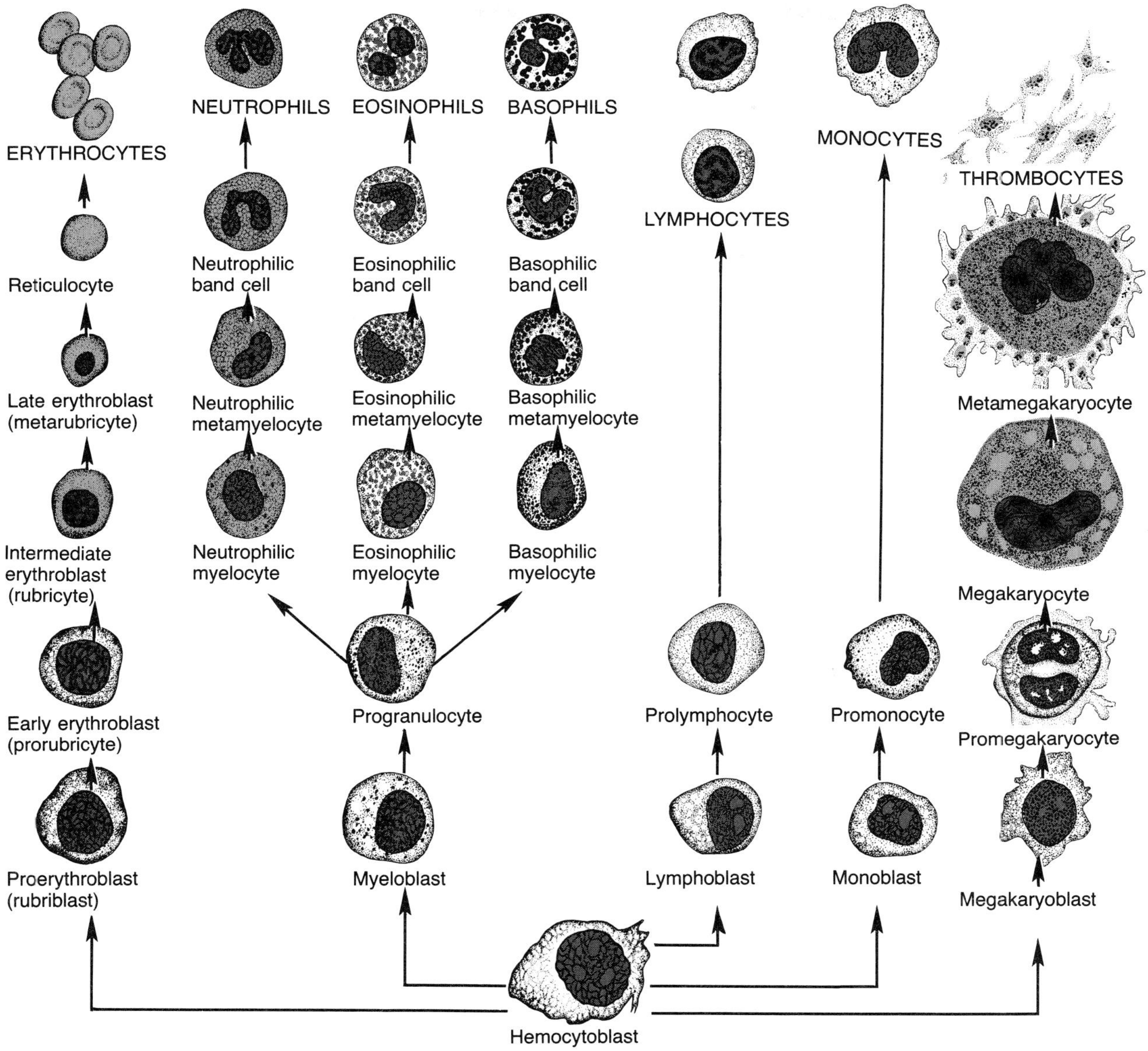

FIGURE 16.2 Hemopoiesis.

tion C, "Precautions Related to Working with Reagents," in Chapter 1 before you begin any of the exercises in this chapter. You should also read the exercises before you perform them to be sure you understand all of the procedures and safety precautions. Remember that it is absolutely required that you wear latex gloves when you come into contact with blood, blood products, or other body fluids.

1. Using a graduated cylinder, place 5 ml of plasma in a test tube. Note the color of the plasma.

2. Dip the end of a length of pH paper into the plasma and determine the pH by comparing the paper color with the color scale on the pH paper container.

3. Add three drops of 0.1N HCl to the plasma and stir to mix. Determine the pH by the procedure in step 2.

4. *Drop the test tube and plasma into the container of fresh bleach solution. Dispose of the pH paper per your instructor's direction.*

5. Record your observations in the LABORATORY REPORT RESULTS at the end of the chapter.

Did the addition of HCl change the pH of the plasma significantly? Explain. ____________

____

EXERCISE 2. Blood Cell Counts

OBJECTIVES

To define normal standards for blood cell counts

To name some causes of abnormal blood counts

To distinguish leucocytes morphologically

To determine the percentages of the five types of leucocytes in normal circulating blood

Normal levels of the formed elements of blood are essential to health. A healthy male has about 5.4 million (±0.8) erythrocytes per cu mm (mm^3) of blood, a healthy female has about 4.8 million (±0.6). RBCs carry oxygen, so a reduction in their number will result in ***anemia***, a decrease in the oxygen-carrying capacity of blood. Anemias are caused by a variety of conditions, including impaired RBC production, increased RBC destruction, and acute blood loss. When the RBC count is increased above normal limits, the condition is called ***polycythemia***.

Between 250,000 and 400,000 thrombocytes are found in each cu mm (mm^3) of blood. A reduction in their number ***(thrombocytopenia)*** causes blood loss through small vessels; this condition can result from pernicious anemia and irradiation.

Leucocytes are less numerous than RBCs and platelets, averaging from 5,000 to 9,000 cells per cu mm (mm^3) of blood. The ratio of RBCs to WBCs is thus about 700:1. An increase in number ***(leucocytosis)*** may result from bacterial or viral infection, metabolic disorders, and malignancies. A decrease in number ***(leucopenia)*** may result from some infections, cirrhosis of the liver, hereditary disorders, and irradiation.

The relative proportion of the different leucocytes is important because a significant change in proportion is often diagnostic of a specific pathological condition. Leukemias, for example, are characterized by abnormal types and numbers of the different WBCs. Leucocytes can be differentiated morphologically by their size, appearance of their nuclei, and presence of differentially stained cytoplasmic granules (see Figure 16.2).

Granulocytes, which mature in red bone marrow, contain lobed nuclei and large cytoplasmic granules that can be seen with a light microscope. There are three types of granulocytes.

Neutrophils. These WBCs are also called polymorphonuclear leucocytes ("polys") because their nuclei have 3 to 7 lobes that may appear disconnected from each other. The cytoplasmic granules stain pale lavender or gray. The neutrophil count increases in acute bacterial infections.

Eosinophils. The nuclei of these cells are usually bilobular, and their cytoplasmic granules stain orange-red. An increase in the eosinophil count is typical of allergic and parasitic conditions.

Basophils. These WBCs contain S-shaped nuclei, and their large cytoplasmic granules stain blue-purple. The basophil count increases in some cases of inflammation.

Agranulocytes, which mature in lymphoid tissue, have spherical nuclei and possess small cytoplasmic granules that cannot be seen with a light microscope. There are two types of agranulocytes.

Lymphocytes. These WBCs have spherical or indented nuclei that stain dark blue. The cytoplasm appears as a pale rim around the nucleus. Lymphocytes predominate in some viral infections, e.g., infectious mononucleosis.

Monocytes. These cells are the largest WBCs. They contain a large round or kidney-shaped nucleus that stains dark blue and may be slightly irregular in outline. The monocyte count increases during chronic infection.

A normal differential white count would be in the following ranges.

Neutrophils	60–70%
Eosinophils	2–4%
Basophils	0.5–1%
Lymphocytes	20–25%
Monocytes	3–8%

MATERIALS

Microscope
Immersion oil
Prepared slide of stained blood
Histology references (optional)

PROCEDURE

1. Using an oil-immersion lens, start at the edge of the prepared slide and examine it by moving the slide as indicated in Figure 16.3. Record each white blood cell you observe by making a mark in the chart below until you have recorded 100 cells. To differentiate the types of leucocytes, use Figure 16.2 and any references available.

2. Calculate the percentage of each cell type you observed (number observed/100) and record your calculations in the LABORATORY REPORT RESULTS at the end of the chapter.

What calculated percentages will be the least accurate? Why? ____________________

____

____

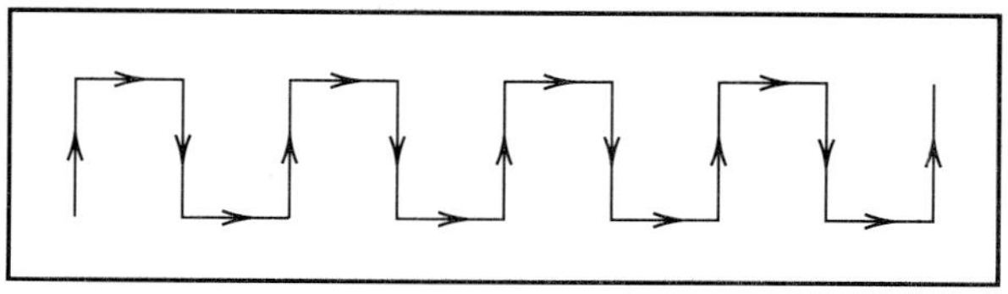

FIGURE 16.3 Scanning pattern for a differential white blood count.

EXERCISE 3. Hematocrit

OBJECTIVES
To identify the percent of blood volume occupied by erythrocytes (hematocrit) To describe the clinical use of this test

The percentage of total blood volume occupied by red blood cells is called the ***hematocrit (Hct)*** or ***packed cell volume (PCV)***. Its measurement is a good routine test for anemia. Normal values for the hematocrit are 47% ± 5% for males and 42% ± 5% for females.

When a tube of blood is centrifuged, the erythrocytes, the heaviest elements, are packed at the bottom of the tube. On top of them will lie a layer of leucocytes and platelets (the buffy coat), and the plasma separates as the top layer. Since the hematocrit consists almost entirely of erythrocytes (about 98%), it is generally considered equivalent to the RBC volume.

MATERIALS

Latex gloves
Lancet
Alcohol wipes
Heparinized capillary tubes
Seal-ease® or clay
Centrifuge
Hematocrit tube reader (Figure 16.6)
Container of fresh 10% bleach solution
Safety goggles
Laboratory apron or coat

Leucocyte		Total Number
Neutrophil		
Eosinophil		
Basophil		
Lymphocyte		
Monocyte		
	Sum =	100

PROCEDURE

CAUTION! *The various blood tests which will be described shortly require several punctures because samples must be taken at different times. In order to avoid each student providing blood samples for all the tests, each student should provide blood for only one or two tests from a single puncture.* The results of the various tests can be tabulated on the blackboard and shared by the entire class. The subject in these procedures, of course, cannot wear a latex glove on the hand to be punctured.

1. Using the finger puncture technique described at the end of this chapter, produce a free flow of blood from your own finger.

CAUTION! *Immediately dispose of the used lancet in a container of fresh bleach solution.*

2. Place the unmarked (clear) end of the capillary tube into the drop of blood (see Figure 16.4). Hold the tube slightly below the level of the blood and do not move the tip from the blood or an air bubble will enter the column.

CAUTION! *If an air bubble is present, immediately dispose of the capillary tube in a fresh bleach solution and begin again.*

3. Allow blood to flow about two-thirds of the way into the tube. The tube will fill easily if you hold the open end below the blood source.

4. Place your finger over the marked (red) end of the tube and keep it in that position as you seal the blood end of the tube with Seal-ease®, clay, or similar sealing material.

5. According to the direction of your laboratory instructor, place the tube into the centrifuge (see Figure 16.5) making sure that the sealed end is against the rubber ring at the circumference. Have your laboratory instructor make sure that the tubes are properly balanced. Write the number that indicates the placement of your tube. ____

6. When all the tubes from your laboratory section are in place, secure the inside cover of the centrifuge and close the outside cover. Centrifuge on high speed for four minutes.

7. Remove your tube and determine the hematocrit value by reading the length of the packed cells on Figure 16.6. To use this figure, place the base of the clay on the base line and move the tube until the top of the plasma is at the line marked 100. The hematocrit can then be read at the level on top of the packed cells.

CAUTION! *Immediately dispose of your capillary tube in a fresh bleach solution.*

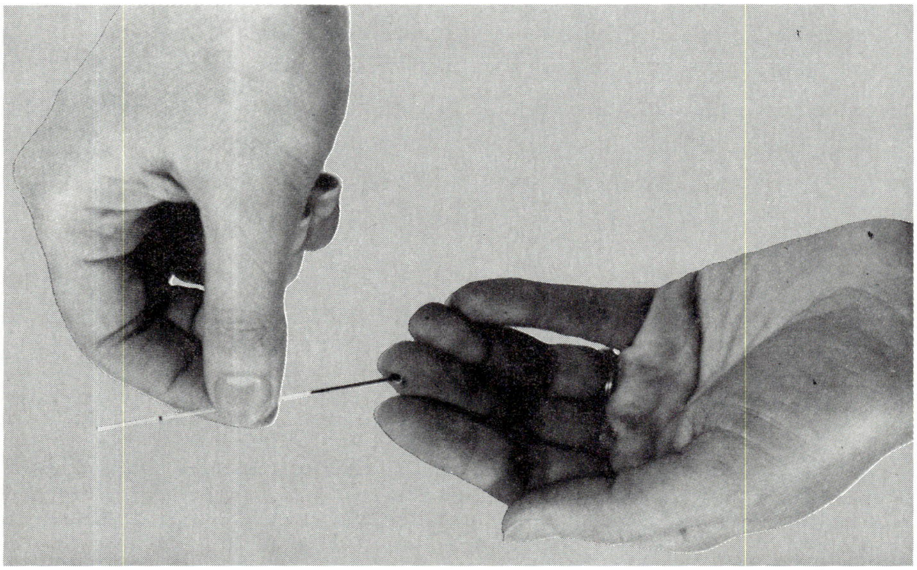

FIGURE 16.4 Filling a capillary tube with blood.

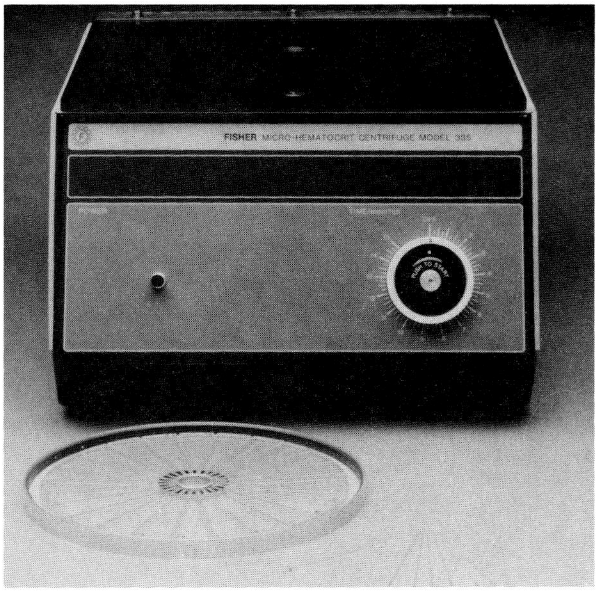

FIGURE 16.5 One type of centrifuge.

8. Record your observations in the LABORATORY REPORT RESULTS at the end of the chapter.

What effect would you expect dehydration to have on the hematocrit? ____________________

EXERCISE 4. Hemoglobin Determination

> OBJECTIVES
>
> To determine the grams (g) of hemoglobin per 100 ml of blood
>
> To describe the clinical application of determining hemoglobin levels

A normal erythrocyte count is possible in anemia if the RBCs are deficient in hemoglobin *(hypochromic anemia)* or if the cells are smaller than normal *(microcytic anemia)*. Thus, the amount of hemoglobin per unit volume of blood (and not necessarily the number of RBCs) is the determining factor in anemia. The hemoglobin content of blood is expressed in grams (g) per 100 ml. The normal ranges depend on the technique used. An average range is 13–16 gm/100 ml in males and 12–15 gm/100 ml in females. The hemoglobin level is higher at birth, declines in childhood and rises at adolescence.

The Tallqvist measurement of hemoglobin is an old and somewhat inaccurate technique, although it is quick and inexpensive. The hemoglobinometer gives more accurate (±5%) results.

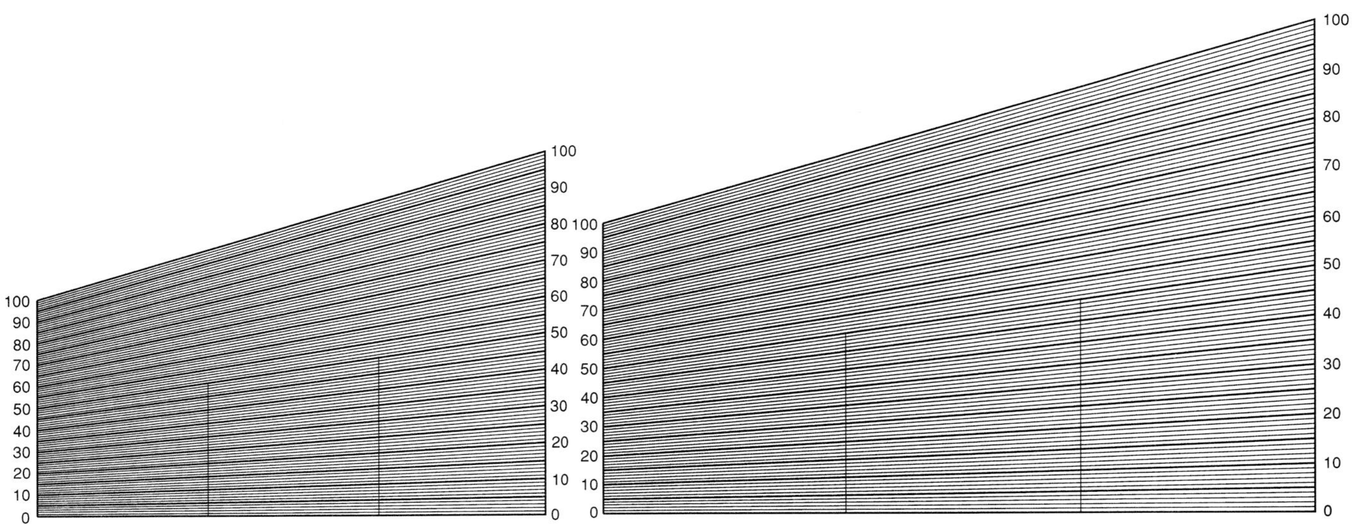

FIGURE 16.6 Hematocrit scale.

A. Tallqvist Method

MATERIALS

Latex gloves
Lancet
Alcohol swab
Tallqvist® paper and scale
Container of fresh 10% bleach solution
Safety goggles
Laboratory apron or coat

PROCEDURE

1. Using the finger puncture technique at the end of this chapter, produce a free flow of blood from your own finger.

CAUTION! *Dispose of the used lancet immediately in a fresh bleach solution.*

2. Place one drop of blood on the Tallqvist® paper.
3. As soon as the blood no longer appears shiny, match its color with the scale provided. Record your observations in the LABORATORY REPORT RESULTS at the end of the chapter.

B. Use of the Hemoglobinometer

MATERIALS

Isopropyl alcohol
Lens paper
Latex gloves
Lancet
Alcohol swabs
Hemoglobinometer
Hemolysis applicator
Container of fresh 10% bleach solution
Safety goggles
Laboratory apron or coat

PROCEDURE

1. Remove the two pieces of glass from the blood chamber assembly (see Figure 16.7a). The piece that contains the moat will receive the blood sample; the other piece serves as a cover glass.
2. Clean the glass pieces with alcohol and wipe with lens paper.
3. Replace the glass piece halfway into the clip with the moat plate on the bottom.
4. Obtain your own blood via the finger puncture technique described at the end of this chapter.

CAUTION! *Dispose of the lancet immediately in the container of fresh bleach solution.*

5. Touch the finger to the moat and completely cover the raised surface of the plate with the blood (see Figure 16.7b).
6. Hemolyze the blood by stirring it with the tip of a hemolysis applicator for about 30–45 seconds; hemolysis is complete when the appearance of the blood changes from cloudy to transparent. This change reflects the lysis of the RBC membranes and the consequent liberation of the hemoglobin.
7. Push the chamber into the clip and push the clip into the hemocytometer (see Figure 16.7c).
8. Holding the hemocytometer in the left hand, look through the eyepiece and turn on the light switch with the left thumb (see Figure 16.7d). You will see a split field.
9. Move the slide button back and forth with the right index finger until the two sides of the field match in color and shading.
10. Determine the grams of hemoglobin per 100 ml of the blood sample by reading the number above the index mark on the hemocytometer.
11. Record your results in the LABORATORY REPORT RESULTS at the end of the chapter.

CAUTION! *Remove the glass pieces from the chamber and wash in a fresh bleach solution.*

Dry the glass pieces with lens paper.

What type of anemia would reveal a normal or slightly low hematocrit and a significantly reduced hemoglobin level? ____________

EXERCISE 5. Sedimentation Rate

OBJECTIVES

To measure the sedimentation rate of blood
To describe the clinical use of this test

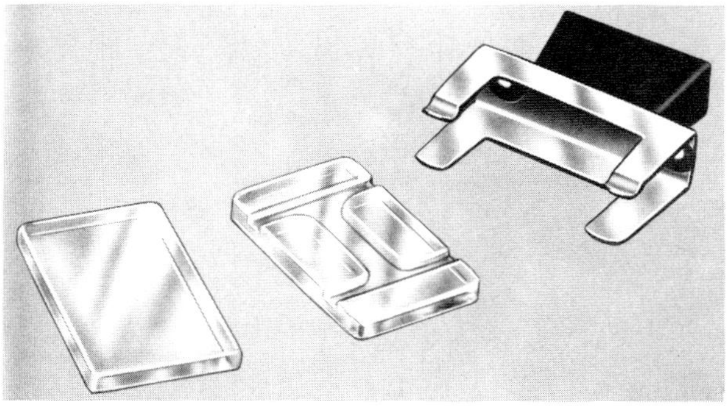

(a)

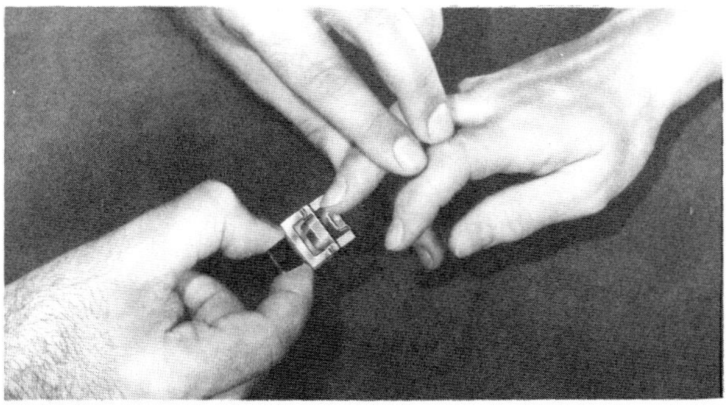

(b)

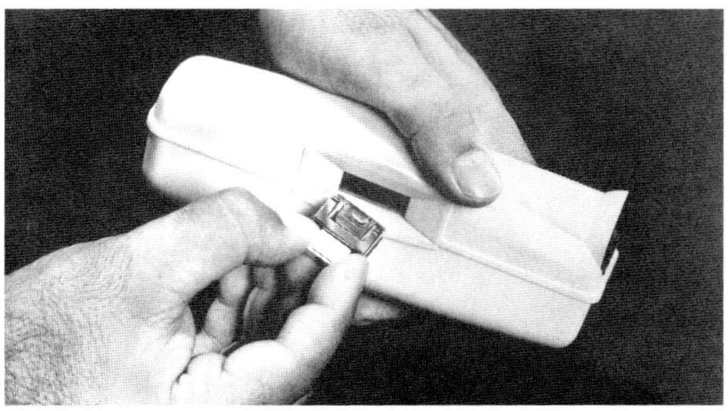

(c)

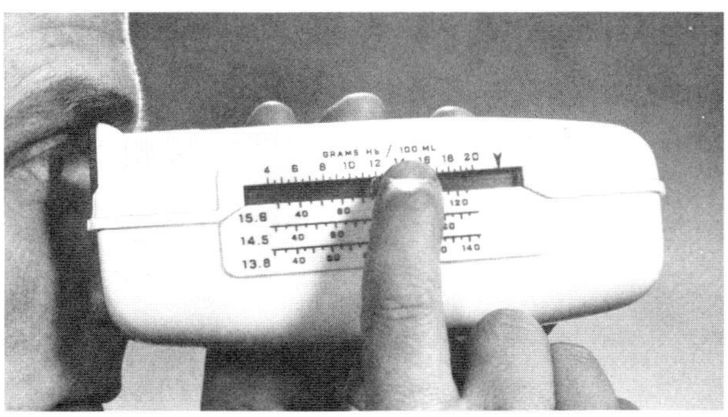

(d)

FIGURE 16.7 Use of the hemoglobinometer. (a) Specimen chamber. (b) Obtaining a specimen. (c) Inserting the sample. (d) Examining the specimen.

If citrated blood is allowed to stand, the heavier erythrocytes fall and leave clear plasma above them. (Citrate binds calcium and thereby prevents coagulation). The distance through which the cells fall for one hour is called the ***sedimentation rate***. The rate is a function of the amount of fibrinogen and gamma globulin present in the blood and the tendency of the RBCs to adhere to each other. The rate is elevated during menstruation, pregnancy, malignancy, and most infections. An increased sedimentation rate is used as a nonspecific indicator of infection or tissue destruction. The rate is affected by the height of the blood column, the lumen diameter of the sedimentation tube, and the type of anticoagulant used. Using the method in this exercise yields a normal adult sedimentation rate of 0 to 6 mm/hour.

MATERIALS

Latex gloves
Lancet
Alcohol wipe
Sed-rate pipette and suction device
5% sodium citrate
Pipette rack
Millimeter ruler (if rack is unscaled)
Two containers of 10% bleach solution
Glass slides
Medicine dropper
Container of fresh 10% bleach solution
Safety goggles
Laboratory apron or coat

PROCEDURE

1. Using the finger puncture technique at the end of this chapter, produce a free flow of blood from your own finger.

CAUTION! *Dispose of the used lancet immediately in a container of fresh bleach solution.*

2. Using a mechanical suction device, draw up sodium citrate solution to the first line that encircles the pipette.

3. Draw free-flowing blood into the pipette to the second line. Do not remove the tip of the pipette from the blood or air bubbles will enter the column.

CAUTION! *If air bubbles are drawn into the blood, carefully expel the mixture onto a clean microscope slide, dispose of the slide in a container of fresh bleach solution, place the pipette into a container of fresh bleach solution, and begin again.*

4. Draw the mixture of fluids up into the bulb and mix by expelling it into the lumen of the tube. Draw and mix the fluids six times. If any air bubbles appear, use the procedure described in step 3.

5. Adjust the level of blood as close to zero as possible.

6. Remove the suction device by placing the lower end of the pipette on the *gloved* index finger of the left hand before removing the device from the other end. The blood will leave the pipette if the end is not held closed.

7. Place the lower end of the pipette on the base of the pipette rack. The tube must be exactly perpendicular to the base (see Figure 16.8). Record the time at which the tube was placed into the rack. ____

8. One hour later, measure the distance from the top of the plasma to the top of the red cell layer with a millimeter scale and record your results in the LABORATORY REPORT RESULTS at the end of the chapter.

CAUTION! *Dispose of the pipette in the container of fresh bleach solution. Using a medicine dropper, rinse the base of the pipette rack with fresh bleach solution.*

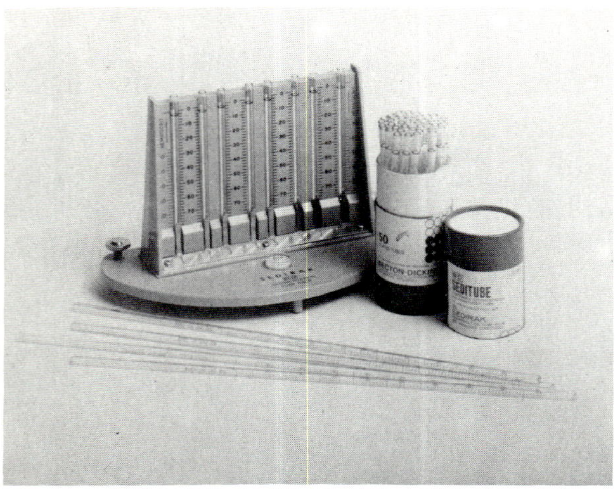

FIGURE 16.8 One type of sedimentation tube rack.

EXERCISE 6. Blood Clotting

OBJECTIVES

To determine the time required for coagulation of blood

To name the factors required for coagulation

To explain the clinical tests for coagulation

When a blood vessel is damaged (or when blood is removed from the body), blood will clot. The clot consists of insoluble fibers that trap the formed elements in the blood. This process, ***coagulation***, utilizes several circulating proteins called ***clotting factors***. The substance remaining after clot formation is called ***serum*** (blood minus formed elements = plasma; plasma minus clotting factors = serum).

Coagulation prevents blood loss when a blood vessel is damaged. It is a complex process involving many clotting factors that can be simplified by dividing it into three stages. In stage 1, ***thromboplastin*** is formed by mechanisms not yet fully understood. In stage 2, thromboplastin converts ***prothrombin***, a circulating alpha globulin produced in the liver, to ***thrombin***. In stage 3, thrombin converts ***fibrinogen***, another circulating plasma protein produced in the liver, to ***fibrin*** monomer. These fibrin molecules then polymerize, that is, form long molecules of fibrin threads that trap the formed elements and thereby form the clot.

A blood clot that forms at the site of vascular damage is called a ***thrombus***; a dislodged thrombus that is transported elsewhere in the body is called an ***embolus*** or ***embolism***.

The time required for blood to coagulate when exposed to air, usually about 2–10 minutes, is known as ***clotting time***; this time is increased in cold temperatures, by some drugs, and in clotting disorders. Clotting time is used to evaluate coagulation defects and to monitor anticoagulation therapy. Two modifications of clotting time, partial thromboplastin time (PTT) and prothrombin time (PT) give more specific information.

MATERIALS

Latex gloves
Lancet
Alcohol swab
Paper towels
Glass slide
Dissection pin
Stop watch or watch with second hand
Container of fresh 10% bleach solution
Safety goggles
Laboratory apron or coat

PROCEDURE

1. Using the finger puncture technique at the end of this chapter, produce a free flow of blood from your own finger.

CAUTION! *Dispose of the used lancet immediately in the container of fresh bleach solution.*

2. Discard the first drop of blood, as it will clot faster than the second drop. At the appearance of the second drop of blood, record the time. ____

3. Put a glass slide on several thicknesses of paper toweling and place 3–4 large drops of blood on the slide.

4. At four minutes and at 60 second intervals after that time, *slowly* pass an applicator stick or a dissection pin through the blood and raise it *slowly* about 5 mm above the blood. Coagulation has occurred when threads of fibrin can be detected between the blood and the end of the stick or pin.

5. Measure the time required for coagulation to occur and record it in the LABORATORY REPORT RESULTS at the end of the chapter.

6. CAUTION! *Promptly dispose of the stick or pin and slide in the container of fresh bleach. Also dispose of the paper towels in the plastic bag provided.*

Vitamin K is required for the formation of prothrombin. What would be a result of Vitamin K deficiency? ____________

Vitamin K is fat soluble; how would fat deprivation affect blood clotting? ____________

____

EXERCISE 7. Blood Typing

OBJECTIVES

To determine your ABO and Rh blood type
To define the principles of agglutination
To explain the relationship of blood typing to blood transfusion

The plasma membranes of red blood cells contain genetically determined antigens (proteins) called ***agglutinogens*** (ag′-loo-TIN-ō-jens). Blood plasma may contain antibodies (gamma globulins) called ***agglutinins*** (a-GLOO-ti-nins). The antibodies cause the ***agglutination (clumping)*** of red blood cells that carry antigens corresponding to plasma antibodies.

The classification of blood groups is based on the presence or absence of the antigens. The two major blood groups are the ***ABO system*** and the ***Rh system***.

A. ABO Typing

The ABO system is based on two antigens symbolized *A* and *B*. Persons whose RBC membranes bear only antigen *A* have blood type A; those with only antigen *B* have blood type B. If both *A* and *B* are present, the blood type is AB; the absence of both *A* and *B* antigens results in type O blood.

The antibodies in this system are antibody *a* (anti-A), which agglutinates cells bearing antigen *A*, and antibody *b* (anti-B), which clumps cells bearing antigen *B*. These antibodies develop shortly after birth. The antigens and antibodies present in each of the four blood types in this system and the various agglutinization reactions that can occur are shown in Figure 16.9 and summarized in Table 16.1. Table 16.2 lists the incidence of ABO blood types in various U.S. ethnic groups.

The ABO antigens and antibodies are of critical importance in blood transfusions. The main danger in unmatched transfusion lies in the possibility of the *recipient's antibody* agglutinating the *donor antigen* (the RBCs) causing clogging of capillaries, kidney damage, and possible death.

Because cells of type O blood contain neither of the two antigens (*A* nor *B*), moder-

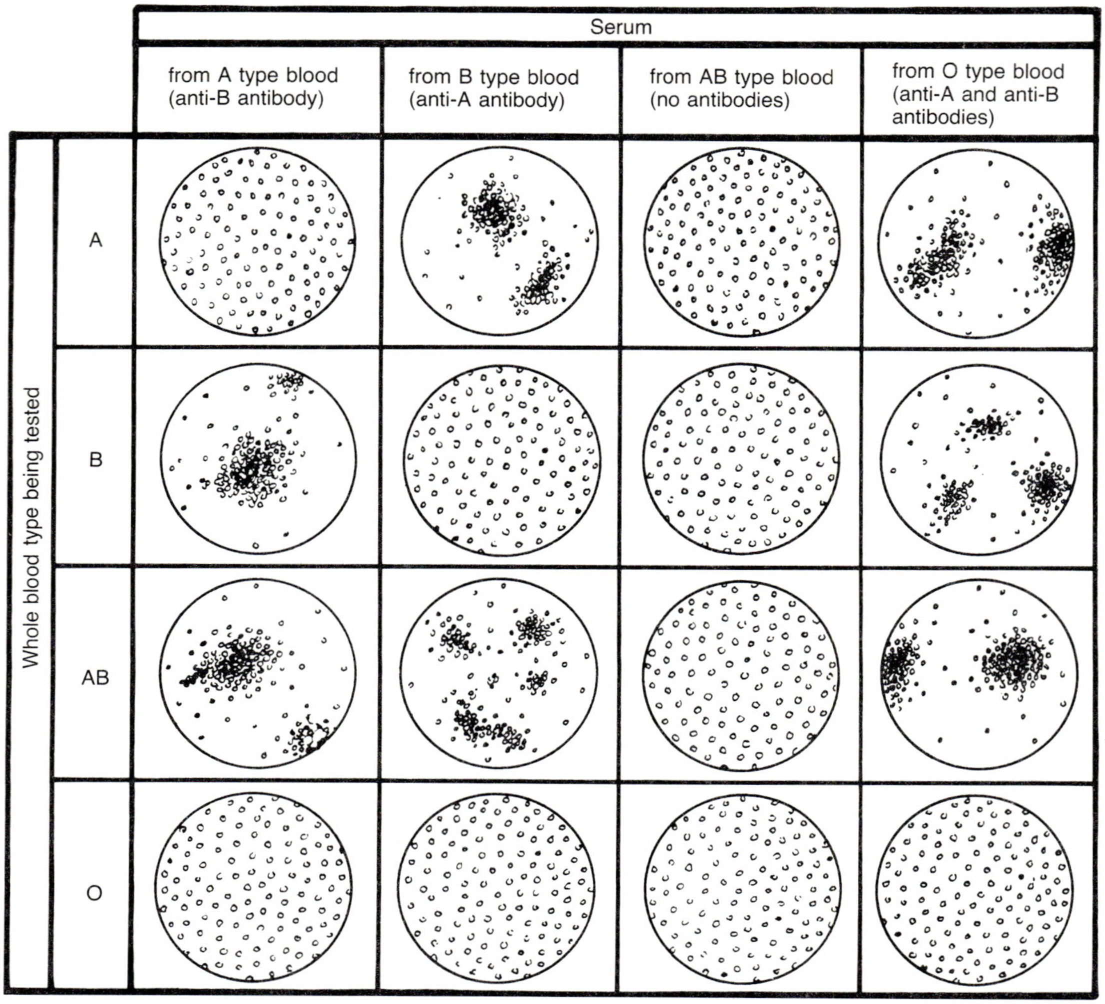

FIGURE 16.9 Agglutination reactions.

ate amounts of this blood can be transfused into a recipient of any ABO blood type without *immediate* agglutination. For this reason, type O blood is referred to as the ***universal donor***. However, transfusing large amounts of type O blood into a recipient of Type A, B, or AB can cause *delayed* agglutination of the recipient's erythrocytes because the transfused antibodies (type O blood contains anti-A or anti-B antibodies) are not sufficiently diluted to prevent the reaction.

Persons with type AB blood are sometimes

TABLE 16.1
INTERREACTIONS OF CELLS AND PLASMA OF ABO SYSTEM

Blood Type	Agglutinogen	Agglutinin	Plasma Causes Agglutination of	Cells Agglutinated by Plasma of
A	*A*	*b*	B, AB	B, O
B	*B*	*a*	A, AB	A, O
AB	*AB*	None	None	A, B, O
O	None	*a, b*	A, B, AB	None

TABLE 16.2
INCIDENCE OF HUMAN BLOOD GROUPS IN THE UNITED STATES

	Blood Groups (Percentages)				
	O	**A**	**B**	**AB**	**Rh⁺**
Caucasians	45	41	10	4	85
Blacks	48	27	21	4	88
Japanese	31	38	22	9	about 100
Chinese	36	28	23	13	about 100
American Indians	23	76	0	1	about 100
Hawaiians	37	61	1.5	0.5	about 100

called ***universal recipients*** because their blood contains no antibodies to agglutinate donor RBCs. *Small quantities* of blood from all other ABO types can be transfused into type AB blood without adverse reaction. However, again, if *large quantities* of type A, B, or O blood are transfused into type AB, the antibodies in the donor blood might be sufficient to clump the recipient's RBCs.

Table 16.3 lists possible donors and recipients of various blood types. Bear in mind the volume cautions detailed in the preceding two paragraphs. In clinical practice, before a transfusion donor and recipient blood is cross-matched small samples are mixed to test for compatibility.

MATERIALS

- Latex gloves
- Lancet
- Alcohol swabs
- Wax pencil and slides OR paper slides
- Anti-A and Anti-B sera
- Two mixing sticks
- Container of fresh 10% bleach solution
- Safety goggles
- Laboratory apron or coat

PROCEDURE

1. Using a wax pencil, draw a line down the middle of a clean glass slide (or use a paper slide). On the left side, place a large drop of anti-A serum; on the right, a large drop of anti-B serum.
2. Using the finger puncture technique at the end of this chapter, produce a free flow of blood from your own finger.

CAUTION! *Dispose of the used lancet immediately in the container of fresh bleach solution.*

3. Place a drop of blood next to both drops of antisera. Be careful not to mix the samples on the left and right sides of the slide.
4. Using a mixing stick, mix the blood on the left with the anti-A serum, and, *using another stick*, mix the drop on the right with the anti-B serum. *Hold the stick at about 30° to the paper if you are using paper slides, as the pointed end will lift paper fibers*.
5. CAUTION! *Immediately dispose of the mixing sticks in the container of fresh bleach solution.*
6. *Gently* tilt the slide back and forth and observe it for about one minute.
7. Record your observations in the LABORATORY REPORT RESULTS at the end of the

TABLE 16.3
POSSIBLE RECIPIENTS AND DONORS OF BLOOD TYPES

Blood Type	Can Be Recipient of	Can Be Donor to
A	A, O	A, AB
B	B, O	B, AB
AB	A, B, AB, O	AB
O	O	A, B, AB, O

chapter. Identify your ABO type based on your observations. If you are so directed, note your blood type in the chart provided in the laboratory and calculate the class distribution of blood types.

CAUTION! *Dispose of your slide in the container of bleach solution.*

B. Rh Typing

As in the ABO system, the ***Rh system*** is based on an antigen which may be present on the membrane of RBCs. The designation Rh^+ (positive) is given to blood that has the antigen; blood without the antigen is termed Rh^- (negative). Estimated incidence of the Rh factor is given in Table 16.2.

Anti-Rh, the antibody against the Rh antigen, is produced only after exposure to blood containing that antigen. Exposure may occur through mismatched transfusion or through the mixing of maternal and fetal blood at delivery or in late pregnancy. If neither of these conditions has occurred, no anti-Rh antibody can be present; by contrast, antibodies in the ABO system arise even without exposure to ABO antigens in blood.

If Rh^+ blood is transfused into an Rh^- recipient with no prior exposure to the Rh antigen, no transfusion reaction will occur. However, such a transfusion will elicit the production of anti-Rh antibody and subsequent exposure to Rh^+ blood will cause serious agglutination.

The Rh factor is of great significance for Rh^- women pregnant with Rh^+ fetuses. If maternal blood is exposed to fetal blood, the mother will produce anti-Rh antibodies. The first pregnancy of this type is rarely affected. However in subsequent pregnancies with an Rh^+ fetus, maternal anti-Rh antibody can enter the fetal circulation and cause ***hemolytic disease of the newborn (erythroblastosis fetalis)***. This fetal-maternal incompatibility is sometimes fatal. It is characterized by hemolysis of the fetal erythrocytes, resulting in anemia and brain damage due to deposition of the RBC breakdown products in the neural tissue. A drug called RhoGAM®, given to Rh^- mothers immediately after delivery or abortion, prevents the production of maternal anti-Rh antibodies, so that children of subsequent pregnancies are unaffected. Without RhoGAM®, 3% of the second pregnancies with an Rh^+ child are affected; 10% of such third pregnancies are affected.

NOTE: The exercise below is less accurate than the ABO determination, since the anti-Rh (anti-D) serum deteriorates at room temperature, and the anti-Rh antigens are less potent in their agglutinizing capability than anti-A or anti-B antigens.

MATERIALS

- Latex gloves
- Lancet
- Alcohol swabs
- Wax pencil and slides OR paper slides
- Anti-Rh (anti-D) serum
- Mixing stick
- Warming box (optional)
- Container of fresh 10% bleach solution
- Safety goggles
- Laboratory apron or coat

PROCEDURE

1. On a clean glass slide (or a paper slide) place a large drop of anti-Rh (anti-D) serum.
2. Using the finger puncture technique at the end of this chapter, produce a free flow of blood from your own finger.

CAUTION! *Dispose of the used lancet immediately in the container of fresh bleach solution.*

3. Using a mixing stick, mix the blood with the anti-Rh serum. *Hold the stock at about 30° to the paper if you are using paper slides, as the pointed end will lift paper fibers.*
4. CAUTION! *Immediately dispose of the mixing sticks in a container of fresh bleach solution.*
5. Place the slide on a preheated warming box and *gently* rock back and forth for 2 minutes. If no warming box is provided, hold the slide in your hand to heat it.
6. Record your observations in the LABORATORY REPORT RESULTS at the end of the chapter. Identify your Rh type based on your observations. If you are so directed, note your blood type in the chart provided in the laboratory and calculate the class distribution of blood types.

7. CAUTION! *Dispose of your slide in the container of fresh bleach.*

How does agglutination differ from clotting?

____

____

EXERCISE 8. Blood Pathology

> OBJECTIVES
>
> To identify some of the morphological characteristics of selected blood diseases
>
> To explain hemopoiesis

Diseases of the blood are characterized by numerical and/or morphological changes in blood cells. Many of them are also characterized by immature forms of blood cells. Consequently, in order to identify cells typical of certain diseases, it is necessary to understand ***hemopoiesis*** (hē′-mō-poy-Ē-sis), the origin and development of the formed elements of the blood. Consult your textbook and Figure 16.2 to understand the development of mature blood cells from hemocytoblasts in the bone marrow.

MATERIALS

- Microscope
- Lens paper
- Immersion oil
- Slide of normal blood
- Slides of various blood pathologies such as sickle-cell anemia, granulocytic (myeloid) leukemia, agranulocytic (lymphoid) leukemia, mononucleosis

PROCEDURE

1. Examine the prepared slides of blood pathologies. Compare them with a prepared slide of normal blood.

2. Note abnormalities in the number, size, and shape of the blood cells. Look at the red blood cells to see if there are reticulocytes or normoblasts (metarubricytes) present. These immature forms are present in diseases involving anemia. Inspect the shape of the leucocyte nuclei; the nuclei of immature WBCs are less lobular than those of mature WBCs.

3. Record your observations in the LABORATORY REPORT RESULTS at the end of the chapter.

What is the most apparent difference between normal and leukemic blood? ______________

____

FINGER PUNCTURE PROCEDURE

In this procedure you cannot wear a glove on the hand from which you are drawing your own blood.

MATERIALS

- Latex gloves
- Lancet
- Alcohol swab
- Adhesive bandages
- Container of fresh 10% bleach solution
- Safety goggles
- Laboratory apron or coat

PROCEDURE

1. To enhance your chances for a successful finger puncture the first time, warm your finger if it is cold, and shake your finger several times to force blood into it.

2. *Thoroughly* cleanse the end of the third or fourth finger with alcohol.

3. Open the lancet packet at the blunt end; *do not touch the sharp end.*

4. *Take a sample of YOUR OWN BLOOD as follows.* Remove the rubber glove from the hand from which you will take blood. Holding your finger firmly, take the lancet and puncture the finger using a quick, jabbing motion. The puncture is made toward the side of the finger rather than in the full fleshy part. (Do not begin the motion from a great distance away from the finger. The closer you are and the quicker the motion, the less the discomfort that results.)

5. If the puncture is made properly, the blood should flow freely from the wound. If not, squeeze the finger moving from its base toward its tip.

6. If an additional puncture is required, discard the first lancet and *use a new sterile one*.

CAUTION! *Make sure the used lancets are discarded immediately in a container of fresh bleach solution to prevent subsequent injury, and to prevent passage of diseases.*

7. Do not use the first drop, which usually coagulates fast.

8. Finally, place a piece of cotton between the finger and the thumb and press them together firmly.

9. *Use an adhesive bandage to cover the puncture site.*

COMPLETE THE LABORATORY REPORT QUESTIONS AT THE END OF THE CHAPTER

LABORATORY REPORT RESULTS

HEMATOLOGY 16

Student ______________________ Date ______________________

Laboratory Section ______________________ Score/Grade ______________________

EXERCISE 1. Blood Plasma

1. Plasma color ______________________
2. Plasma pH ______________________
3. pH of plasma + 0.1 HCl ______________________ Would you expect the same result if you had added three drops of 0.1 HCl to 5 ml water? Explain. ______________________

____

EXERCISE 2. Blood Cell Counts

Differential white blood cell count results: _____ % neutrophils

_____ % eosinophils

_____ % basophils

_____ % lymphocytes

_____ % monocytes

EXERCISE 3. Hematocrit

Hematocrit = _____ %

EXERCISE 4. Hemoglobin Determination

1. Estimation with Tallqvist® paper: _____ g/100 ml blood
2. Estimation with hemoglobinometer: _____ g/100 ml blood

EXERCISE 5. Sedimentation Rate

Sedimentation rate = _____ mm/hr

EXERCISE 6. Blood Clotting

Clotting time = _____ minutes

EXERCISE 7. Blood Typing

In which situation was your blood agglutinated?

_____ by anti-A serum only

_____ by anti-B serum only

_____ by anti-A and anti-B sera

_____ neither by anti-A nor by anti-B serum

Based on your observations, what is your ABO blood type? _____

Was your blood agglutinated by anti-Rh (anti-D) serum? _____

Is your observed blood type Rh^+ or Rh^-? _____

EXERCISE 8. Blood Pathology

Describe and draw the various slides you viewed.

LABORATORY REPORT QUESTIONS

HEMATOLOGY 16

Student ______________________ Date ______________________

Laboratory Section ______________________ Score/Grade ______________________

PART I. MULTIPLE CHOICE

_____ 1. To measure blood glucose levels, one would test (a) erythrocytes (b) leucocytes (c) thrombocytes (d) plasma

_____ 2. In what condition would the hematocrit fail to reflect red blood cell volume accurately? (a) polycythemia (b) anemia (c) leukemia (d) thrombocytopenia

_____ 3. Which of the following would NOT be appropriate for diagnosing anemia? (a) RBC count (b) hematocrit (c) hemoglobin estimation (d) sedimentation rate determination

_____ 4. Hemolytic disease of the newborn (erythroblastosis fetalis) could occur in (a) the Rh^+ child of an Rh^- mother (b) the Rh^- child of an Rh^+ mother (c) the Rh^+ mother of an Rh^- child (d) the Rh^- mother of an Rh^+ child (e) more than one of the above

_____ 5. Agglutinins (a) are on the surface of the RBC membrane (b) are located in the blood plasma (c) are antigens

_____ 6. Clotting time would be longer than normal in an individual with (a) thrombocytosis (b) a Vitamin K deficiency (c) anemia

PART II. MATCHING

_____ 7. Number of RBC/cu mm blood in male

_____ 8. Number of WBC/cu mm blood

_____ 9. Number of thrombocytes/cu mm blood

_____ 10. Percent of WBC that are lymphocytes

_____ 11. Normal hematocrit in males

_____ 12. Normal number of g of hemoglobin/100 ml blood

_____ 13. Normal sedimentation rate

_____ 14. Normal clotting time

_____ 15. Percent of Caucasians who are Rh^+

_____ 16. Percent of blood composed of plasma

A. 15.5
B. 600
C. 7000
D. 300,000
E. 5,400,000
F. 2%
G. 25%
H. 46%
I. 55%
J. 85%
K. 1 mm/hour
L. 20 mm/hour
M. 10 minutes

PART III. TRUE OR FALSE. IF THE STATEMENT IS FALSE, CHANGE IT TO A TRUE STATEMENT.

_____ 17. Erythrocytes are an integral part of the immune response.

_____ 18. The most abundant leucocyte is the lymphocyte.

______ 19. AB^+ is the most common blood type.

______ 20. If type A and type AB blood are mixed, agglutination will occur.

______ 21. Type O blood contains anti-a and anti-b antibodies.

______ 22. Thromboplastin converts fibrinogen to fibrin.

______ 23. Neutrophils are phagocytes.

______ 24. Thrombocytes are cell fragments of metamegakaryocytes.

______ 25. Anemia is a reduction in the clotting capacity of blood.

______ 26. All granulocytes have lobed nuclei.

______ 27. The life span of an RBC is about one week.

______ 28. A thrombus is a clot that has dislodged from its site of formation.

______ 29. Serum is the liquid portion of blood without the formed elements.

______ 30. A high reticulocyte count is characteristic of sickle-cell anemia.

DISCUSSION: With regard to hemolytic disease of the newborn (erythroblastosis fetalis), A. Why are erythroblasts present? B. Why is jaundice characteristic of the disease? C. Give possible reasons for this occurring in the first child born to an Rh^- mother and an Rh^+ father.

CARDIOVASCULAR PHYSIOLOGY 17

KNOW BLOOD FOLOW

EXERCISE 1. The Conduction System of the Heart and the Electrocardiogram

EXERCISE 2. The Cardiac Cycle

- *A. Observation of the Normal Cardiac Cycle*
- *B. Recording the Cardiac Cycle*
- *C. Intrinsic Control of the Cardiac Cycle*
- *D. Extrinsic Control of the Cardiac Cycle*
  - *1. Effect of vagal stimulation*
  - *2. Effect of acetylcholine*
  - *3. Effect of atropine sulfate*
  - *4. Effect of epinephrine*
- *E. Demonstration of the Refractory Period*

EXERCISE 3. Auscultation of the Heart

EXERCISE 4. Pulse Rate

EXERCISE 5. Blood Pressure

EXERCISE 6. Vascular Physiology

WORD ROOTS

brady- = slow

cardio-, -cardium = heart

endo- = within

myo- = muscle

peri- = around

sphygmo- = pulse

tachy- = swift

The ***heart*** (see Figure 17.1) is a muscular pump, located in the ***mediastinum*** (mē-dē-as-TĪ-num), with two-thirds of its mass lying to the left of the body's midline. Its pointed ***apex*** projects inferiorly to the left; its broad ***base*** projects superiorly to the right. The heart is roughly the size of the clenched fist and its adult weight is about 250 grams (8.8 ounces) in females and 300 grams (10.6 ounces) in males.

A loose-fitting serous membrane called the ***pericardium (pericardial sac)*** encloses the heart. The membrane is composed of two parts, the fibrous pericardium and the serous pericardium. The outer ***fibrous pericardium*** is tough connective tissue that adheres to the parietal pleura and anchors the heart in the mediastinum. The inner ***serous pericardium***, like all serous membranes, is a double layered structure. The outer ***parietal layer*** of the serous pericardium lies directly beneath the fibrous pericardium. The inner ***visceral layer*** of the serous pericardium (also called the ***epicardium***) adheres to the heart muscle. Between the parietal and visceral layers of the serous pericardium is a potential space, the ***pericardial cavity***, into which pericardial fluid is secreted. This fluid functions to reduce friction between the visceral and parietal membranes as the heart beats.

The heart muscle or ***myocardium*** forms the bulk of the heart and is responsible for contraction. The irregular inner surface of the ventricular myocardium bears ridges called ***trabeculae carneae*** (tra-BEK-yoo-lē KAR-nē-ē). The surface is lined with ***endocardium***, a thin layer of endothelium that also covers the heart valves and the tendons attached to them. The endocardium is continuous with the lining of all the blood vessels.

The interior of the heart is divided into four chambers which receive circulating blood. The two superior chambers are known as the ***left***

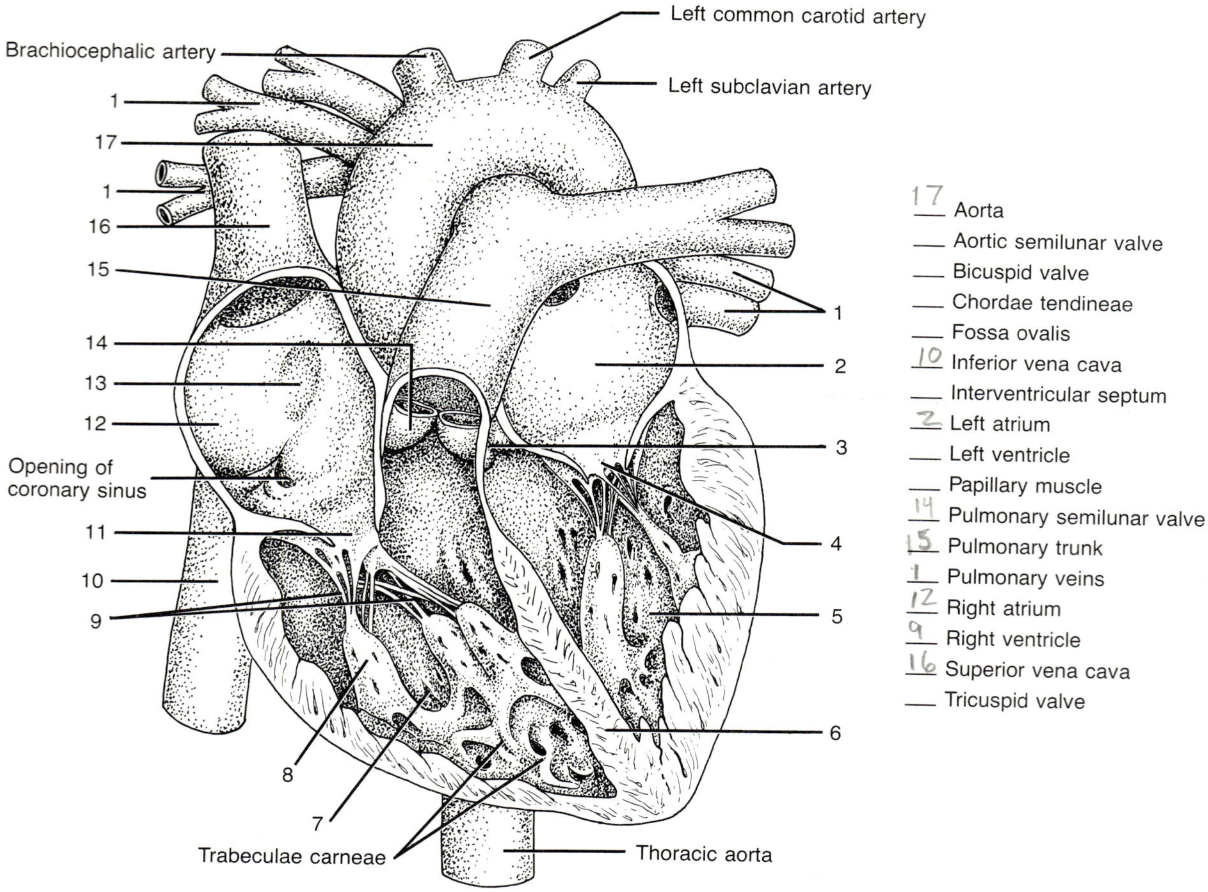

FIGURE 17.1 Internal structure of the human heart.

and ***right atria*** (singular: atrium) and are separated internally by a partition known as the ***interatrial septum***. This septum bears a shallow depression, the ***fossa ovalis***, which corresponds to the site of the ***foramen ovale*** (for-Ā-men ō-VA-lē), an opening in the fetal heart which allows blood to bypass the nonfunctional lungs. Each atrium has an appendage known as an ***auricle***.

The two larger inferior chambers of the heart are the ***left*** and ***right ventricles***, separated internally by a partition called the ***interventricular septum***. The left ventricle is larger and has a thicker wall than the right ventricle.

The right atrium receives blood from systemic circulation through three veins: ***superior vena cava*** draining the upper body, ***inferior vena cava*** draining the lower body, and ***coronary sinus*** draining the heart wall. Blood passes from the right atrium into the right ventricle through the ***tricuspid valve***. The right atrium pumps blood through the ***pulmonary semilunar valve*** within the ***pulmonary trunk*** to the lungs where the blood releases its carbon dioxide and takes up oxygen. The oxygenated blood returns to the heart through four ***pulmonary veins*** which empty into the left atrium. It then passes through the ***bicuspid (mitral) valve*** into the left ventricle. The left ventricle pumps blood through the ***aortic semilunar valve*** into the ***ascending aorta*** and then it is distributed to all areas of the body, except the lung tissue where gas exchange occurs.

The valves of the heart prevent backflow of blood because they are constructed so as to allow blood flow in one direction only. The cuspid valves could evert into the atria and permit backflow were they not attached to fibrous structures called ***chordae tendineae*** (KŌR-dē TEN-din-ē-ē) which hold the cusps within the ventricles. The chordae tendineae are anchored to projections of the ventricular wall called ***papillary muscles***.

The myocardium is supplied with blood through the ***left*** and ***right coronary arteries***, which are branches of the ascending aorta. Most of the deoxygenated blood from the heart drains into the coronary sinus.

Review your knowledge of heart anatomy by labeling Figure 17.1.

EXERCISE 1. The Conduction System of the Heart

OBJECTIVES

To describe the conduction system of the heart
To interpret a normal electrocardiogram (ECG)
To measure cardiac depolarization

The heart is innervated by the autonomic nervous system (ANS) which modulates but does not initiate contraction. The heart can contract even if it is separated from the ANS because specialized muscle fibers (cells) in the right atrium known as the ***sinoatrial (SA) node*** initiate spontaneous action potentials (nerve impulses). These cells have lost their ability to contract and have become specialized for nerve impulse conduction. The SA node, the normal pacemaker of the heart, is never stabilized at an electrically resting state. As soon as the cells have repolarized they begin to depolarize, due to spontaneous changes in their membrane permeability to cations.

Once a nerve action potential is initiated by the SA node, it spreads over both atria, causing them to contract and, at the same time, depolarizing the ***atrioventricular (AV) node*** near the inferior portion of the interatrial septum. From the AV node, a tract of conducting fibers called the ***atrioventricular (AV) bundle*** extends to the top of the interventricular septum and continues down both sides of the septum as the ***right*** and ***left bundle branches***. The atrioventricular bundle distributes electrical impulses over the medial surfaces of the ventricles. Actual contraction of the ventricles is stimulated by ***conduction myofibers (Purkinje fibers)*** that emerge from the bundle branches and pass into fibers of the ventricular myocardium. Ventricular contraction begins about 0.1 second after atrial contraction.

Label the components of the conduction system of the heart in Figure 17.2.

A. The Electrocardiogram

The ***electrocardiograph (ECG*** or ***EKG)*** is an instrument that measures the electrical activity of the heart, *not* its contractile activity. The ECG measures the voltage between pairs of electrodes, which may be placed at two points on the body (bipolar leads) or at one place on the body and another in the electrocardiograph itself (unipolar leads).

The ECG records ***deflection waves*** that indicate the magnitude and direction of the electrical impulses generated by the heart. A normal ECG, drawn in Figure 17.3, shows three deflection waves.

1. ***P wave***, the result of depolarization of the atria, occurring just prior to atrial contraction.
2. ***QRS wave (complex)***, the result of depolarization of the ventricles occurring just prior to ventricular contraction.
3. ***T wave***, the result of ventricular repolarization.

Atrial repolarization is not usually recorded as a deflection wave by surface electrodes because it is masked by the QRS wave that occurs simultaneously with it.

The ***P-R interval*** lasts from the beginning of the P wave to the beginning of the QRS wave and represents the time needed for impulses to pass from the SA node to the ventricular myocardium. It is lengthened in conditions such as atherosclerotic heart disease and rheumatic fever that cause damage to the conduction pathways to the ventricles.

The ***P-R segment*** from the end of the P wave to the beginning of the QRS wave is normally at the baseline, indicating no change in the electrical potential of the surface of the heart. During this time, nerve impulses are traveling within the atrial myocardium, from the AV node to the conduction myofibers (Purkinje fibers).

The ***S-T segment*** represents the time between the end of ventricular depolarization and ventricular repolarization. During this time,

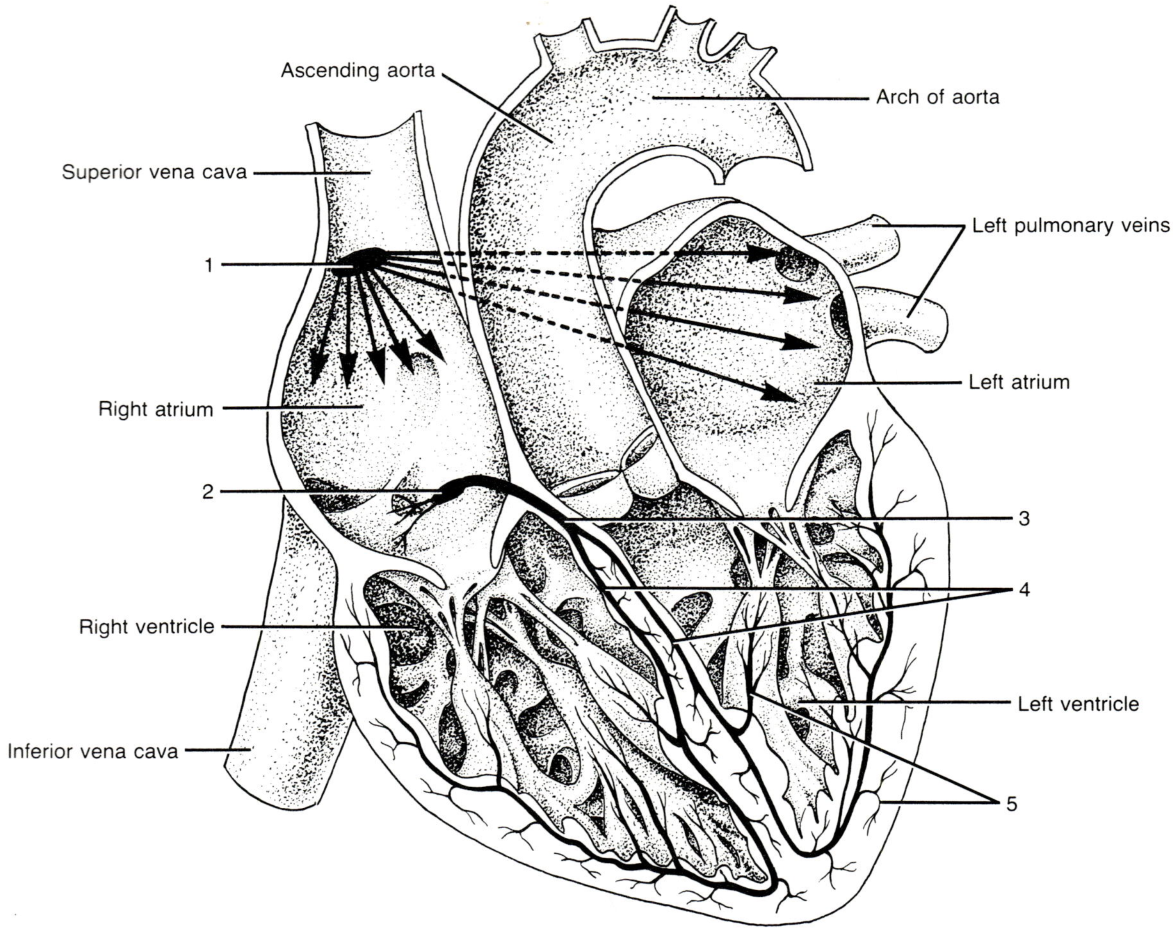

FIGURE 17.2 Conduction system of the heart.

there is no electrical change so the record is at the baseline. The S-T segment lengthens when the ventricular muscle is damaged by events such as myocardial infarction (MI).

Fibrillation is an arrhythmia caused by the irregular and uncoordinated spread of impulses throughout the myocardium. ECGs depicting atrial and ventricular fibrillation are shown in Figure 17.4.

MATERIALS

Cot or table

Recording apparatus (Physiograph or electrocardiograph)

Electrode cream, jelly, or saline paste

Cables and plate electrodes

Recording paper

Alcohol wipes

PROCEDURE

1. Follow the directions from your laboratory instructor for the use of the recording instrument in your laboratory. Before you begin this exercise, make certain that you understand

a. The calibration of the device. Generally, 1 centimeter of deflection = 1 millivolt of potential difference.

b. How to set paper speed. By convention, paper speed is set at 2.5 centimeters/second.

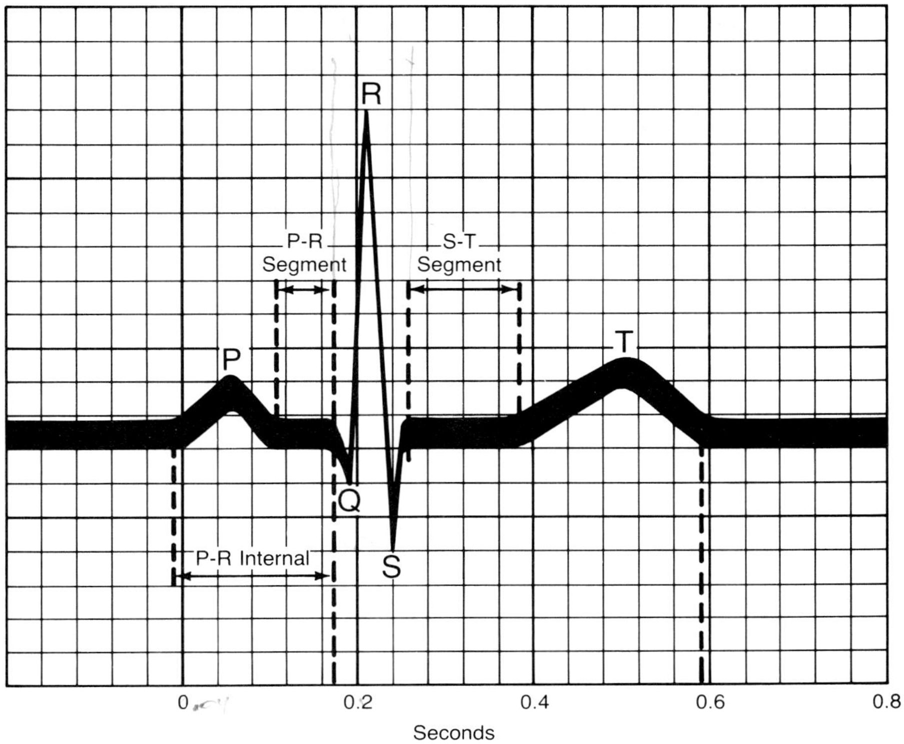

FIGURE 17.3 A normal electrocardiogram (ECG).

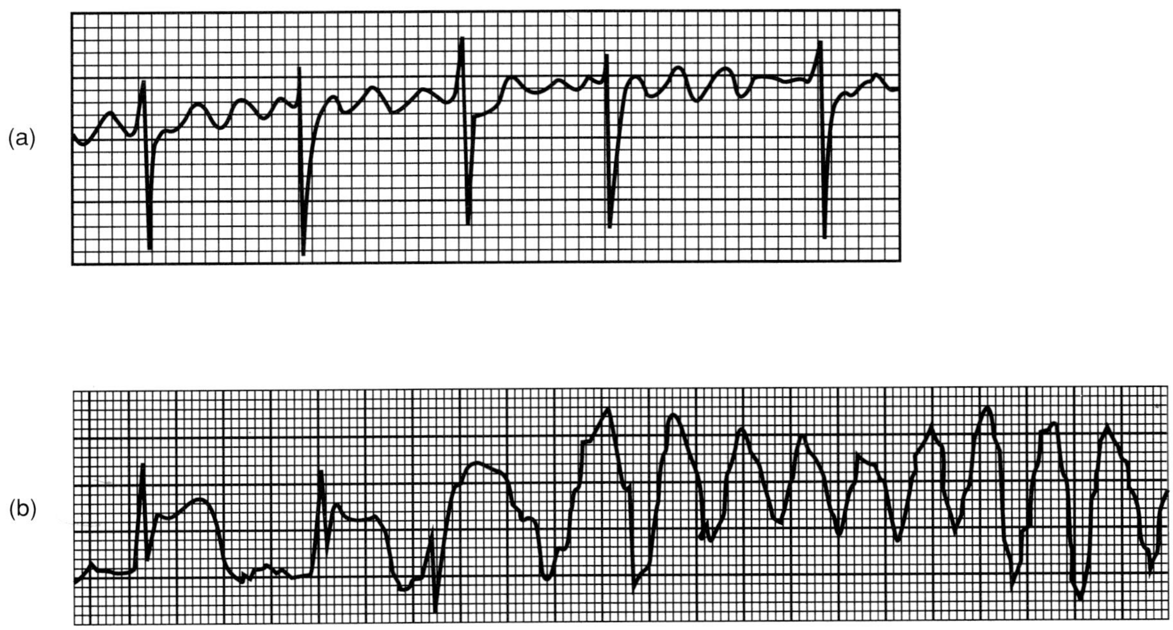

FIGURE 17.4 Fibrillation. (a) Atrial fibrillation. (b) Ventricular fibrillation.

c. The setting of the various switches.

d. The initial positioning of the recording stylus.

e. The connection of the leads to the electrode plates. Leads record the potential differences between a pair of electrodes.

2. Have your laboratory partner lie down on a table or cot, uncover the left ankle, and *remove all metal jewelry*.

3. Swab the skin with an alcohol pad and apply electrode cream, jelly, or saline paste where electrodes will be applied to the subject's inner forearms just above the wrist and to the inside of the leg just above the left ankle. Also apply it to the concave surface of the electrode plates.

4. Fasten the electrode plates securely to the limb area surfaces with rubber straps. *They must fit snugly but not so tight as to impede blood flow*.

5. Connect the proper end of the electrode cables to the electrode plates, using the standard limb leads below.

Lead	Electrodes Used
I	Right wrist to left wrist
II	Right wrist to left ankle
III	Left wrist to left ankle

6. Connect the other end of the electrode cables to the recording instrument, if they are not already in place.

7. Before recording, ascertain that the

a. Recording power switch is on.

b. Paper is sufficient for recording and the pen is properly centered with ink flowing freely (or that the heated stylus is properly adjusted).

c. Subject is lying quietly and relaxed.

8. Turn the instrument on and record for 30 seconds from each lead. Obtain directions from your laboratory instructor on the procedure to be followed when switching from lead to lead. When the recording leads are switched, note the change by marking it on the electrocardiogram. *The subject must remain very still during the recording period*.

9. Turn off the recording instrument and disconnect the leads from the subject. Clean the excess paste from the electrodes and the subject. The skin can be washed with water to remove the electrode cream.

10. Fasten a sample of the electrocardiogram in the LABORATORY REPORT RESULTS at the end of the chapter. Identify the P wave, QRS wave, T wave, P-R interval, and P-R and S-T segments.

11. Calculate the heart rate and record the calculations in the LABORATORY REPORT RESULTS at the end of the chapter. Begin by measuring the time between successive QRS complexes. (At a speed of 2.5 centimeters/second, each small square on the recording paper usually represents 0.4 seconds.) Then divide this time into 60, as in the example below.

$$60\ \frac{\text{seconds}}{\text{minute}} \div 0.83\ \frac{\text{seconds}}{\text{beat}} = 72\ \frac{\text{beats}}{\text{minute}}$$

What heart abnormalities would not be detected by the electrocardiograph? ____________

____

EXERCISE 2. The Cardiac Cycle

OBJECTIVES

To observe and record a normal cardiac cycle

To identify intrinsic and extrinsic factors that control the cardiac cycle

To describe the refractory period in cardiac muscle

When the cardiac muscle fibers (cells) in the atria or ventricles are stimulated, contraction or ***systole*** (SIS-tō-lē) occurs. After contraction, the heart chambers relax during ***diastole*** (dī-AS-tō-lē). A ***cardiac cycle***, or complete heartbeat, consists of atrial systole and diastole plus ventricular systole and diastole. The relationship of these parts of the cycle is shown in Figure 17.5a. In a complete cardiac cycle, the atria are in systole for 0.1 second and in diastole 0.7 second. By contrast, ventricular systole lasts 0.3 seconds and ventricular diastole 0.5 seconds. The average cardiac cycle requires about 0.8 seconds when the heart rate is 75 beats per minute (60 seconds/minute ÷ .75 beats/minute).

The cardiac cycle is usually subdivided into four phases (see Figure 17.5a). The first is the period of ***ventricular filling***, which begins with the opening of the atrioventricular valves, that is, the tricuspid and bicuspid valves (see Figure

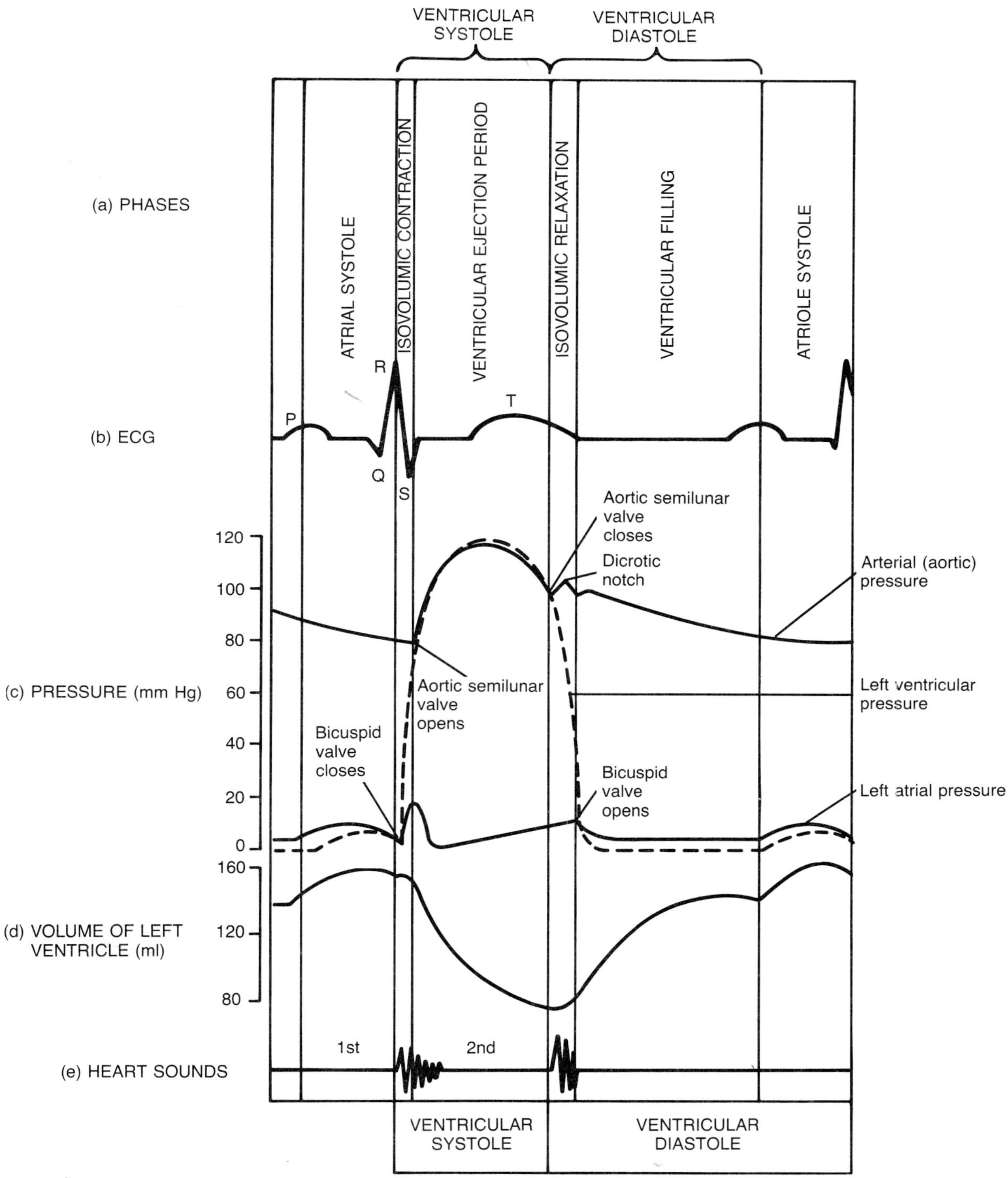

FIGURE 17.5 Cardiac cycle. (a) Phases. (b) ECG. Tracing of the lead II electrocardiogram recording related to cardiac cycle. (c) Left atrial, left ventricular, and arterial (aortic) pressure changes along with opening and closure of valves during cardiac cycle. (d) Volume of left ventricle. (e) Heart sounds related to cardiac cycle.

17.5c). The initial filling of the ventricles is fast; 70% of the blood moves into the ventricles by venous pressure. The last 30% of the blood is pumped into the ventricles by the force of atrial contraction (systole).

The second phase of the cardiac cycle is ***isovolumic ventricular contraction***. During this phase, the ventricles start to contract, thereby increasing ventricular pressure. The rising pressure causes the atrioventricular valves to close. The semilunar valves remain closed due to the pressure gradient between the ventricles and the great vessels leaving the heart.

Ventricular ejection, the third phase of the cardiac cycle, starts when the pressure within the ventricles exceeds that in the aorta and pulmonary trunk, thereby causing the semilunar valves to open and blood to leave the ventricles. Initially, blood leaves the ventricles at a very high velocity. As ventricular pressure decreases, the rate of blood flow out of the ventricles decreases considerably.

When the ventricular pressure falls below that within the aorta and pulmonary artery, the respective semilunar valves close, initiating the period of ***isovolumic ventricular relaxation***. Since the ventricular pressure is still greater than atrial pressure, the atrioventricular valves remain closed. When the ventricular pressure drops below atrial pressure, the atrioventricular valves open, initiating ventricular filling once again. The atria are filling constantly because there are no valves between the venae cavae and right atrium and the pulmonary veins and left atrium.

A. Observation of the Normal Cardiac Cycle

MATERIALS

Living frog or turtle
Frog board
Dissecting tools
Frog Ringer's solution
Safety goggles
Laboratory apron or coat

PROCEDURE

CAUTION! *Please reread Section D, "Precautions Related to Dissection" in Chapter 1 before you begin.*

NOTE: It is strongly suggested that either your instructor or a laboratory assistant perform the following pithing procedure since it requires some practice and may prove difficult for inexperienced individuals.

1. Depending on the specimen of choice, obtain a pithed frog (or turtle). The frog and turtle hearts are shown in Figure 17.6a and b. They differ from the mammalian heart anatomically in that they have only a *single* ventricle from which all blood exits. The large dorsal sinus venosus serves as the pacemaker.
2. Fasten the specimen to a board ventral side up, and expose the heart by cutting through the body wall of the thoracic region.

Frog	**Turtle**
Make a midline incision from the abdomen to the jaw and extend the incision laterally. Pin the body flaps to the board. Carefully remove the pericardial sac.	Using a saw and scalpel, remove the ventral shell and associated musculature according to the directions of your laboratory instructor. Carefully remove the mediastinum and pericardial sac.

3. *Throughout this exercise keep the heart moist with frog Ringer's solution.*
4. Observe the sequence of contraction of the atria and the ventricle and determine the rate of contraction for 30 seconds. Calculate the heart rate per minute and record it in the LABORATORY REPORT RESULTS at the end of the chapter.

Estimate the relationship of atrial and ventricular cycles by shading in a portion of the bars below to indicate systole and leaving the portion representing diastole unshaded.

Atrial	
Ventricular	

B. Recording the Cardiac Cycle

MATERIALS

Recording device
Living frog or turtle
Frog Ringer's solution
Thread and hook
Safety goggles
Laboratory apron or coat

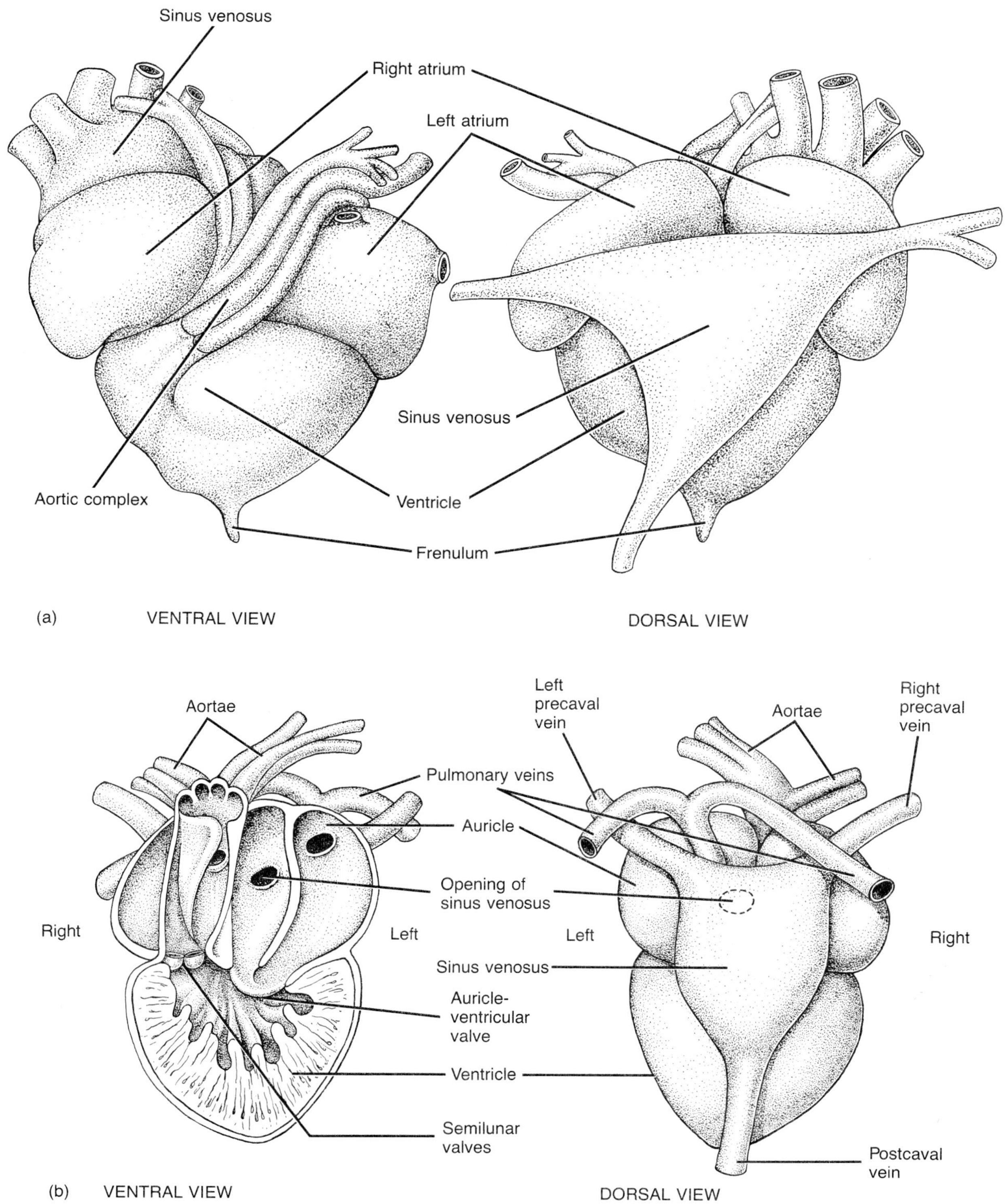

FIGURE 17.6 (a) Turtle heart. (b) Frog heart.

PROCEDURE

1. Review the use of the physiograph (or kymograph) in Chapter 9, Section A. *Throughout this exercise keep the heart moist with frog Ringer's solution.*

2.

Frog	Turtle
Tie a thread to a small metal hook and carefully insert the hook into the tip of the ventricular myocardium. *Do not* penetrate the chamber.	Tie a thread ligature tightly around the cardiac frenulum at the ventricular apex and cut the frenulum *distal* to the thread.

3. Connect the loose end of the thread to a force transducer with just enough tension to keep the thread taut so that the contracting ventricle pulls on the thread.

4. Connect an atrium to a second force transducer by inserting a small metal hook or bent pin through the atrium and connecting it to the transducer with a thread. Again regulate the tension as directed in step 3.

5. Record several cardiac cycles and paste a strip of the recording paper in the LABORATORY REPORT RESULTS at the end of the chapter. Label atrial (smaller) and ventricular (larger) systolic waves. Calculate and record the heart rate per minute.

Why do the ventricular waves have greater amplitude than the atrial waves? ___________

____

C. Intrinsic Control of the Cardiac Cycle

Intrinsic control of the cardiac cycle refers to mechanisms arising totally within the heart, devoid of external influence from nerves or hormones. The major intrinsic control mechanism is ***Starling's Law of the Heart*** which says that the heart will pump out all of the blood it receives, within physiological limits. In other words, the more the heart is stretched, the stronger will be the contraction of the myocardium.

MATERIALS

Recording device
Living frog or turtle
Frog Ringer's solution
Safety goggles
Laboratory apron or coat

PROCEDURE

1. *Throughout this exercise keep the heart moist with frog Ringer's solution.* While continuously recording the cardiac cycle, increase the tension on the ventricle in stepwise increments by one of the following:

   a. Raising the heart level or the transducer.
   b. Adding weights to the muscle lever.
   c. Turning the tension adjuster.

Allow several beats at each tension setting.

2. Return the heart to its original tension setting when the contraction strength starts to diminish.

3. Graph the relationship between the tension and amplitude of ventricular contraction in the LABORATORY REPORT RESULTS at the end of the chapter. Explain your results.

What normal physiological event is mimicked by artificially increasing tension on the heart?

____

D. Extrinsic Control of the Cardiac Cycle

Extrinsic control of the cardiac cycle is exerted through the autonomic nervous system (ANS) and hormones of the adrenal medulla. Before beginning this exercise, review the use of the stimulator in Chapter 9.

1. Effect of Vagal Stimulation

MATERIALS

Recording device
Living frog or turtle
Ligature
Dissecting tools
Four medicine droppers
Stimulator
Solutions in frog Ringer's:
  1:1000 solution of acetylcholine
  1:1000 solution of atropine sulfate
  1:1000 solution of epinephrine
Safety goggles
Laboratory apron or coat

PROCEDURE

a. *Throughout this exercise keep the heart moist with frog Ringer's solution*. Expose the vagus (X) nerve in the neck and pass a ligature beneath it but *do not tie the ligature*.

Frog	Turtle
The vagus (X) nerve lies beside the external jugular vein. Use blunt dissection with a glass probe to separate the left or right nerve.	The vagus (X) nerve lies deep in the neck muscles beside the carotid artery. Use dissection scissors to expose the muscles of the neck and blunt dissection with a glass probe to isolate the left or right nerve.

b. While continuously recording, stimulate the vagus (X) nerve with various strengths of stimuli from an electronic stimulator at a frequency of 25 per second and a duration of 2 milliseconds (msec). Stimulate for approximately 30 seconds at each strength.

c. Attach the tracing in the LABORATORY REPORT RESULTS at the end of the chapter and explain your observations.

2. Effect of Acetylcholine

a. After allowing several minutes for recovery, use a medicine dropper to apply three drops of a 1:1000 solution of acetylcholine in frog Ringer's solution to the surface of the heart.

b. Monitor any changes in the cardiac cycle for 2 to 3 minutes, and then use a medicine dropper to rinse with frog Ringer's solution. Allow several minutes for recovery. Using a medicine dropper, gently aspirate any accumulated fluid.

c. Attach the tracing in the LABORATORY REPORT RESULTS at the end of the chapter and explain your observations.

3. Effect of Atropine Sulfate

a. After allowing several minutes for recovery, use a medicine dropper to apply three drops of a 1:1000 solution of atropine sulfate in frog Ringer's solution to the surface of the heart.

b. Monitor any changes in the cardiac cycle for 2 to 3 minutes, and then use a medicine dropper to rinse with frog Ringer's solution. Allow several minutes for recovery. Using a medicine dropper, *gently* aspirate any accumulated fluid.

c. Attach the tracing in the LABORATORY REPORT RESULTS at the end of the chapter and explain your observations.

4. Effects of Epinephrine

a. After allowing several minutes for recovery, use a medicine dropper to apply three drops of a 1:1000 solution of epinephrine in frog Ringer's solution to the surface of the heart.

b. Monitor any changes in the cardiac cycle for 2 to 3 minutes, and then use a medicine dropper to rinse with frog Ringer's solution. Allow several minutes for recovery. Using a medicine dropper, *gently* aspirate any accumulated fluid.

c. Attach the tracing in the LABORATORY REPORT RESULTS at the end of the chapter and explain your observations.

Which of the solution(s) mimics the effect of the sympathetic stimulation? ____________

of parasympathetic stimulation? ____________

E. Demonstration of the Refractory Period

The ***absolute refractory period*** is the time during which a muscle will not respond to a stimulus, regardless of strength. In other words, the threshold stimulus is infinity. The ***relative refractory period*** is the time during which it takes a greater than normal stimulus to elicit contraction. Compared to skeletal muscle, cardiac muscle has a longer duration of contraction and a longer refractory period. Normally, the fibers (cells) cannot be stimulated again until the end of the refractory period. Thus, summation and tetany are not possible, and the heart pumps rhythmically.

Stimulation of the cardiac muscle at some points in the cycle may produce an extra beat (extrasystole) followed by a compensatory pause.

MATERIALS

Recording instrument
Living frog or turtle
Frog Ringer's solution
Safety goggles
Laboratory apron or coat

PROCEDURE

1. Use the frog or turtle heart preparation from the preceding exercises, and *remember to keep the heart moist with frog Ringer's solution.*
2. Set the paper drive of the physiograph to its highest speed.
3. While continuously recording, stimulate the ventricle with a single stimulus of about 50 volts for 2 milliseconds (msec). Make sure that both electrodes touch the ventricle.
4. Allowing several contractions between stimuli, stimulate the ventricle at the following five points of the ventricular systole.

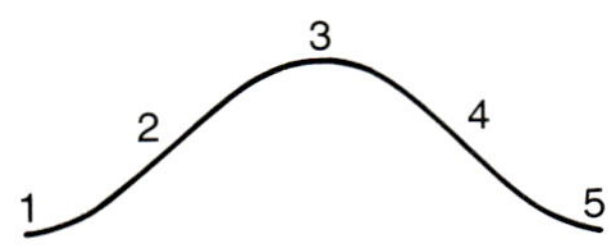

5. Note whether an extrasystole occurs at any or all of the five points, and, if so, whether it is followed by a compensatory pause.
6. Continuously stimulate the ventricle for 10 seconds to see if you can elicit tetany.
7. Record your observations in the LABORATORY REPORT RESULTS at the end of the chapter.

When in the cardiac cycle does the absolute refractory period occur? ______________________

____

EXERCISE 3. Auscultation of the Heart

> OBJECTIVE
>
> To hear the heart sounds and explain their causes

Two well-defined sounds occurring during the adult human cardiac cycle can be easily heard with the stethoscope. The first sound (lubb) is caused by the closure of the atrioventricular valves soon after ventricular systole begins (see Figure 17.5e). This sound is lower, duller, and longer than the second heart sound. This second sound (dupp) is caused by the closure of the semilunar valves near the end of ventricular systole.

The heart sounds provide information about the valves. Peculiar sounds are called ***murmurs*** and may be caused by blood backflow into a chamber because of improper valve closure or by stenosis (narrowing) of a valve or other anomalies such as septal defects. Many murmurs are not pathologic and have no clinical significance.

Listening to the sounds of the body is called auscultation. Figure 17.7 illustrates the areas where the heart sounds are best heard.

MATERIALS

Stethoscope

Alcohol wipes

PROCEDURE

1. The stethoscope should be used in a quiet room.
2. *Clean the earpieces of the stethoscope with alcohol.* Direct them slightly forward in your ears.
3. Listen to the heart sounds of your laboratory partner by placing the diaphragm of the stethoscope next to the skin in the positions illustrated in Figure 17.7.
4. The first sound is best heard at the apex of the heart, located approximately at the fifth intercostal space at the midline.
5. The second heart sound is best heard over the area between the second costal cartilage and the second intercostal space on the left side.
6. CAUTION! *If your partner has no known cardiac or other health problems and is capable of such an activity,* ask her/him to run in place about 25 steps. Listen to the heart sounds again.
7. Record your observations in the LABORATORY REPORT RESULTS at the end of the chapter.

What factors could make auscultation of heart sounds difficult? ______________________

____

____

EXERCISE 4. Pulse Rate

> OBJECTIVE
>
> To determine pulse rate and understand the factors that affect it

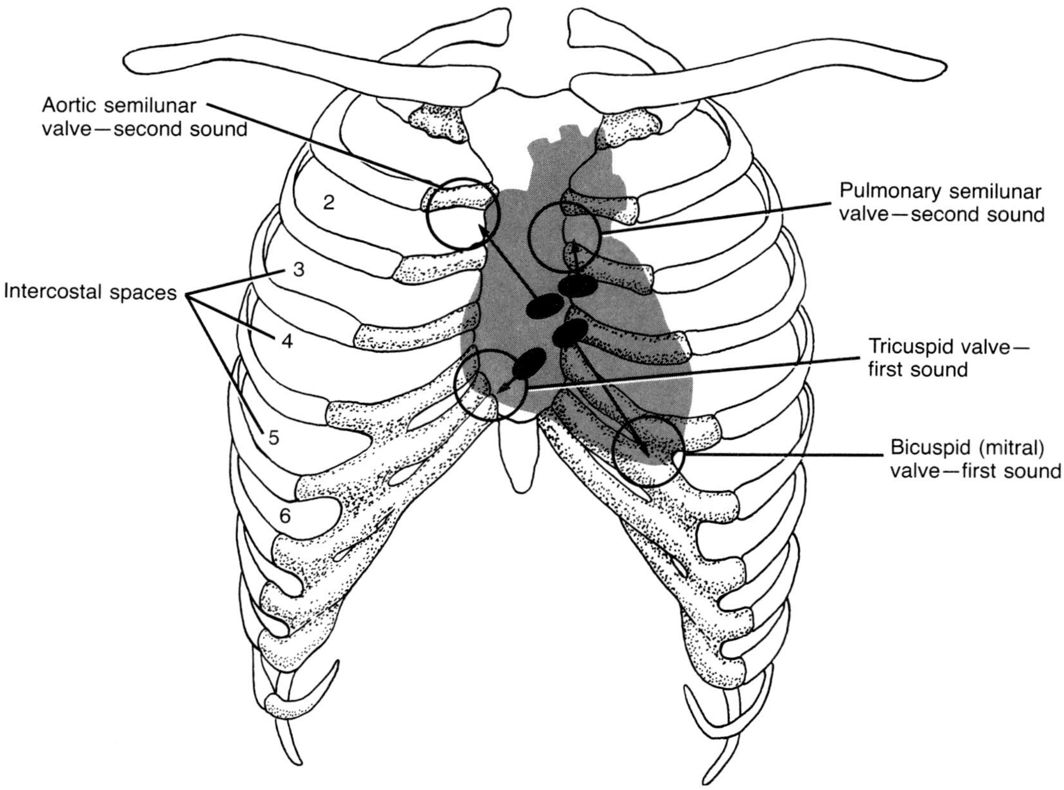

FIGURE 17.7 Surface areas where heart valve sounds are heard best.

During ventricular systole, a wave of pressure, called ***pulse***, is produced in the arteries due to ventricular contraction. Pulse rate and the heart rate are essentially the same. Pulse can be felt readily where an artery is near the surface of the skin. Pulse rates vary considerably in individuals, depending on the time of day, temperature, emotions, stress, and other factors. The normal adult pulse rate of the heart at rest is within a range of 72–80 beats per minute. A rapid rate (over 100 beats/minute) is called ***tachycardia*** (tak′-e-KAR-dē-a); an abnormally slow rate (below 50 beats/minute) is called ***bradycardia*** (brād′-e-KAR-dē-a).

MATERIALS

Watch with a second hand

PROCEDURE

1. Using your index and middle fingers, palpate your partner's radial artery. The thumb should never be used because it has its own prominent pulse.

2. Count the pulse for 30 seconds; change positions and record your results in the LABORATORY REPORT RESULTS at the end of the chapter.

3. Place your index and middle fingers on one side of your partner's larynx and *gently* press posteriorly until you feel the carotid pulse with two fingers.

4. Calculate the pulse rate for 10 seconds and change positions.

5. Obtain a radial pulse rate under the following conditions.
   a. Sitting quietly.
   b. Standing quietly.
   c. Right after walking 60 steps.
   d. Right after running in place 60 steps.

CAUTION! *Perform (d) only if your laboratory partner has no known cardiac or other health problem and is capable of such activity.*

Note how long it takes for the pulse to return to the resting rate after the running exercises.

6. Record your results in the LABORATORY REPORT RESULTS at the end of the chapter.

EXERCISE 5. Blood Pressure

> OBJECTIVE
>
> To measure blood pressure and explain factors that affect it

Clinically, ***blood pressure*** refers to the pressure exerted by blood on the walls of the large vessels. Arterial pressure is most commonly measured, and it is reported in millimeters of mercury (mm Hg), i.e., the height of a column of mercury that is held up by a given pressure.

The highest pressure in the artery, occurring during ventricular systole, is termed ***systolic blood pressure***.

The lowest pressure, occurring during ventricular diastole and reflecting the elastic recoil and peripheral resistance of the arterial walls, is termed ***diastolic blood pressure***.

The difference between the systolic and diastolic pressures is termed ***pulse pressure***. The normal value is about 40 mm Hg.

Arterial pressure can be measured in a variety of ways. This exercise employs the auscultatory method, in which the sounds of blood flow are heard with a stethoscope. Blood flow in an artery is impeded with a ***sphygmomanometer*** (SFIG-mō-man-om′-et-er), a device consisting of an inflatable cuff, a rubber bulb which introduces air into the cuff, and a manometer, which measures cuff pressure.

When the cuff of the sphygmomanometer applies sufficient pressure to completely occlude blood flow, no sounds can be heard distal to the cuff because no blood flows through the artery. When cuff pressure drops just below the maximal (systolic) pressure in the artery, blood is heard passing through the vessel. When cuff pressure drops below the lowest (diastolic) pressure in the vessel, the sound becomes muffled and disappears.

Blood pressure can be taken in any artery which can be occluded easily. The brachial artery is at approximately the same level as the heart, so brachial pressure closely reflects aortic pressure.

Blood pressures are usually expressed as a ratio of systolic/diastolic, for example, 120/80 (read 120 over 80). If the muffling is reported as well, the blood pressure would read, for example, 120/80/76. These figures are normal for a 20 year old male. Blood pressure is usually higher in males, in the elderly, and in the obese.

MATERIALS

Stethoscope
Alcohol wipes
Sphygmomanometer

PROCEDURE

1. Have your laboratory partner sit comfortably with the arm bared, slightly flexed, abducted (see Figure 17.8).

2. Wrap the deflated cuff of the sphygmomanometer around the arm with the lower edge about 1 inch above the antecubital space.

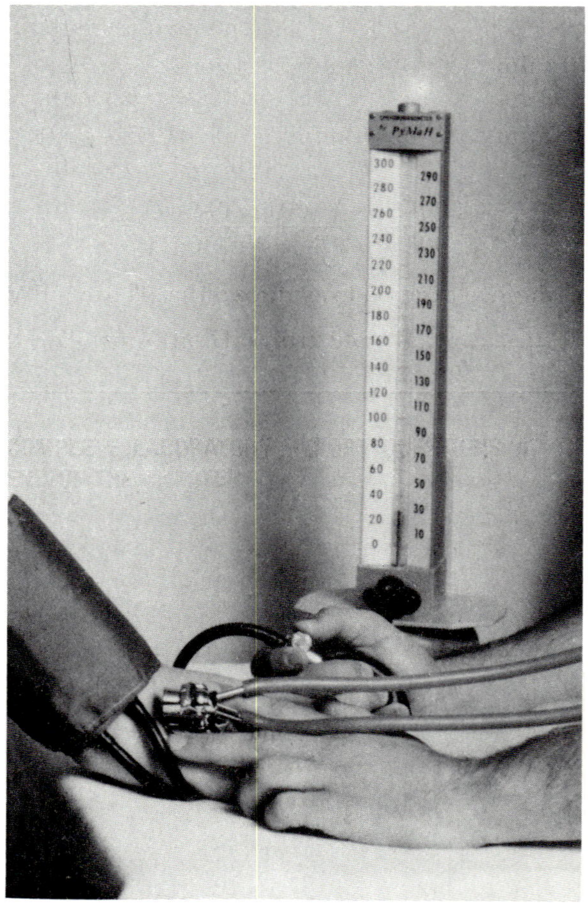

FIGURE 17.8 Use of sphygmomanometer.

3. Close the valve on the neck of the rubber bulb.

4. *Clean the earpieces of the stethoscope with alcohol* and listen for the brachial pulse in the antecubital space on the inner margin of the biceps brachii muscle.

5. Inflate the cuff by squeezing the bulb until the pressure slightly exceeds 170 mm Hg. At this point the wall of the brachial artery should be compressed so tightly that no blood can flow through.

6. Place the diaphragm of the stethoscope firmly over the brachial artery and, while watching the pressure gauge, slowly turn the valve, releasing air from the cuff. Listen carefully as you watch the pressure fall and note the reading on the gauge when you hear a loud rapping noise. This is the systolic pressure reading.

7. Continue listening as the pressure falls. When the sounds become muffled or disappear, take the diastolic pressure reading.

8. Allowing a few minutes for recovery, repeat this procedure to see if you get consistent results.

9. Repeat the procedure when your partner is standing.

10. Repeat the procedure after your partner has run in place 50 times, *if your laboratory partner has no known cardiac or other health problem and is capable of such activity.*

11. Record your measurements in the LABORATORY REPORT RESULTS at the end of the chapter.

Would the *measured* blood pressure in an obese individual be abnormally high or low? ____

EXERCISE 6. Vascular Physiology

> OBJECTIVE
>
> To observe blood flow and to demonstrate factors that affect blood vessel diameter and velocity of blood in vessels

Blood flows from the heart through arteries to arterioles to capillaries. Capillaries join to form venules which lead to veins which return blood to the heart. The greatest cross-sectional area of the circulatory system is occupied by capillaries. Capillary blood flow can be observed in the fish tail and the webbing of a frog foot.

MATERIALS

- Living fish or frog
- Frog board and paper towels
- Frog Ringer's solution OR amphibian Ringer's solution
- Dissecting pins
- Light microscope
- Rubber bands
- Four medicine droppers
- Ice water
- Room temperature water
- 1:1000 epinephrine solution
- 1:10,000 histamine solution
- Methyl salicylate (oil of wintergreen)
- Safety goggles
- Laboratory apron or coat

PROCEDURE FOR USE OF FROG

1. *NOTE: It is strongly suggested that either your instructor or a laboratory assistant perform the procedure for pithing a frog since it requires some practice and may prove difficult for inexperienced individuals.*

2. Tie a pithed frog dorsal side up on the frog board with the feet at the hole end. Cover the body with moist paper towel and secure the frog to the board with string or rubber bands (see Figure 17.9a).

3. Spread the web of the foot over the opening in the board and secure it with dissecting pins. Keep the web moist with frog Ringer's solution.

4. Attach the board to the microscope stage with a heavy rubber band and place the web under the low-power objective.

PROCEDURE FOR USE OF FISH

1. Saturate two paper towels with goldfish Ringer's solution. Place one on the frog board adjacent to the hole.

2. Position the fish on the paper towel with the tail extending over the hole and cover the fish with the other towel. If the paper towel does not have sufficient weight to hold the fish in place, tie it with string.

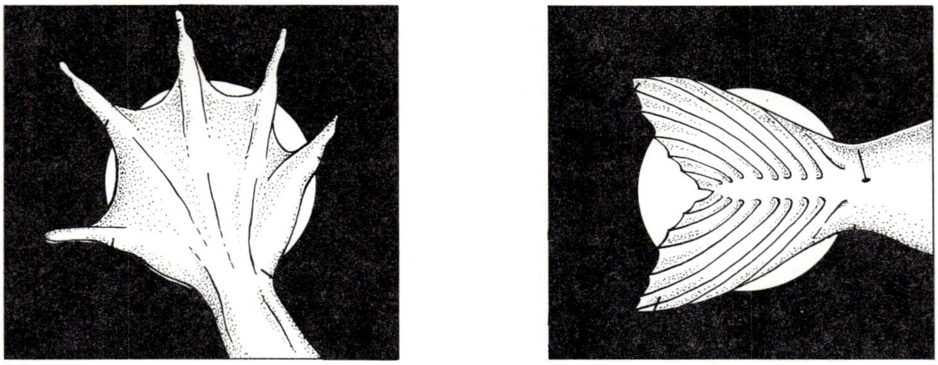

(a) (b)

FIGURE 17.9 (a) Placement of frog leg on frog board. (b) Placement of fish tail on board.

3. Spread the tail over the hole and fasten on each side with dissecting pins (see Figure 17.9b).

4. Attach the board to the microscope stage with a heavy rubber band and place the tail under the low-power objective.

PROCEDURE FOR OBSERVATION OF CIRCULATION

1. Examine the vessels and distinguish between an arteriole and venule by noting the direction of blood flow.

2. Note in which type of vessel pulsations occur.

3. Describe the movement of blood cells within a capillary.

4. Describe the rate of blood flow in the vessels observed.

5. Using a medicine dropper, bathe the specimen with the following solutions. Observe any resultant changes. Rinse the specimen with Ringer's solution. Repeat with another solution.

   a. Ice water.

   b. Room temperature water.

   c. 1:1000 epinephrine solution.

   d. 1:10,000 histamine solution.

   e. Methyl salicylate.

6. Record your observations in the LABORATORY REPORT RESULTS at the end of the chapter.

In which vessel is the velocity the fastest?

____

Is the velocity faster at the margin or at the center of this vessel? ________________

RESPIRATORY PHYSIOLOGY 18

EXERCISE 1. Mechanics of Respiration
A. Artificial Thorax
B. Chest and Abdominal Measurement
EXERCISE 2. Respiratory Sounds
EXERCISE 3. Use of Pneumograph
EXERCISE 4. Measurement of Respiratory Volumes
A. Use of Wet Spirometer
B. Use of Handheld Spirometer
C. Use of Collins Respirometer
EXERCISE 5. Chemical Regulation of Respiration

WORD ROOTS

pneum-, pneuma-, pneumato- = air, breath
pulmo- = lung
spiro- = breathe

The respiratory system, shown in Figure 18.1, consists of organs involved in the exchange of gases between the blood and atmosphere. The mouth, nose, pharynx (throat), larynx (voice box), trachea (windpipe), and bronchial tubes transport air to and from the alveoli of the lungs. In the alveoli, oxygen (O_2) diffuses from the alveolar air into blood, and carbon dioxide (CO_2) diffuses from the blood into alveolar air. This process is called ***external respiration***. The cardiovascular system then transports oxygenated blood to the tissues where ***internal respiration*** occurs. In this process, oxygen is delivered to the systemic tissues from blood and carbon dioxide diffuses from the tissues into blood.

The movement of gases into and out of the lungs is the result of changes in the volume of the thoracic cavity. These changes are brought about by the muscles of respiration, the diaphragm and external intercostal muscles, for the most part. During heavy breathing, the external intercostals, sternocleidomastoid, scalenes, and serratus anterior muscles affect inspiration, and the rectus abdominis and internal intercostals affect expiration.

Control of the rate and depth of respiration is mediated by reflex centers in the medulla oblongata.

EXERCISE 1. Mechanics of Respiration

OBJECTIVES

To visualize the mechanical factors responsible for respiratory movements
To correlate the mechanics of respiration with volume changes in the thorax and abdomen

A. Artificial Thorax

Contraction of the muscles of respiration increases the size of the thorax. Since the pressure of a gas is inversely proportional to its volume (Boyle's Law: $P \propto 1/V$), an increase in thoracic size results in a decrease in intrapulmonic pressure (pressure within lungs). If intrapulmonic pressure falls below atmospheric pressure (760 mm Hg at sea level), air will move down its pressure gradient and enter the lungs until equilibration with atmospheric pressure is reached.

At expiration, the muscles of respiration relax, causing a decrease in thoracic size, a consequent increase in intrapulmonic pressure, and movement of air out of the lungs until equilibration with atmospheric air is reached.

The pressure in the intrapleural space (the space between the parietal and visceral pleura) is always slightly negative, slightly less than

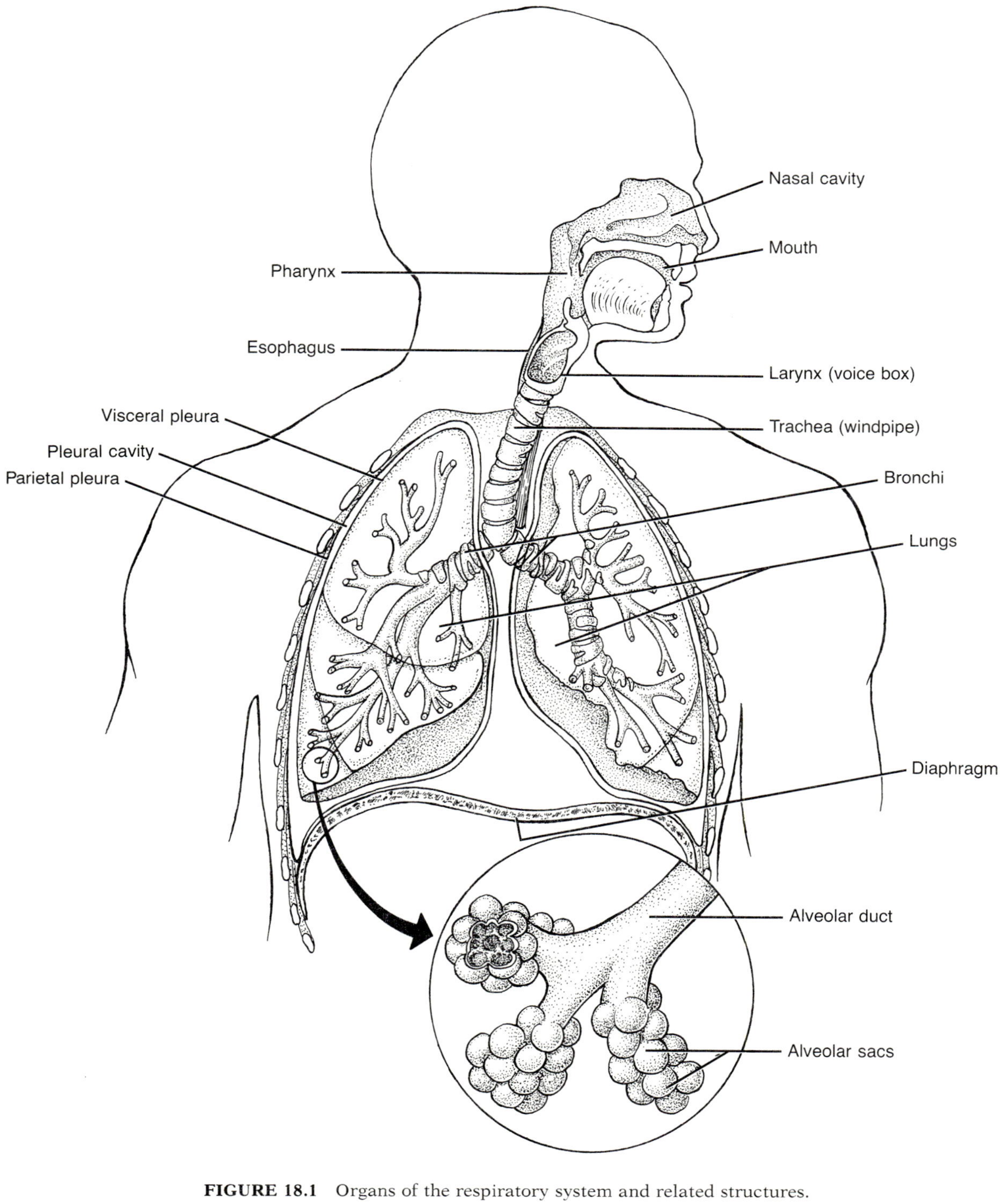

FIGURE 18.1 Organs of the respiratory system and related structures.

intrapulmonic pressure. This negative pressure counterbalances the tendency of the lungs to recoil. The recoil tendency is the result of (1) the elasticity of pulmonary tissue, and (2) the surface tension of water in the liquid which lines the alveoli.

Because of the inherent elasticity of the lungs, they would collapse if intrapleural pressure equalled atmospheric pressure. This condition, called ***pneumothorax***, results if a chest wound or alveolar rupture allows air to enter the intrapleural space and raise the pressure therein.

If water were the only liquid to line the alveoli, they would collapse since water molecules have a greater affinity for each other than they do for air. However, some alveolar cells (septal cells) secrete ***surfactant*** (ser-FAK-tant), a phospholipid which reduces the surface tension and hence the recoil tendency of the alveoli.

The pressure changes that occur during respiration are diagrammed in Figure 18.2.

An artificial thorax is a device which mimics the organs of the respiratory system and allows the pressure/volume relationships to be manipulated. A diagram of such a device is shown in Figure 18.3. Some models will not have a stopcock "glottis"; some will not have a tube opening into the intrapleural space.

MATERIALS

Artificial thorax

PROCEDURE

1. Label the diagram in Figure 18.3 with the anatomical structures represented by the following parts: glottis, thoracic wall, primary bronchus, lungs, intrapulmonic space, intrapleural space, and diaphragm.

2. Pull on the rubber membrane (diaphragm) to simulate inspiration. What changes occur in intrapleural pressure? ____________

in intrapulmonic pressure? ____________

3. Push the rubber membrane upward to simulate expiration. What changes occur in intrapleural pressure? ____________

in intrapulmonic pressure? ____________

4. Open the clamp on the tube leading to the intrapleural space. This simulates pneumothorax. Try to cause inspiration and expiration. Explain your results. ____________

____

____

5. Close the stopcock (glottis) and simulate expiration. This procedure mimics the Valsalva maneuver (forced expiration against a closed glottis). What changes occur in intrathoracic and intrapulmonic pressure? ____________

____

B. Chest and Abdominal Measurement

When the diaphragm contracts, the dome shape of this muscle flattens; the flattening pushes against the abdominal viscera and increases thoracic volume which, in turn, decreases intrapulmonic pressure. The volume changes in the abdomen and chest can easily be measured.

MATERIALS

Tape measure

PROCEDURE

1. Place a tape measure at the level of the fifth rib (about armpit level) and determine the size of the chest immediately after a
   a. Normal inspiration.
   b. Normal expiration.
   c. Maximal inspiration.
   d. Maximal expiration.

2. Repeat step 1 with the tape measure at the level of the waist to determine abdominal size.

3. Record your results in the LABORATORY REPORT RESULTS at the end of the chapter.

Which measurement increased during inspiration? ____________

Which increased during expiration? ____________

____

EXERCISE 2. Respiratory Sounds

OBJECTIVE

To identify the sounds heard during breathing and to explain their origin

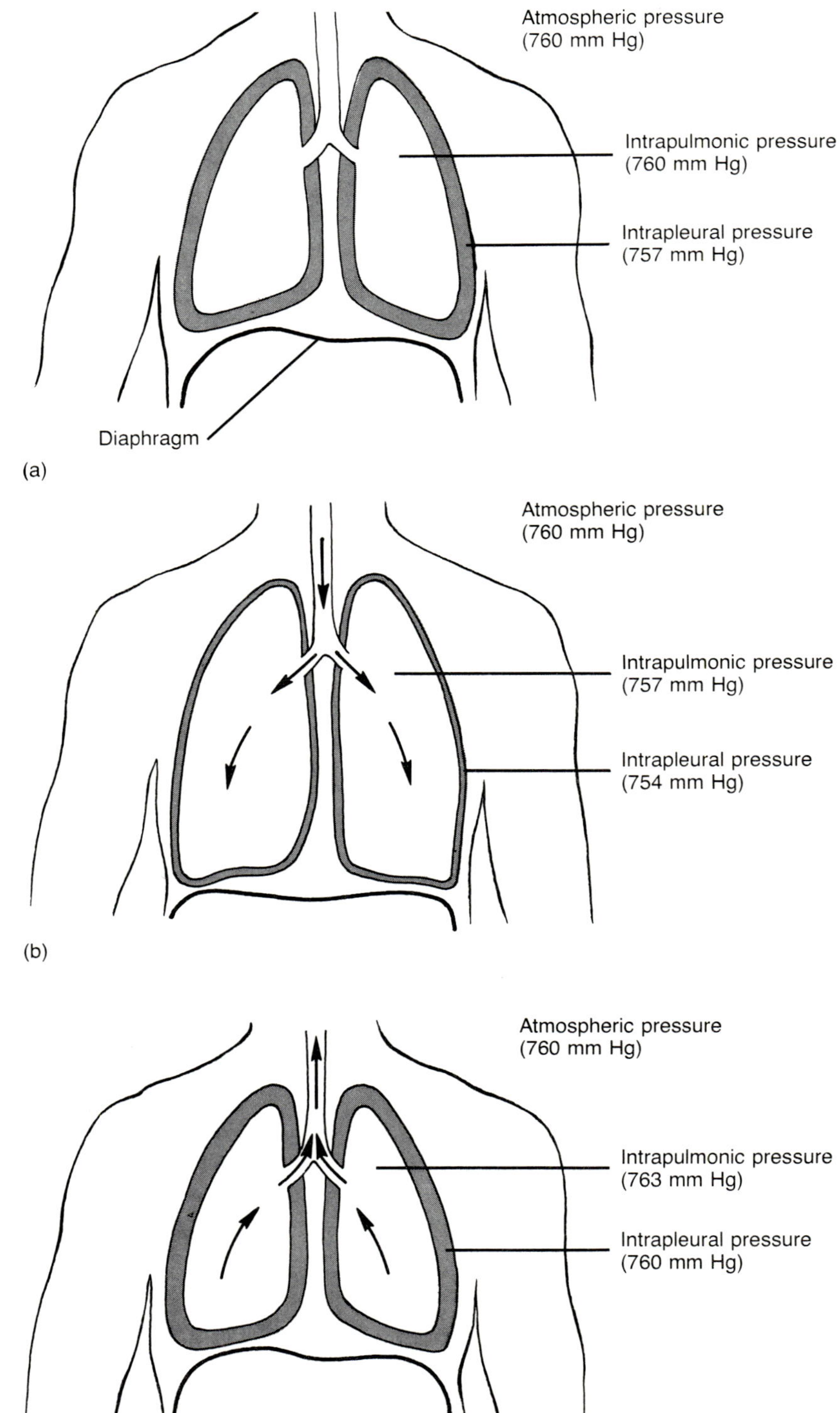

FIGURE 18.2 The mechanics of pulmonary ventilation. (a) Pressures between breaths. (b) Pressures at inspiration when thoracic size increases. (c) Pressures at expiration when thoracic size decreases.

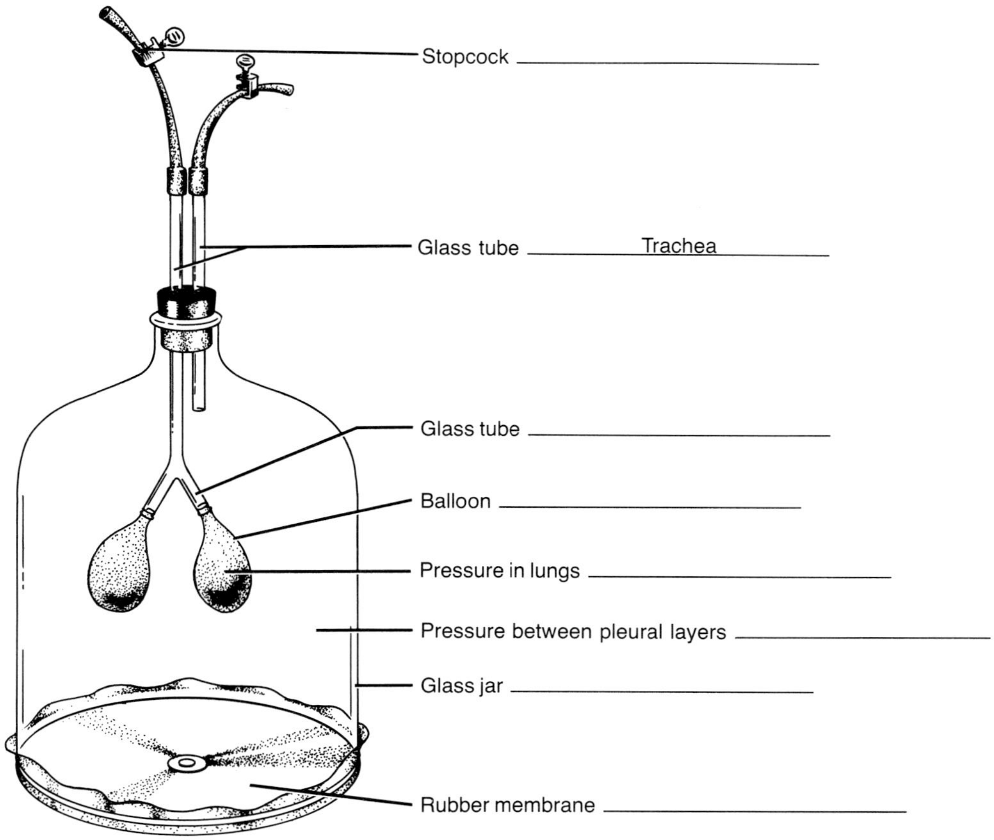

FIGURE 18.3 "Artificial thorax."

Normal breathing sounds include a soft-breezy inspiration as air fills the lungs, followed by a shorter, lower-pitched expiration.

MATERIALS

Stethoscope

Alcohol wipes

PROCEDURE

1. *Clean the earplugs of the stethoscope with alcohol.*
2. Listen to the breathing sounds when the stethoscope diaphragm is placed
   a. Just below larynx.
   b. At various intercostal spaces (spaces between ribs).
   c. Just below the clavicle.
   d. In the interscapular space.
3. Record your observations in the LABORATORY REPORT RESULTS at the end of the chapter.

Which sounds are heard only during inspiration? ______________________

____

EXERCISE 3. Use of Pneumograph

OBJECTIVE

To demonstrate various respiratory movements

The ***pneumograph*** is an instrument that measures variations in breathing patterns. As the subject breathes, chest movements cause changes in the air pressure within the pneumograph that are transmitted to the recorder. Normal inspiration and expiration can thus be recorded, and the effects of a wide range of physical and chemical factors on these movements can be studied.

Follow the instructions for setting up your particular pneumograph.

MATERIALS

Pneumograph

Paper cup

PROCEDURE

1. Seat a subject in a position where the pneumograph recording is not visible.

2. Record normal quiet breathing ***(eupnea)*** for about 30 seconds.

3. Have the subject inhale maximally and hold the breath as long as possible. Record the breathing pattern for 30 seconds after this procedure.

4. Record breathing pattern during the following activities.

   a. Reading.

   b. Swallowing water.

   c. Laughing.

   d. Yawning.

   e. Coughing.

   f. Sniffing.

5. Label the inspiratory and expiratory phases; determine the duration of each; calculate the respiratory rate. Record this information in the LABORATORY REPORT RESULTS at the end of the chapter.

How does the respiratory rate change after hyperventilation? ______________________

____

____

EXERCISE 4. Measurement of Respiratory Volumes

> OBJECTIVES
>
> To define the components of total lung capacity
>
> To measure these volumes by spirometry

The ***respiratory rate*** of a normal adult is about 14–18 respirations per minute. Each cycle of inspiration and expiration involves the exchange of specific volumes of air between the atmosphere and the lungs. The volumes given in this exercise are those normal for a tall, healthy adolescent male.

The volume of air which is exchanged in normal, quiet breathing is the ***tidal volume***, usually about 500 ml (cc) of air. Each inspiration pulls about 500 ml of air into the respiratory passageways and alveoli, and the same amount moves out with each expiration. Only about 350 ml of this tidal volume actually reaches the alveoli. The other 150 ml, which remains in the nose, pharynx, larynx, trachea, and bronchial tubes, is called the ***dead air volume*** because it is not available for exchange.

A very deep breath (forced inspiration) can move about 3600 ml of air into the body. The air which can be inspired above the tidal volume is termed the ***inspiratory reserve volume***. It is usually about 3100 ml (3600 ml of forced inspiration minus 500 ml of tidal volume).

If we inspire a normal tidal volume and then expire with maximal force, we can push about 1200 ml of air out of the body in addition to the 500 ml tidal volume. The amount of air which can be forcibly expired after expiration of the tidal volume is the ***expiratory reserve volume***. Even after this forcible expiration, about 1200 ml of air remains in the lungs because the lower intrapleural pressure keeps the alveoli slightly inflated. This air, the ***residual volume***, amounts to about 1200 ml. Even if pneumothorax results from opening the chest cavity and atmospheric pressure forces most of the residual volume out of the lungs, a small amount of air, the ***minimal volume***, remains. This can be demonstrated by floating a piece of lung in water.

Lung capacities can be calculated by summing various volumes. The ***inspiratory capacity***, the total amount of air which can be inspired, is equal to the tidal volume plus the inspiratory reserve volume (500 ml + 3100 ml = 3600 ml). This capacity can be measured directly. The ***functional residual capacity***, the amount of air left after a normal exhalation of tidal volume, is the sum of the expiratory reserve volume and the residual volume (about 2400 ml). The ***vital capacity***, the total amount of air which can be moved in or out of the lungs, is the sum of the inspiratory reserve volume, the tidal volume, and the expiratory reserve volume (about 4800 ml). Finally, ***the total lung capacity*** is the sum of all volumes (about 6000 ml).

The residual volume cannot be measured directly since it cannot be exhaled. Consequently, neither the functional residual capacity nor the total lung capacity can be measured directly. However, the residual volume can be predicted on the basis of the measured vital capacity. Estimation factors are given for this purpose in Table 18.1. To determine a predicted residual volume, multiply the vital capacity by the age appropriate factor, e.g., if the vital capacity of a 16 year old is 4800 ml, the predicted residual capacity would be 4800 × .25 or 1200 ml.

Standards for the various volumes and capacities vary with height, age, and sex. The values given above, for example, are for an 18 year old male about 6 ′1½″. In general, female values are about 25% less than the values for a male of comparable height. These standards are obviously greater in athletes.

A ***respirometer (spirometer)*** is an instrument which is commonly used to measure these volumes and some capacities of the air exchanged in breathing. Three different types of respirometer are shown in Figure 18.4. The results of spirometry are graphed as a ***spirogram***; a simple spirogram is shown in Figure 18.5.

Spirometry can also measure the rate of air flow. If expired volume is measured per unit of time, it is called the ***forced expiratory volume (FEV_T)***. The T indicates that the volume of air is timed, FEV_1 is the volume of air forcibly expired in 1 second, FEV_2, the volume expired in 2 seconds, and so forth. A normal individual should be able to expire 83% of the total capacity during the first second, 94% in two seconds, and 97% in 3 seconds. Disorders such as emphysema and asthma can reduce the FEV_T considerably.

A. Use of Wet Spirometer

The wet spirometer, shown in Figure 18.4b, works by measuring the displacement of water by exhaled air. Inspiratory volumes must be calculated indirectly.

TABLE 18.1

Age	Residual volume estimation factor	Total lung capacity estimation factor
16–34	0.250	1.250
35–49	0.305	1.305
50–69	0.445	1.445

MATERIALS

Wet spirometer

Disposable mouthpieces

PROCEDURE

1. Examine the graduated scale on the spirometer and determine how it is read. Usually the scale will be calibrated in liters and tenths of liters.

2. Move the rubber indicator or the needle indicator to zero.

3. Place a mouthpiece in the spirometer tube and hold the tube in your hand while you breathe normally for a few respirations.

4. After a normal inspiration of the tidal volume, place the mouthpiece in your mouth and exhale normally through it to measure your ***tidal volume***.

5. Record the volume expired and *return the scale indicator to zero and make sure the bell is returned to its resting position in the water.*

6. Repeat steps 4 and 5 three times and average the results. Record in the LABORATORY REPORT RESULTS at the end of the chapter.

7. Breathe normally for a few respirations. Following a normal expiration of tidal volume, forcibly exhale as much air as possible into the spirometer tube to measure your ***expiratory reserve volume***.

8. Repeat steps 5 and 7 twice. Average your results and record in LABORATORY REPORT RESULTS at the end of the chapter.

9. To determine ***vital capacity***, breathe deeply a few times and inhale as much air as possible. Exhale as fully and as steadily as possible into the spirometer tube.

10. Repeat steps 5 and 9 twice. Average your results. *Dispose of the mouthpiece*.

11. Calculate your ***inspiratory reserve volume*** by substituting the known volumes in this equation.

Vital capacity = inspiratory reserve volume
+ tidal volume
+ expiratory reserve volume

Record this value in the LABORATORY REPORT RESULTS at the end of the chapter.

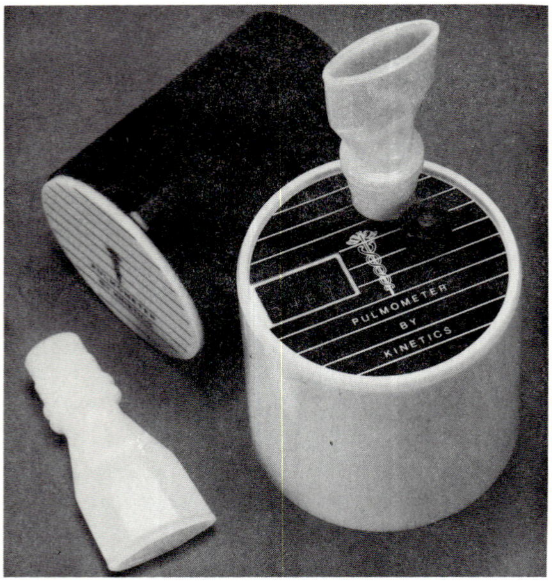

(a)

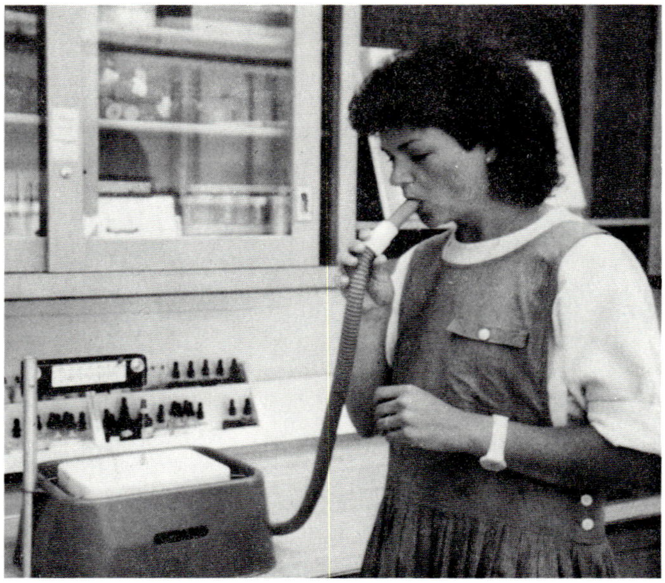

(b)

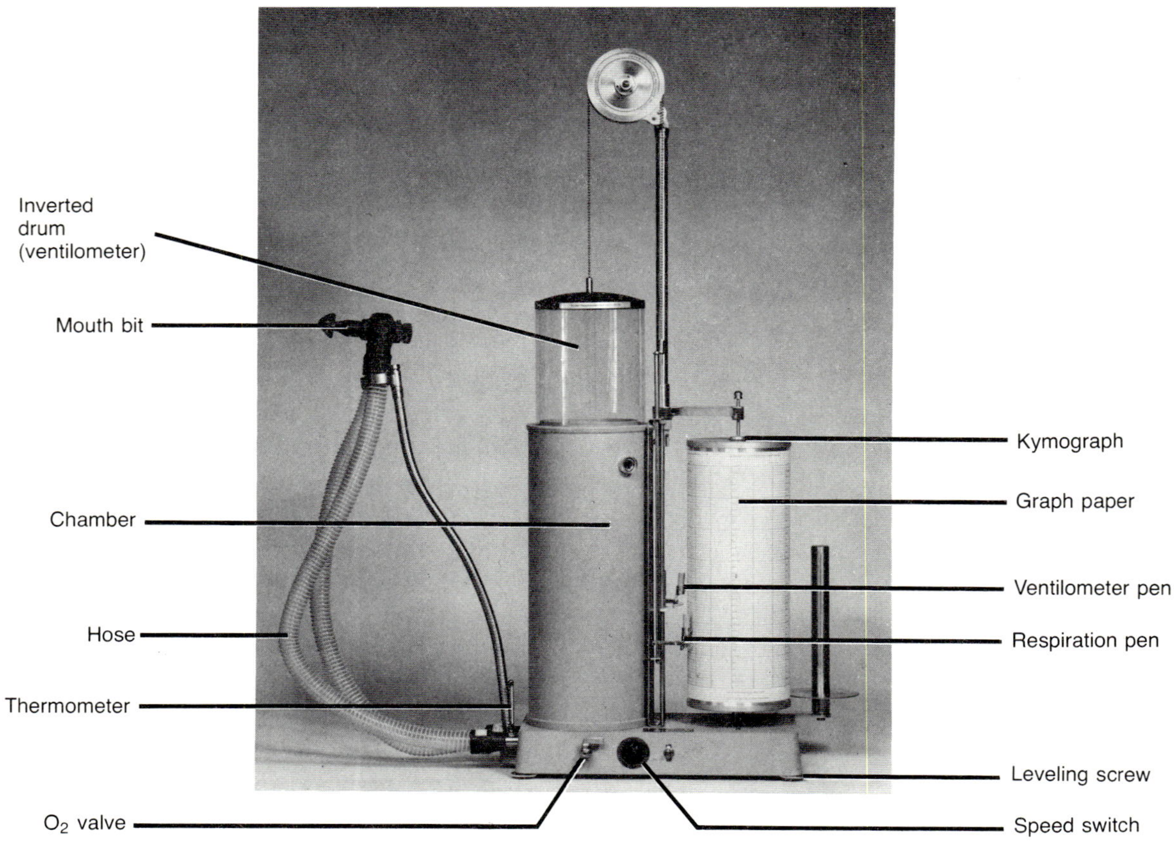

(c)

FIGURE 18.4 Respirometers. (a) Handheld respirometer. (b) Wet spirometer. (c) Collins respirometer.

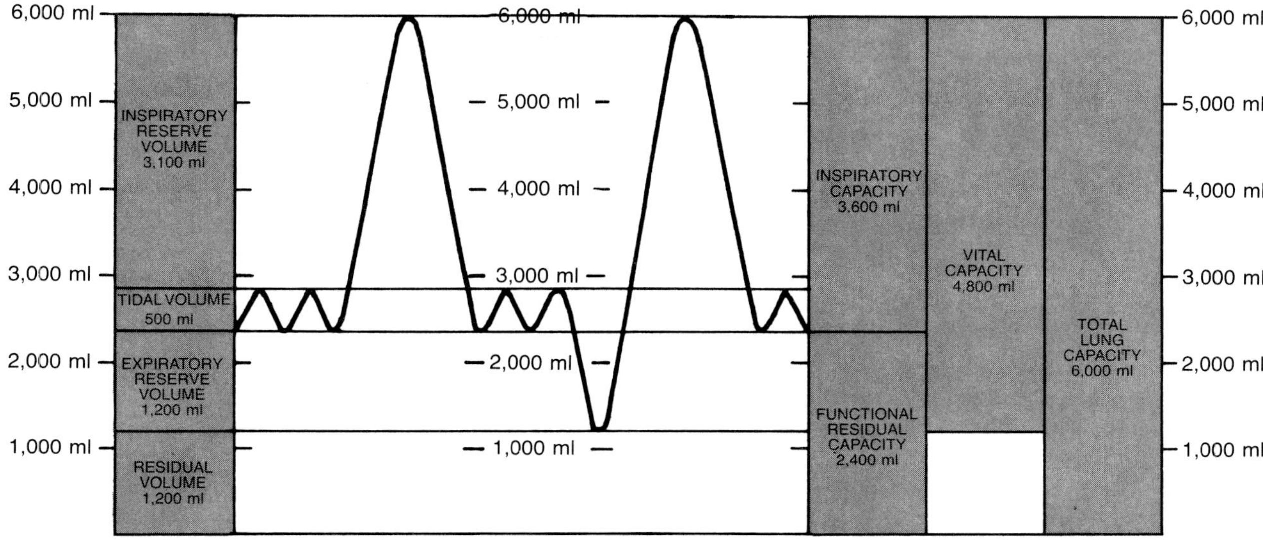

FIGURE 18.5 Spirogram of lung volumes and capacities.

12. Compare your vital capacity with the normal values shown in Tables 18.2 and 18.3.

13. Determine your ***residual volume*** by the use of Table 18.1 and your measured vital capacity. Calculate your total lung capacity. Record this value in the LABORATORY REPORT RESULTS at the end of the chapter.

14. Sit quietly and count your respirations per minute. Calculate your ***minute respiratory volume*** by multiplying the breaths per minute by your tidal volume.

$$\frac{\text{number breaths}}{\text{minute}} \times \frac{\text{number ml}}{\text{breath}} = \frac{\text{number ml}}{\text{minute}}$$

Record this value in the LABORATORY REPORT RESULTS at the end of the chapter.

B. Use of Handheld Spirometer

MATERIALS

Handheld spirometer
Disposable mouthpieces
Stopwatch

PROCEDURE

1. Set the needle or the digital indicator to zero.

2. *Place a clean mouthpiece in the spirometer tube* and hold the tube in your hand while you breathe normally for a few respirations. *NOTE: Inhale through the nose and exhale through the mouth.*

3. Place the mouthpiece in your mouth and inhale; exhale three normal breaths through the mouthpiece.

4. Divide the total volume of air expired by three to determine your average ***tidal volume***. Record in the LABORATORY REPORT RESULTS at the end of the chapter.

5. Return the scale indicator to zero.

6. Breathe normally for a few respirations. Following a normal expiration of tidal volume, forcibly exhale as much air as possible into the mouthpiece.

7. Repeat step 6 twice. Divide the total amount of air expired by three to determine your average ***expiratory reserve volume***. Record this value in the LABORATORY REPORT RESULTS at the end of the chapter.

8. To determine ***vital capacity***, breathe deeply a few times and inhale as much air as possible. Exhale as fully and as steadily as possible into the spirometer tube.

9. Repeat step 8 twice. Divide the total volume of expired air by three to determine your average vital capacity. Record this value in the LABORATORY REPORT RESULTS at the end of the chapter.

10. Calculate your ***inspiratory reserve volume*** by substituting the known volumes in this equation.

TABLE 18.2
PREDICTED VITAL CAPACITIES FOR FEMALES

	Height in centimeters and inches																		
	cm	152	154	156	158	160	162	164	166	168	170	172	174	176	178	180	182	184	186	188
Age	in.	59.8	60.6	61.4	62.2	63.0	63.7	64.6	65.4	66.1	66.9	67.7	68.5	69.3	70.1	70.9	71.7	72.4	73.2	74.0
16		3,070	3,110	3,150	3,190	3,230	3,270	3,310	3,350	3,390	3,430	3,470	3,510	3,550	3,590	3,630	3,670	3,715	3,755	3,800
17		3,055	3,095	3,135	3,175	3,215	3,255	3,295	3,335	3,375	3,415	3,455	3,495	3,535	3,575	3,615	3,655	3,695	3,740	3,780
18		3,040	3,080	3,120	3,160	3,200	3,240	3,280	3,320	3,360	3,400	3,440	3,480	3,520	3,560	3,600	3,640	3,680	3,720	3,760
20		3,010	3,050	3,090	3,130	3,170	3,210	3,250	3,290	3,330	3,370	3,410	3,450	3,490	3,525	3,565	3,605	3,645	3,695	3,720
22		2,980	3,020	3,060	3,095	3,135	3,175	3,215	3,255	3,290	3,330	3,370	3,410	3,450	3,490	3,530	3,570	3,610	3,650	3,685
24		2,950	2,985	3,025	3,065	3,100	3,140	3,180	3,220	3,260	3,300	3,335	3,375	3,415	3,455	3,490	3,530	3,570	3,610	3,650
26		2,920	2,960	3,000	3,035	3,070	3,110	3,150	3,190	3,230	3,265	3,300	3,340	3,380	3,420	3,455	3,495	3,530	3,570	3,610
28		2,890	2,930	2,965	3,000	3,040	3,070	3,115	3,155	3,190	3,230	3,270	3,305	3,345	3,380	3,420	3,460	3,495	3,535	3,570
30		2,860	2,895	2,935	2,970	3,010	3,045	3,085	3,120	3,160	3,195	3,235	3,270	3,310	3,345	3,385	3,420	3,460	3,495	3,535
32		2,825	2,865	2,900	2,940	2,975	3,015	3,050	3,090	3,125	3,160	3,200	3,235	3,275	3,310	3,350	3,385	3,425	3,460	3,495
34		2,795	2,835	2,870	2,910	2,945	2,980	3,020	3,055	3,090	3,130	3,165	3,200	3,240	3,275	3,310	3,350	3,385	3,425	3,460
36		2,765	2,805	2,840	2,875	2,910	2,950	2,985	3,020	3,060	3,095	3,130	3,165	3,205	3,240	3,275	3,310	3,350	3,385	3,420
38		2,735	2,770	2,810	2,845	2,880	2,915	2,950	2,990	3,025	3,060	3,095	3,130	3,170	3,205	3,240	3,275	3,310	3,350	3,385
40		2,705	2,740	2,775	2,810	2,850	2,885	2,920	2,955	2,990	3,025	3,060	3,095	3,135	3,170	3,205	3,240	3,275	3,310	3,345
42		2,675	2,710	2,745	2,780	2,815	2,850	2,885	2,920	2,955	2,990	3,025	3,060	3,100	3,135	3,170	3,205	3,240	3,275	3,310
44		2,645	2,680	2,715	2,750	2,785	2,820	2,855	2,890	2,925	2,960	2,995	3,030	3,060	3,095	3,130	3,165	3,200	3,235	3,270
46		2,615	2,650	2,685	2,715	2,750	2,785	2,820	2,855	2,890	2,925	2,960	2,995	3,030	3,060	3,095	3,130	3,165	3,200	3,235
48		2,585	2,620	2,650	2,685	2,715	2,750	2,785	2,820	2,855	2,890	2,925	2,960	2,995	3,030	3,060	3,095	3,130	3,160	3,195
50		2,555	2,590	2,625	2,655	2,690	2,720	2,755	2,785	2,820	2,855	2,890	2,925	2,955	2,990	3,025	3,060	3,090	3,125	3,155
52		2,525	2,555	2,590	2,625	2,655	2,690	2,720	2,755	2,790	2,820	2,855	2,890	2,925	2,955	2,990	3,020	3,055	3,090	3,125
54		2,495	2,530	2,560	2,590	2,625	2,655	2,690	2,720	2,755	2,790	2,820	2,855	2,885	2,920	2,950	2,985	3,020	3,050	3,085
56		2,460	2,495	2,525	2,560	2,590	2,625	2,655	2,690	2,720	2,755	2,790	2,820	2,855	2,885	2,920	2,950	2,980	3,015	3,045
58		2,430	2,460	2,495	2,525	2,560	2,590	2,625	2,655	2,690	2,720	2,750	2,785	2,815	2,850	2,880	2,920	2,945	2,975	3,010
60		2,400	2,430	2,460	2,495	2,525	2,560	2,590	2,625	2,655	2,685	2,720	2,750	2,780	2,810	2,845	2,875	2,915	2,940	2,970
62		2,370	2,405	2,435	2,465	2,495	2,525	2,560	2,590	2,620	2,655	2,685	2,715	2,745	2,775	2,810	2,840	2,870	2,900	2,935
64		2,340	2,370	2,400	2,430	2,465	2,495	2,525	2,555	2,585	2,620	2,650	2,680	2,710	2,740	2,770	2,805	2,835	2,865	2,895
66		2,310	2,340	2,370	2,400	2,430	2,460	2,495	2,525	2,555	2,585	2,615	2,645	2,675	2,705	2,735	2,765	2,800	2,825	2,860
68		2,280	2,310	2,340	2,370	2,400	2,430	2,460	2,490	2,520	2,550	2,580	2,610	2,640	2,670	2,700	2,730	2,760	2,795	2,820
70		2,250	2,280	2,310	2,340	2,370	2,400	2,425	2,455	2,485	2,515	2,545	2,575	2,605	2,635	2,665	2,695	2,725	2,755	2,780
72		2,220	2,250	2,280	2,310	2,335	2,365	2,395	2,425	2,455	2,480	2,510	2,540	2,570	2,600	2,630	2,660	2,685	2,715	2,745
74		2,190	2,220	2,245	2,275	2,305	2,335	2,360	2,390	2,420	2,450	2,475	2,505	2,535	2,565	2,590	2,620	2,650	2,680	2,710

From: *Archives of Environmental Health,* February, 1966, Vol. 12, pp. 146–189, E. A. Gaensler, MD and G. W. Wright, MD.

TABLE 18.3
PREDICTED VITAL CAPACTITIES FOR MALES

	Height in centimeters and inches																		
	cm	152	154	156	158	160	162	164	166	168	170	172	174	176	178	180	182	184	186	188
Age	in.	59.8	60.6	61.4	62.2	63.0	63.7	64.6	65.4	66.1	66.9	67.7	68.5	69.3	70.1	70.9	71.7	72.4	73.2	74.0
16		3,920	3,975	4,025	4,075	4,130	4,180	4,230	4,285	4,335	4,385	4,440	4,490	4,540	4,590	4,645	4,695	4,745	4,800	4,850
18		3,890	3,940	3,995	4,045	4,095	4,145	4,200	4,250	4,300	4,350	4,405	4,455	4,505	4,555	4,610	4,660	4,710	4,760	4,815
20		3,860	3,910	3,960	4,015	4,065	4,115	4,165	4,215	4,265	4,320	4,370	4,420	4,470	4,520	4,570	4,625	4,675	4,725	4,775
22		3,830	3,880	3,930	3,980	4,030	4,080	4,135	4,185	4,235	4,285	4,335	4,385	4,435	4,485	4,535	4,585	4,635	4,685	4,735
24		3,785	3,835	3,885	3,935	3,985	4,035	4,085	4,135	4,185	4,235	4,285	4,330	4,380	4,430	4,480	4,530	4,580	4,630	4,680
26		3,755	3,805	3,855	3,905	3,955	4,000	4,050	4,100	4,150	4,200	4,250	4,300	4,350	4,395	4,445	4,495	4,545	4,595	4,645
28		3,725	3,775	3,820	3,870	3,920	3,970	4,020	4,070	4,115	4,165	4,215	4,265	4,310	4,360	4,410	4,460	4,510	4,555	4,605
30		3,695	3,740	3,790	3,840	3,890	3,935	3,985	4,035	4,080	4,130	4,180	4,230	4,275	4,325	4,375	4,425	4,470	4,520	4,570
32		3,665	3,710	3,760	3,810	3,855	3,905	3,950	4,000	4,050	4,095	4,145	4,195	4,240	4,290	4,340	4,385	4,435	4,485	4,530
34		3,620	3,665	3,715	3,760	3,810	3,855	3,905	3,950	4,000	4,045	4,095	4,140	4,190	4,225	4,285	4,330	4,380	4,425	4,475
36		3,585	3,635	3,680	3,730	3,775	3,825	3,870	3,920	3,965	4,010	4,060	4,105	4,155	4,200	4,250	4,295	4,340	4,390	4,435
38		3,555	3,605	3,650	3,695	3,745	3,790	3,840	3,885	3,930	3,980	4,025	4,070	4,120	4,165	4,210	4,260	4,305	4,350	4,400
40		3,525	3,575	3,620	3,665	3,710	3,760	3,805	3,850	3,900	3,945	3,990	4,035	4,085	4,130	4,175	4,220	4,270	4,315	4,360
42		3,495	3,540	3,590	3,635	3,680	3,725	3,770	3,820	3,865	3,910	3,955	4,000	4,050	4,095	4,140	4,185	4,230	4,280	4,325
44		3,450	3,495	3,540	3,585	3,630	3,675	3,725	3,770	3,815	3,860	3,905	3,950	3,995	4,040	4,085	4,130	4,175	4,220	4,270
46		3,420	3,465	3,510	3,555	3,600	3,645	3,690	3,735	3,780	3,825	3,870	3,915	3,960	4,005	4,050	4,095	4,140	4,185	4,230
48		3,390	3,435	3,480	3,525	3,570	3,615	3,655	3,700	3,745	3,790	3,835	3,880	3,925	3,970	4,015	4,060	4,105	4,150	4,190
50		3,345	3,390	3,430	3,475	3,520	3,565	3,610	3,650	3,695	3,740	3,785	3,830	3,870	3,915	3,960	4,005	4,050	4,090	4,135
52		3,315	3,353	3,400	3,445	3,490	3,530	3,575	3,620	3,660	3,705	3,750	3,795	3,835	3,880	3,925	3,970	4,010	4,055	4,100
54		3,285	3,325	3,370	3,415	3,455	3,500	3,540	3,585	3,630	3,670	3,715	3,760	3,800	3,845	3,890	3,930	3,975	4,020	4,060
56		3,255	3,295	3,340	3,380	3,425	3,465	3,510	3,550	3,595	3,640	3,680	3,725	3,765	3,810	3,850	3,895	3,940	3,980	4,025
58		3,210	3,250	3,290	3,335	3,375	3,420	3,460	3,500	3,545	3,585	3,630	3,670	3,715	3,755	3,800	3,840	3,880	3,925	3,965
60		3,175	3,220	3,260	3,300	3,345	3,385	3,430	3,470	3,500	3,555	3,595	3,635	3,680	3,720	3,760	3,805	3,845	3,885	3,930
62		3,150	3,190	3,230	3,270	3,310	3,350	3,390	3,440	3,480	3,520	3,560	3,600	3,640	3,680	3,730	3,770	3,810	3,850	3,890
64		3,120	3,160	3,200	3,240	3,280	3,320	3,360	3,400	3,440	3,490	3,530	3,570	3,610	3,650	3,690	3,730	3,770	3,810	3,850
66		3,070	3,110	3,150	3,190	3,230	3,270	3,310	3,350	3,390	3,430	3,470	3,510	3,550	3,600	3,640	3,680	3,720	3,760	3,800
68		3,040	3,080	3,120	3,160	3,200	3,240	3,280	3,320	3,360	3,400	3,440	3,480	3,520	3,560	3,600	3,640	3,680	3,720	3,760
70		3,010	3,050	3,090	3,130	3,170	3,210	3,250	3,290	3,330	3,370	3,410	3,450	3,480	3,520	3,560	3,600	3,640	3,680	3,720
72		2,980	3,020	3,060	3,100	3,140	3,180	3,210	3,250	3,290	3,330	3,370	3,410	3,450	3,490	3,530	3,570	3,610	3,650	3,680
74		2,930	2,970	3,010	3,050	3,090	3,130	3,170	3,200	3,240	3,280	3,320	3,360	3,400	3,440	3,470	3,510	3,550	3,590	3,630

From: *Archives of Environmental Health,* February, 1966, Vol. 12, pp. 146–189, E. A. Gaensler, MD and G. W. Wright, MD.

Vital capacity = inspiratory reserve volume
+ tidal volume
+ expiratory reserve volume

Record this volume in the LABORATORY REPORT RESULTS at the end of the chapter.

11. Compare your vital capacity with the normal values shown in Tables 18.2 and 18.3.

12. Determine your ***residual volume*** by the use of Table 18.1 and your measured vital capacity. Calculate your ***total lung capacity***. Record this value in the LABORATORY REPORT RESULTS at the end of the chapter.

13. Sit quietly and count your respirations per minute. Calculate your ***minute respiratory volume*** by multiplying the breaths per minute by your tidal volume.

$$\frac{\text{number breaths}}{\text{minute}} \times \frac{\text{number ml}}{\text{breath}} = \frac{\text{number ml}}{\text{minute}}$$

Record this value in the LABORATORY REPORT RESULTS at the end of the chapter.

C. Use of Collins Respirometer

The Collins respirometer, pictured in Figure 18.4c, is a closed system which allows the measurement of volumes of air inhaled and exhaled. The air volumes are recorded on a spirogram; the horizontal (x) axis of the spirogram is graduated in millimeters and records elapsed time; the vertical (y) axis is graduated in milliliters and records air volumes.

The air in the body is at a different temperature than the air contained in the respirometer; body air is also saturated with water vapor. To make the correction for these differences, one measures the temperature of the respirometer and uses Table 18.4 to obtain a conversion factor (***BTPS factor:*** Body Temperature, atmospheric Pressure, Saturated with water vapor). All measured volumes are then multiplied by this factor.

MATERIALS

Collins respirometer

Disposable mouthpieces or rubber mouthpiece and 70% alcohol and cotton

Nose clamp (optional)

TABLE 18.4
TEMPERATURE VARIATION CONVERSION FACTORS

Temperature °C (°F)	Conversion factor
20 (68.0)	1.102
21 (69.8)	1.096
22 (71.6)	1.091
23 (73.4)	1.085
24 (75.2)	1.080
25 (77.0)	1.075
26 (78.8)	1.068
27 (80.6)	1.063
28 (82.4)	1.057
29 (84.2)	1.051
30 (86.0)	1.045
31 (87.8)	1.039
32 (89.6)	1.032
33 (91.4)	1.026
34 (93.2)	1.020
35 (95.0)	1.014
36 (96.8)	1.007
37 (98.6)	1.000

PROCEDURE

1. *When using the Collins respirometer, the disposable mouthpiece is discarded after use by each subject, and the hose is then detached and rinsed with 70% alcohol.* CAUTION! *This procedure must be repeated by every student using the equipment.*

2. Students should work in pairs, with one student operating the respirometer while the other student is the subject.

3. Before starting the recording, a little practice may be necessary to learn to inhale and exhale only through your mouth and into the hose. A nose clip may be used to prevent nose breathing.

4. Make sure that the respirometer is functioning. Your instructor may have already prepared the instrument for use.

a. The leveling screws must be raised/lowered so that the bell does not rub on the metal body.

b. Paper must be fed from a roll onto the kymograph OR taped onto the kymograph in single sheets.

c. The soda-lime which absorbs carbon dioxide must be pink (fresh) and not purple (saturated with CO_2).

d. Pen reservoirs must be full and primed.

5. Raise and lower the drum several times to flush the respirometer of stale air.

6. Position the ventilometer pen (the upper pen, usually with black ink) so that it will begin writing in the center of the spirogram paper.

7. Set the free-breathing valve so that the opening is seen through the side of the valve.

8. Place a *sterile or disposable mouthpiece* in the mouth and close the nose with a clamp or with the fingers.

9. Breathe several times to become accustomed to the use of this instrument.

10. Have your lab partner close the free-breathing valve (turn it completely to the opposite direction so that no opening is seen) and turn on the respirometer to the slow speed. At this setting, the kymograph moves 32 mm (the distance between two vertical lines) each minute.

11. Breathe normally for 1 minute to record ***tidal volumes***.

12. At the end of 1 minute, have your lab partner instruct you to expire maximally at the end of a normal (tidal) expiration, in order to chart your ***expiratory reserve volume***. Breathe normally for five more breaths.

13. Inspire maximally and expire maximally to record your ***vital capacity***.

14. After five tidal respirations, inspire maximally and hold your breath while your partner sets the recording switch to fast speed (1920 mm/min.). At this speed, the kymograph moves the distance between two adjacent vertical lines each second.

15. To measure your ***FEV**$_T$*, exhale as rapidly and forcibly as possible until you can no longer expire any air.

16. Turn off the spirometer and remove the spirogram. If you are using a rubber mouthpiece, follow your instructor's directions for cleaning; if you are using a disposable mouthpiece, discard it.

17. Evaluate the spirogram as described in the following section.

EVALUATION OF THE SPIROGRAM

a. Study the spirogram carefully. The recording is made from right to left. Inhalation causes upward movement of the recording pen; exhalation results in downward movement. A sample spirogram is depicted in Figure 18.6.

b. To measure ***tidal volume***, measure the distance of five breaths made in the first minute (right-hand portion of the spirogram). Subtract the measurement at each trough from the measurement of the corresponding (right-hand) peak. Sum the five volumes and average by dividing by 5. Multiply your result by the BTPS factor. In all sample calculations, the temperature will be assumed to be 21°C; hence, a BTPS factor of 1.096 will be used. Record your results in the LABORATORY REPORT RESULTS at the end of the chapter.

EXAMPLE from Figure 18.6

$$
\begin{aligned}
2510 \text{ ml} - 2000 \text{ ml} &= 510 \text{ ml} \\
2590 \text{ ml} - 2070 \text{ ml} &= 520 \text{ ml} \\
2600 \text{ ml} - 2100 \text{ ml} &= 500 \text{ ml} \\
2650 \text{ ml} - 2140 \text{ ml} &= 510 \text{ ml} \\
2710 \text{ ml} - 2200 \text{ ml} &= 510 \text{ ml} \\
\hline
& \quad 2550 \text{ ml}/5 \\
&= 510 \text{ ml} \times 1.096 \\
&= 559
\end{aligned}
$$

c. To calculate your ***expiratory reserve volume***, measure the column recorded during step 12 and subtract your average tidal volume from it. Multiply this volume by the BTPS factor and record your measurement in the LABORATORY REPORT RESULTS at the end of the chapter.

EXAMPLE from Figure 18.6

$$
\begin{aligned}
2850 \text{ ml} - 1250 \text{ ml} &= 1600 \text{ ml} \\
1600 \text{ ml} \times 1.096 &= 1754 \text{ ml} - 559 \text{ ml} \\
&= 1195 \text{ ml}
\end{aligned}
$$

d. To calculate your ***inspiratory reserve volume***, measure the maximal inspiration recorded in step 13 and subtract from it the previous tidal inspiration. Multiply this volume by the BTPS factor and record your measurement in the LABORATORY REPORT RESULTS at the end of the chapter.

EXAMPLE from Figure 18.6

$$
\begin{aligned}
4210 \text{ ml} - 420 \text{ ml} &= 3790 \text{ ml} \\
3790 \text{ ml} \times 1.096 &= 3458 \text{ ml}
\end{aligned}
$$

e. To calculate your ***vital capacity***, measure the volumes recorded in steps 13 and 15; average them and multiply the average by the BTPS factor. Record the average in the LABORA-

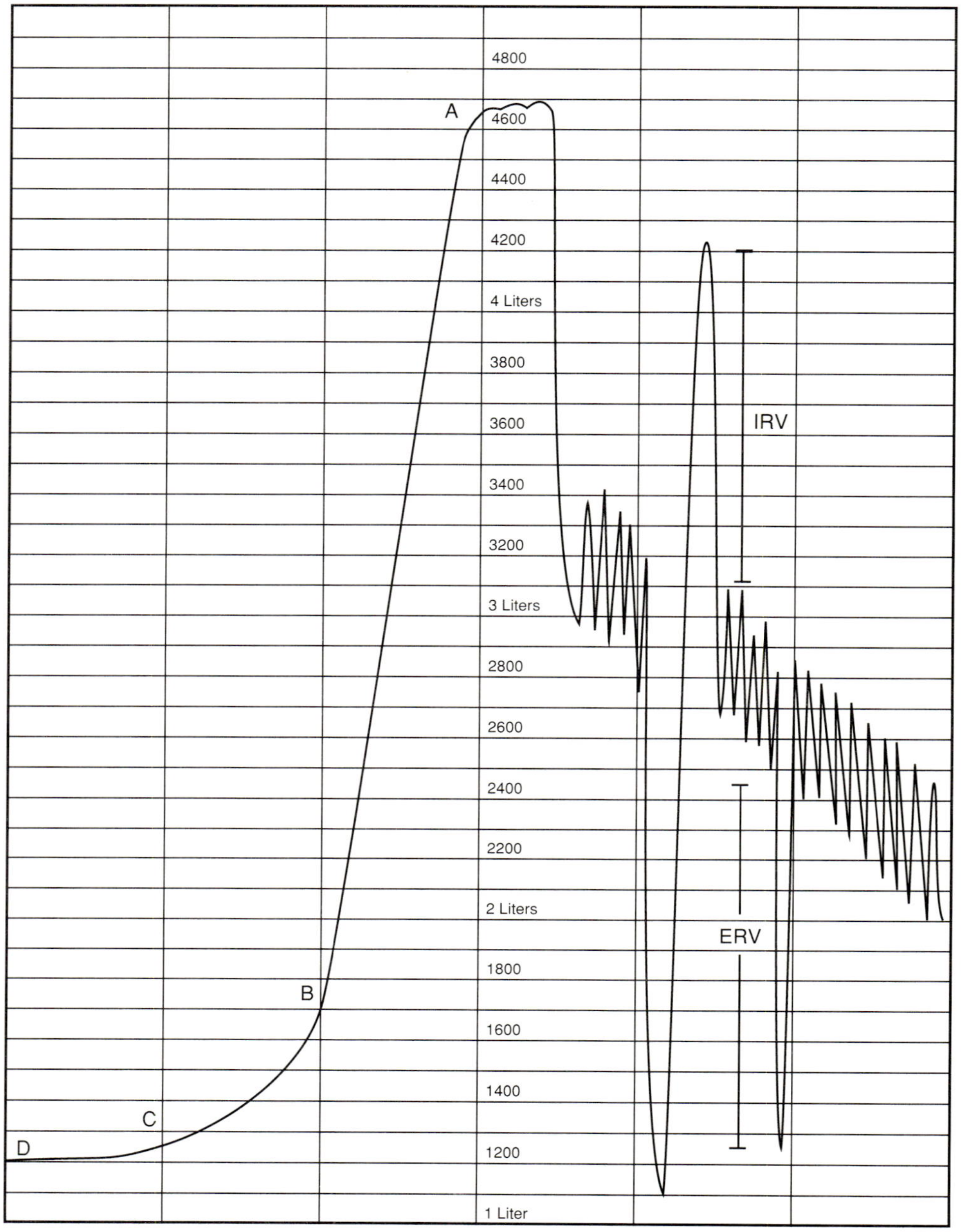

FIGURE 18.6 Spirogram from Collins respirometer.

TORY REPORT RESULTS at the end of the chapter.

EXAMPLE from Figure 18.6

4210 ml − 1100 ml = 3110 ml
4650 ml − 1200 ml = <u>3450 ml</u>
6560 ml ÷ 2
= 3280 ml × 1.096
= 3595 ml

f. Compare your vital capacity with the normal values shown in Tables 18.2 and 18.3.

g. To determine your ***FEV***$_T$

1. Obtain your total vital capacity from step 12 (and calculated in step e).

2. Determine the FEV_1 by marking the beginning of expiration (just left of the plateau resulting from breath holding) as

Point A and then measuring 3.2 cm to the left (mark this Point B).

3. Measure the volume exhaled during this 1 second interval (the distance from Point A to Point B).

EXAMPLE from Figure 18.6

$$4650 \text{ ml} - 1700 \text{ ml} = 2950 \text{ ml}$$

4. Divide by the total vital capacity and multiply by 100 to derive the ***FEV***$_1$, the percent of vital capacity exhaled in the first second.

EXAMPLE from Figure 18.6

$$2950 \text{ ml} \div 3595 \text{ ml} = .82$$
$$.82 \times 100 = 82\%$$

5. Measure 3.2 cm to the left of Point B and mark it Point C. Measure the volume exhaled during the first two second interval (Point A to Point C).

EXAMPLE from Figure 18.6

$$4650 \text{ ml} - 1250 \text{ ml} = 3400 \text{ ml}$$

6. Divide this volume by the total vital capacity and multiply by 100 to derive the ***FEV***$_2$, the percent of vital capacity exhaled in the first two seconds.

EXAMPLE from Figure 18.6

$$3400 \text{ ml} \div 3595 \text{ ml} = .946 \times 100 = 94.6\%$$

7. Measure 3.2 cm to the left of Point C and mark it Point D. Measure the volume expired in the first three seconds (Point A to Point D).

EXAMPLE from Figure 18.6

$$4650 \text{ ml} - 1200 \text{ ml} = 3450 \text{ ml}$$

8. Divide this volume by the total vital capacity and multiply by 100 to derive the ***FEV***$_3$, the percent of vital capacity exhaled in the first three seconds.

EXAMPLE from Figure 18.6

$$3450 \text{ ml} \div 3595 \text{ ml} = .96 \times 100$$
$$= 96\%$$

9. Record these forced expiratory volumes in the LABORATORY REPORT RESULTS at the end of the chapter.

h. Determine your ***residual volume*** by the use of Table 18.1 and your measured vital capacity. Calculate your ***total lung capacity*** (TLC = RV + VC). Record the result in the LABORATORY REPORT RESULTS at the end of the chapter.

i. Sit quietly and count your respirations per minute. Calculate your ***minute respiratory volume*** by multiplying the breaths per minute by your tidal volume.

$$\frac{\text{number breaths}}{\text{minute}} \times \frac{\text{number ml}}{\text{breath}} = \frac{\text{number ml}}{\text{minute}}$$

Record this value in the LABORATORY REPORT RESULTS at the end of the chapter.

EXERCISE 5. Chemical Regulation of Respiration

OBJECTIVES

To test the effects of hyperventilation, rebreathing air, and exercise on the respiratory rate

To measure the CO_2 content of exhaled air

The rate and depth of respiration are controlled by respiratory centers in the medulla oblongata which send nerve impulses to the muscles of respiration. Inspiration is stimulated when the pH falls, to a lesser extent by a rise in the PCO_2, and when there is a gross reduction in the PO_2 of arterial blood.

The gas composition and pH of arterial blood are reflections of the metabolic activity of the body and of respiration. *In vivo*, the pH and the PCO_2 are intimately connected, since carbon dioxide (CO_2) combines with water (H_2O) in the presence of carbonic anhydrase to form carbonic acid (H_2CO_3), which then dissociates into hydrogen (H^+) ions and bicarbonate (HCO_3^-) ions.

$$CO_2 + H_2O \xrightarrow{\text{carbonic anhydrase}} H_2CO_3 \rightarrow H^+ + HCO_3^-$$

Thus, the pH of blood, the measurement of the H^+ ion concentration, is a direct function of the PCO_2 of the blood.

The respiratory centers in the medulla are also controlled by cerebral input, as well as input from (1) chemoreceptors in the aortic arch and carotid body and (2) chemoreceptors in the medulla oblongata itself.

The aortic arch and carotid body contain cells that are sensitive to very small changes in the pH and the PCO_2 of arterial blood. In addition they are also triggered by gross reductions in the PO_2 of arterial blood.

The chemoreceptors in the medulla are primarily sensitive to the pH of cerebrospinal fluid (CSF). Since CSF is manufactured from arterial blood in the choroid plexi, its PCO_2 is equivalent to the PCO_2 of arterial blood. The CO_2 in CSF yields hydrogen ions as described previously. An increase in H^+ ion content (measured by a reduction in pH) then triggers the inspiratory center to increase its rate of stimulation to the muscles of inspiration.

Increased respiration increases excretion of carbon dioxide, hence it also increases the pH of arterial blood and of CSF. In a typical negative feedback pattern, stimulation of the inspiratory center is decreased, and the respiratory rate decreases.

We can measure the effect of various factors on respiration by measuring (1) the rate of respiration, or (2) the CO_2 content of exhaled air. In order to measure CO_2 content, a gas is bubbled through lime water and the time is measured until the liquid becomes cloudy. Lime water is a solution of calcium hydroxide ($Ca(OH)_2$). The cloudiness occurs because carbon dioxide combines with calcium hydroxide to form calcium carbonate, a white precipitate, in the following reaction.

CO_2	+	$Ca(OH)_2$	→	$CaCO_3$	+	H_2O
Carbon dioxide		Calcium hydroxide		Calcium carbonate		Water

MATERIALS

Four Pyrex test tubes
Test tube rack
Marking pencil
Paper bag
Nose clamp (optional)
Straw or pipette
Calcium hydroxide (lime water) solution
Stopwatch
Safety goggles
Laboratory apron or coat

PROCEDURE

1. Label three test tubes N, H, and E (Normal, Hyperventilation, Exercise). Fill each about half full of calcium hydroxide ($Ca(OH)_2$) solution.

2. While pinching the nose, start the stopwatch and exhale normal expirations through the straw into tube N. Note the time elapsed until the solution becomes turbid.

3. Hyperventilate about 30 seconds to 1 minute.

CAUTION! *Stop hyperventilation at the first sensation of dizziness or lightheadedness.*

4. Repeat step 2, *exhaling* normally into tube H.

5. CAUTION! *If your partner has no known cardiac or other health problems and is capable of such an activity, ask her/him, after a 2 minute rest, to exercise briskly for 2 minutes.*

6. Repeat step 2, *exhaling* into tube E.

7. Record all times in the LABORATORY REPORT RESULTS at the end of the chapter.

In which situation was the CO_2 content of exhaled air the greatest? ______________

Why? ______________________________

____

COMPLETE THE LABORATORY REPORT QUESTIONS AT THE END OF THE CHAPTER

LABORATORY REPORT QUESTIONS

RESPIRATORY PHYSIOLOGY 18

Student ________________________ Date ________________________

Laboratory Section ________________________ Score/Grade ________________________

EXERCISE 1. Mechanics of Respiration

B. Chest and Abdomen Measurement

Size After	Chest	Abdomen
Normal inspiration		
Normal expiration		
Maximal inspiration		
Maximal expiration		

EXERCISE 2. Respiratory Sounds

Sounds Heard	At Inspiration	At Expiration
Below larynx		
Intercostal space		
Below clavicle		
Interscapular space		

EXERCISE 3. Use of Pneumograph

Attach the record of a breathing pattern on the back of this page. Label the phases and duration of phases. Calculate the respiratory rate.

EXERCISE 4. Measurement of Respiratory Volumes

	Your Average	Normal Value
Tidal volume		
Expiratory reserve volume		
Vital capacity		
Inspiratory reserve volume		
FEV_1		
FEV_2		
FEV_3		
Estimated residual volume		
Estimated total lung capacity		
Resting respiratory rate		
Minute respiratory volume		

EXERCISE 5. Chemical Regulation of Respiration

	Time Until Turbidity	Respiratory Rate
Tidal respirations		
After hyperventilation		
After exercise		

LABORATORY REPORT QUESTIONS

RESPIRATORY PHYSIOLOGY 18

Student ______________________ **Date** ______________________

Laboratory Section ______________________ **Score/Grade** ______________________

PART I. MATCHING

_____ 1. Tidal volume
_____ 2. Inspiratory reserve volume
_____ 3. Inspiratory capacity
_____ 4. Expiratory reserve volume
_____ 5. Vital capacity
_____ 6. Total lung capacity
_____ 7. Dead air volume
_____ 8. Functional residual capacity
_____ 9. Residual volume

A. 350 ml
B. 500 ml
C. 1200 ml
D. 2400 ml
E. 3100 ml
F. 3600 ml
G. 6000 ml

PART II. MULTIPLE CHOICE

_____ 10. Which of the following is increased in emphysema? (a) FEV_1 (b) residual volume (c) vital capacity (d) all of the above (e) none of the above

_____ 11. The respiratory rate increases following (a) exercise (b) hyperventilation (c) increase in PO_2 in arterial blood (d) all of the above (e) none of the above

_____ 12. The primary stimulus for the inspiratory center in the medulla is (a) increased PO_2 in arterial blood (b) increased pH of CSF (c) increased H^+ ion concentration in CSF (d) increased PCO_2 of arterial blood

_____ 13. The FEV_1 is (a) the amount of air exhaled in one second (b) the percent of vital capacity exhaled in one second (c) the percent of total lung capacity exhaled in one second (d) the time required to exhale the vital capacity

_____ 14. The pneumograph measures (a) volumes of air expired (b) the rate and depth of respiration (c) the PO_2 and PCO_2 (d) respiratory capacities (e) all of the above

_____ 15. Pneumothorax (a) can result from a depressed respiratory rate (b) is caused by overinflation of the lung (c) results when intrapleural pressure equals atmospheric pressure (d) all of the above (d) none of the above

_____ 16. A normal respiratory rate is (a) 4–8/minute (b) 14–18/minute (c) 32–40/minute (d) 72–80/minute

_____ 17. Surfactant (a) is manufactured by alveolar cells (b) covers the outer surface of alveoli (c) causes infant respiratory distress syndrome (hyaline membrane disease) when produced in excess amounts (d) all of the above (e) none of the above

_____ 18. The dead air volume is (a) the air that remains in the lungs after expiring the expiratory reserve volume (b) the air that remains in the lungs following pneumothorax (c) the portion of the tidal volume that is not available for gas exchange

_____ 19. At high altitudes where the atmospheric PO_2 is low (a) respiratory rate will increase (b) respiratory minute volume will increase (c) arterial blood PCO_2 will decrease (d) all of the above (e) none of the above

PART III. COMPARISONS. FILL IN THE BLANKS WITH > (GREATER THAN) OR < (LESS THAN)

20. Intrapleural pressure _____ Intrapulmonic pressure

21. PCO_2 in alveolar air _____ PCO_2 in venous blood

22. PO_2 in alveolar air _____ PO_2 in venous blood

23. Size of thorax at end of inspiration _____ Size of thorax at end of expiration

24. Intrapulmonic pressure at beginning of expiration _____ Intrapulmonic pressure at beginning of inspiration

25. Abdominal diameter at inspiration _____ Abdominal diameter at expiration

26. Respiratory rate after exercise _____ Respiratory rate after hyperventilation

27. Functional residual capacity _____ Residual volume

28. FEV_1 _____ FEV_2

29. Blood pH after hyperventilation _____ Blood pH after tidal respirations

DISCUSSION: A. Hysterical or severely stressed individuals tend to hyperventilate. This may lead to a severe reduction in the respiratory rate and even to fainting. Treatment consists of breathing into a paper bag. Explain the cause of the symptoms and the rationale for the treatment.

DISCUSSION: B. Premature infants may have respiratory distress syndrome (RDS) of the newborn (hyaline membrane disease), since surfactant is not produced until late in fetal life. Explain (1) how a lack of surfactant could cause atelectasis (nonexpansion of the lung) and (2) how treatment with CPAP (continuous positive airway pressure) to keep the airways open might cause the complication of pneumothorax.

EXERCISE PHYSIOLOGY 19

EXERCISE 1. Muscular Flexibility
A. Toe Touch
B. Flexibility Index
C. Effect of Warm-up
EXERCISE 2. Muscular Strength
EXERCISE 3. Muscular Endurance and Aerobic Fitness

Physical fitness is dependent on many interrelated factors. One indicator of physical fitness is ***body composition***, the percent of fat-free body weight that will be determined in Chapter 21, Exercise 1. Fitness also involves factors such as agility, balance, coordination, and reaction time. Important components of fitness include the cardiovascular and respiratory responses to physical stress. The physical fitness of muscle can be measured by three indicators: ***strength***, the ability of muscles to exert force; ***endurance***, the ability of muscles to exert sustained force for a long period of time or for many repetitions of a task; and ***flexibility***, the range of motion available at joints. These parameters can be measured separately or combined to give a general index of muscular fitness.

For this laboratory, you should wear comfortable clothing and athletic shoes. CAUTION! *If you are not feeling well, or if you have ANY condition that could be jeopardized by exercise, do NOT attempt these exercises. If there is ANY question of your fitness, do not participate in these exercises without permission from your physician*. You may obtain the appropriate data by observing others.

EXERCISE 1. Muscular Flexibility

OBJECTIVES

To measure muscular flexibility
To define and measure the effects of warm-up exercise

Movement at joints is limited by the shape of the joint, by tendons and ligaments, and by fascia that covers muscles. Flexibility can be developed through stretching exercises which increase the range of motion available.

Warm-up exercises can be used to increase flexibility and also to prevent injury. The ideal warm-up time for an individual depends on the state of conditioning of their muscles; the maximum effective warm-up time is about 15 minutes.

Muscle contraction produces heat. After warm-up, neural transmission is more rapid and muscles are more flexible because, within limits, the rate of chemical reactions increases with increased temperature.

In this exercise, you will measure the effect of warm-up and determine your flexibility score.

MATERIALS

Ruler or meter stick
Stool
Masking tape

PROCEDURE

A. Toe Touch

1. Tape a ruler or meter stick to a stool with the zero end pointing upward (see Figure 19.1).
2. Remove your shoes and stand on the stool.
3. Let your hands drop and bend down as smoothly and slowly as possible *without bouncing*. Keep your knees straight and reach equally with both hands.
4. Have your laboratory partner measure the distance you stretched and record the measurement in the LABORATORY REPORT RESULTS at the end of the chapter.

B. Flexibility Index

1. Place a 6 inch strip of masking tape on the floor or exercise mat and a yardstick perpendicular to the tape so that the 15 inch mark is on the tape edge.
2. Sit on the floor with legs stretched in front of you and the yardstick between your legs, with the 36 inch end farthest from you and your heels at the tape edge (15 inch mark).
3. Bend at the waist and reach for your toes. Hold the position for 20 seconds. Repeat five times.
4. Slowly reach as far forward as possible without jerking and have your laboratory partner measure the farthest point you can reach. Record the best of three tries in the LABORATORY REPORT RESULTS at the end of the chapter.
5. Determine your flexibility score from Table 19.1. A score of 50 is average for flexibility in a forward bend.

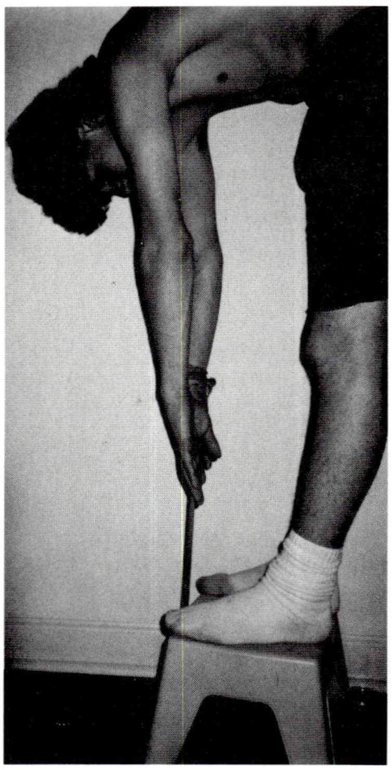

FIGURE 19.1 Position for toe touch. (Courtesy of Bruce Adams.)

C. Effect of Warm-up

1. Repeat steps 2 to 4 of section A three times and average your results. Record the distance in the LABORATORY REPORT RESULTS at the end of the chapter.

Why do you think a 30 minute warm-up would be counterproductive? ____________

____

EXERCISE 2. Muscular Strength

OBJECTIVES

To measure muscular strength
To list some causes of strength
To differentiate isotonic from isometric strength

The maximum strength of muscle is a function of the number of myofilaments and the development of the sarcoplasmic reticulum in white or fast muscle; the more myofilaments, the greater the number of cross bridges available to produce tension.

TABLE 19.1
FLEXIBILITY INDEX

Score	Females Inches	Males Inches
100	24–27	22–23
75	21–23	20–21
50	16–20	14–19
25	13–15	12–13
0	0–12	0–11

Strength is measured in two ways. ***Isometric strength*** is the greatest force that can be exerted against a fixed resistance; ***isotonic strength*** is the greatest weight that can be moved.

Muscular strength can be increased through activity that is forceful enough to cause hypertrophy or growth of the muscle. No enlargement of muscle can occur unless the muscle contracts to at least 75% of its maximal tension. Thus, to increase strength, exercises with a high isometric component such as weight lifting are employed. Even short sessions of isometric exercise are sufficient to cause muscle growth. With muscle growth, the strength of associated tendons and ligaments also increases.

This exercise measures the ability to make a quick burst of muscular power. CAUTION! *Do not perform this exercise without warming up.*

MATERIALS

Masking tape
Step ladder
Measuring stick

PROCEDURE

1. Wrap a piece of masking tape in a circle, sticky side out, and place it lightly on the tip of your middle finger. With your heels on the ground, reach as high as you can and apply the tape to the wall.

2. Place another piece of tape on your middle finger. Facing the wall, crouch down and swinging your arms, jump as high as possible and apply the tape to the wall.

3. Repeat step 2 three times and measure the distance between the highest *jump height* and the first tape applied at the *standing height*. Record this measurement in the LABORATORY REPORT RESULTS at the end of the chapter.

4. Consult Table 19.2 for your score. A score of 50 indicates average ability to summon a burst of muscle strength.

How would you improve a low score in muscular strength? ______________________________

____

____

EXERCISE 3. Muscular Endurance and Aerobic Fitness

Endurance is a property of red or slow muscle fibers. Prolonged mild exercise causes development of the capillary beds in slow muscle and a consequent increase in the levels of oxidative enzymes and myoglobin in slow muscle. Myoglobin is a substance similar to hemoglobin in its ability to hold oxygen inside the muscle cell. The increased oxygen level delays muscle fatigue. Endurance can be increased by prolonged isotonic activity.

Endurance also involves cardiovascular and respiratory fitness. The Harvard Step Test measures all three factors by determining pulse rate after a standardized physical activity.

TABLE 19.2
STRENGTH INDEX

Score	Females Age: 15–25	26–35	36–45	46–over	Score	Males Age: 15–25	26–35	36–45	46–over
	Inches	Inches	Inches	Inches		Inches	Inches	Inches	Inches
100	18	16	14	11.8	100	26.5	25.2	24	19
90	17.5	15.5	13.5	11	90	26	25	23.5	18
80	17	15	13	10	80	25	24	23	16–17
70	15–16	13–14	12	9	70	23–24	22–23	21–22	14–15
60	14	12	10–11	7–8	60	21–22	19–21	18–20	13
50	12–13	9–11	8–9	5–6	50	18–20	16–18	14–16	9–11
40	8–10	6–8	5–7	4	40	14–17	14	10–12	6–7
30	6	4–5	4	2–3	30	10–12	8–12	6–8	4–5
20	3–4	2–3	2–3	1–2	20	6–8	6	3–4	3
10	1–2	1	1	1	10	3–5	2–4	2	2
0	0	0	0	0	0	0–2	1	1	1

MATERIALS

Watch with second hand
Bench or stool

PROCEDURE

1. Review the pulse taking procedure in Chapter 17, Exercise 4, until you are thoroughly familiar with it.

2. Using Table 19.3, determine the bench height appropriate to your height.

3. When your laboratory partner begins timing, step up and down from the bench at the rate of 30 steps per minute (step up requires one second, step down requires one second). Bring both feet onto the bench before stepping back down to the floor. Have your laboratory partner count out the pace.

4. When you can no longer keep up the pace for 15 seconds, the test is terminated. Note the time: ____ seconds. Only about 1/3 of all subjects can complete the full five minutes of this exercise.

5. Upon completion, sit down. One minute after termination, your laboratory partner should take your pulse for 30 seconds. After 30 seconds, the 30-second pulse should be taken again. After another 30-second wait, the pulse should be taken for another 30 seconds. Record the 30-second pulses and their expression as beats per minute in the LABORATORY REPORT RESULTS at the end of the chapter.

6. Calculate your general physical condition index according to the example below and interpret your score according to Table 19.4.

$$\text{Index} = \frac{\text{seconds of exercise} \times 100}{2(\text{sum of three pulse counts})}$$

EXAMPLE

Minutes of exercise: 4

Pulse rate from 1 minute to $1^1/2$ minutes after exercise: 60

Pulse rate from 2 minutes to $2^1/2$ minutes after exercise: 50

Pulse rate from 3 minutes to $3^1/2$ minutes after exercise: 40

$$\text{Index} = \frac{240 \times 100}{2(60 + 50 + 40)} = \frac{24000}{300} = 48.8$$

What are possible sources of error in evaluating scores from the Harvard Step Test? ____

____

TABLE 19.3

Subject Height	Bench Height
5′–5′3″	14″
5′3″–5′9″	16″
5′9″–6′	19″
over 6′	20″

TABLE 19.4
GENERAL PHYSICAL CONDITION INDEX

Greater than 90	=	excellent condition
80–90	=	good condition
50–80	=	average condition
Less than 50	=	poor condition

COMPLETE LABORATORY REPORT QUESTIONS AT THE END OF THE CHAPTER

DIGESTION 20

EXERCISE 1. Deglutition
EXERCISE 2. Observation of the Rat Gastro-intestinal Tract
EXERCISE 3. Physiology of Intestinal Smooth Muscle
A. Inherent Contractile Activity
B. Effect of Oxygen
C. Effect of Temperature
D. Effect of Norepinephrine
E. Effect of Acetylcholine
F. Effect of Atropine
G. Effect of Atropine and Acetylcholine
H. Effect of Atropine, Acetylcholine, and Norepinephrine
I. Effect of Calcium Removal
EXERCISE 4. Enzymatic (Chemical) Digestion
A. Digestion of Proteins
B. Digestion of Fats
1. Emulsification
2. Action of lipase on fats
C. Digestion of Carbohydrates
1. Benedict's test for sugar
2. Lugol's test for starch
3. Digestion of starch
4. Effect of temperature on starch digestion
5. Effect of pH on starch digestion

WORD ROOTS

-ase = enzyme
lip-, lipo- = fat
-lysis = splitting
rect- = straight
saccharo- = sugar
sigmoid = S-shaped

The general functions of the digestive system are ingestion, digestion, absorption, and excretion of solid wastes. Digestion is both a mechanical and a chemical process. In ***mechanical digestion***, teeth effect the physical breakdown of food by chewing ***(mastication)***, and the smooth muscle of the walls of the stomach and small intestine further enhance this breakdown by churning the food and mixing it with enzymes. ***Chemical digestion*** consists of a series of catabolic reactions that break down large carbohydrate, protein, and lipid molecules into end products which are able to be absorbed across the lining of the gastrointestinal tract into blood or lymph.

The digestive organs are those of the accessory structures and the gastrointestinal tract. The ***accessory structures*** include the ***teeth***, ***tongue***, ***salivary glands***, ***liver***, ***gallbladder***, and ***pancreas***.

The ***gastrointestinal (GI) tract*** or ***alimentary canal*** is a continuous tube measuring about 9 m (30 ft) in length. It is composed of the ***mouth***, ***esophagus***, ***stomach***, ***small intestine***, ***large intestine***, and ***anus***. The small intestine includes three regions, the ***duodenum*** (doo′-ō-DĒ-num), ***jejunum*** (je-JOO-num), and ***ileum*** (IL-ē-um). The large intestine has four regions, the ***cecum*** (sē-kum), ***colon***, ***rectum***, and ***anal canal***. The colon is divided into the ***ascending colon***, ***transverse colon***, ***descending colon***, and ***sigmoid colon***.

Chemical and mechanical digestion occur

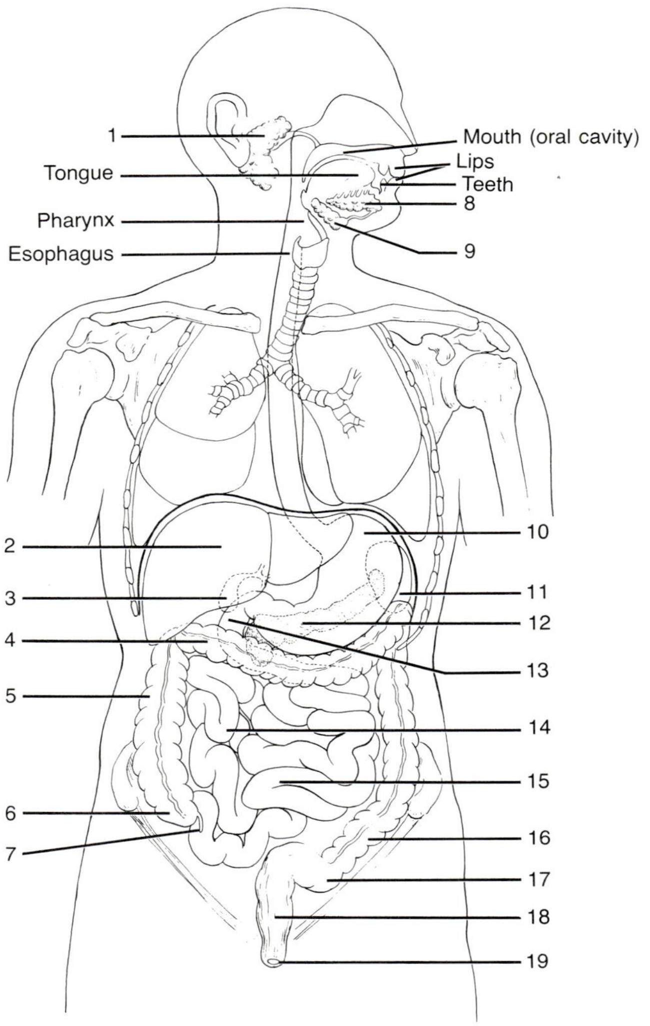

___ Anus
___ Appendix
___ Ascending colon
___ Cecum
___ Descending colon
___ Duodenum
___ Gallbladder
___ Ileum
___ Jejunum
___ Liver
___ Pancreas
___ Parotid gland
___ Rectum
___ Sigmoid colon
___ Spleen
___ Stomach
___ Sublingual gland
___ Submaxillary gland
___ Transverse colon

FIGURE 20.1 Organs of the digestive system and related structures.

in the mouth, stomach, and small intestine; ***absorption*** occurs primarily in the small intestine, although some substances are also absorbed from the stomach and large intestine.

To review the anatomy of the digestive system, label Figure 20.1.

All parts of the gastrointestinal tract secrete mucus. Hormones and enzymes are also secreted by some parts of the digestive system. Enzymatic secretions are listed in Table 20.1 and described in Exercise 4.

EXERCISE 1. Deglutition

OBJECTIVES

To describe the three stages of deglutition
To distinguish voluntary and reflex activity in swallowing
To hear the sounds produced by various phases of deglutition

TABLE 20.1
DIGESTIVE ENZYMES

Enzyme	Source	Substrate	Products	Comments
Enzymes Acting in the Mouth				
Salivary amylase	Parotid and sublingual glands	Starch	Maltose	
Enzymes Acting in the Stomach				
Pepsin	Glands in gastric epithelium	Protein	Polypeptides	Converted from inactive pepsinogen by HCl
Gastric lipase		Emulsified butter fats	Fatty acids and glycerol	Of limited value
Rennin		Milk casein	Paracasein (milk curd)	Functional in infants
Enzymes Acting in Small Intestine				
Trypsin	Acinar cells in pancreas	Protein	Polypeptides	Converted from inactive trypsinogen by enterokinase
Chymotrypsin		Protein	Peptides	Activated by trypsin
Carboxypeptidase		Protein	Peptides and amino acids	Converted from inactive procarb-oxypeptidase by trypsin
Pancreatic lipase		Emulsified fats	Fatty acids, glycerol, and glycerides	
Pancreatic amylase		Starch	Maltose	
Aminopeptidase	Brush border of intestinal epithelial cells		Peptides	Di- and Tripeptides and amino aicds
Dipeptidase			Dipeptides	Amino acids
Lactase			Lactose	Glucose and galactose
Maltase			Maltose	Glucose
Sucrase			Sucrose	Glucose and fructose
Nucleases			RNA and DNA nucleotides	Pentose sugars and nitrogenous bases

Swallowing or ***deglutition*** (dē′-gloo-TI-shun) is the movement of food from the oral cavity through the esophagus to the stomach. It can be divided into three stages.

1. ***The Oral Stage***. This first stage of deglutition is voluntary. Food mixed with saliva is pressed into a ball called a ***bolus***. The tongue is elevated against the palate, forcing the bolus into the pharyngeal opening.

2. ***The Pharyngeal Stage***. As the bolus touches the ***fauces*** (FAW-sez), the opening from the mouth cavity to the pharynx, it stimulates receptors which transmit nerve impulses to the swallowing center in the brain stem. Efferent impulses from the swallowing center cause

a. Movement of the soft palate and uvula to block the entrance of food into the nasal passageways.

b. Partial closure of the pharyngeal entrance to prevent large unmasticated objects from entering the pharynx.

c. Movement of the larynx against the epiglottis to prevent food from entering the glottis. This closure interrupts breathing temporarily.

d. Upward movement of the larynx which stretches the esophageal opening and closes the vocal folds.

e. A constriction of pharyngeal muscles which moves the bolus into the esophagus.

3. ***The Esophageal Stage***. This involuntary stage is a continuation of the peristaltic contraction which begins in the pharynx. ***Peristalsis*** is a reflex action in which a ring of circular muscle contracts rhythmically, forcing the bolus ahead of the contraction. The contractile wave is followed by a wave of relaxation. This stage, initiated by the presence of food in the esophagus, requires about 5–10 seconds for solid food.

The swallowing mechanism can be damaged by failure of the swallowing muscles or of the swallowing center in the brain stem. ***Achalasia***, the failure of the lower esophagus to relax, causes food to remain in the esophagus. This condition is caused by damage to the ***myenteric (Auerbach's) plexus***, the esophageal nerve supply.

MATERIALS

Crackers

Cup

Stethoscope

Alcohol and cotton or alcohol pads

PROCEDURE

1. Chew a cracker and note the movements of your tongue as you begin to swallow. Chew another cracker, lean over your chair, placing your mouth below the level of your pharynx, and attempt to swallow again.

2. Note the movements of your laboratory partner's larynx during the pharyngeal stage of deglutition.

3. *Clean the earpieces of a stethoscope with alcohol*. Using the stethoscope, listen to the sounds which occur when your laboratory partner swallows water. Place the stethoscope just to the left of the midline at the level of the sixth rib. You should hear the sound of water as it makes contact with the lower esophageal sphincter (a ring of circular muscle which serves as a valve) at the junction of the esophagus and stomach. The second sound which follows is the sound of water passing through the sphincter after the sphincter relaxes.

4. Record your observations in the LABORATORY REPORT RESULTS at the end of the chapter.

At what point can deglutition be stopped voluntarily? ____________________

____

EXERCISE 2. Observation of the Rat Gastrointestinal Tract

OBJECTIVES

To locate organs of the digestive system
To observe smooth muscle movement in the gastrointestinal tract of a mammal
To measure the pH of gastric and intestinal contents

Food, semidigested food, and wastes are moved along the entire gastrointestinal tract by ***peristalsis*** at a net rate of about 1–2 cm per minute. Nonpropulsive movements, pendular motion, and segmentation occur as well. These movements serve to mix food with enzymes, to facilitate absorption, and to compact fecal material.

Pendular movements involve alternate contraction and relaxation of longitudinal muscle, shortening and lengthening the intestine, and thus spilling the contents back and forth.

In the small intestine, ***segmentation*** constricts the intestine into small localized segments. Circular muscle fibers in adjacent segments contract and relax alternately, spilling the contents back and forth. As one set of constrictions relaxes, the next set occurs at a point midway between the previous contractions, thus chopping the intestinal contents.

In the large intestine, ***haustral churning***, a type of segmental movement, churns the contents of one pouch (haustrum) and exposes them to the mucosa where absorption can occur.

In addition, strong peristaltic waves, known as ***mass peristalsis***, occur along the length of the large intestine about three or four times each day.

The movement of the contents of the gastrointestinal tract facilitates the chemical digestion of food which occurs when enzymes come into contact with food molecules. The enzymes are pH specific, that is, they function most effectively within a narrow pH range. Oral enzymes function at a pH near neutral (7); gastric enzymes at a highly acidic pH (1); duodenal enzymes at an alkaline pH (8). The pH of the stomach secretions is so low because the gastric mucosa produces hydrochloric acid; the mixture of hydrochloric acid, gastric enzymes, and food is called ***chyme***. As it enters the duodenum, the acidic chyme is neutralized by hepatic, pancreatic, and intestinal secretions.

MATERIALS

Rat which has not been fed for 24 hours
Latex gloves
Laboratory coat or apron
Dissecting pan or frog board
Surgical scissors
Blunt forceps
Gauze sponges
Water bath at 37°C with supply of Locke's solution or isotonic saline
Medicine dropper
pH paper
Safety goggles
Laboratory apron or coat

CAUTION! *Please reread Section D, "Precautions Related to Dissection," in Chapter 1 before you begin any of the exercises in this chapter. You should also read the exercises before you perform them to be sure that you understand all of the procedures and safety precautions.*

PROCEDURE

1. Obtain a rat from your laboratory instructor. The rats will have been sacrificed just prior to the beginning of the laboratory period either by cervical dislocation or by the injection of an air embolism.

2. Using surgical scissors with a blunt point, quickly make a midline incision through the skin and muscle of the abdomen from just below the xiphoid process to the pubis (see Figure 20.2). Hold your scissors parallel to the abdominal wall so that you do not injure the viscera.

3. Make four lateral incisions, two just beneath the diaphragm and two at the level of the pubis. Do not enter the thoracic cavity. Reflect the abdominal skin to expose the viscera.

4. Note the parietal peritoneum which lines the abdominal wall.

5. Identify the stomach. Note any movements of the stomach musculature.

6. Using a blunt forceps, gently squeeze the pyloric sphincter. Gently squeeze a loop of the small intestine. Note any reaction.

7. Identify the greater omentum, a double fold of peritoneum which is suspended from the greater curvature of the stomach.

8. Cover the stomach with a small sponge soaked in Locke's solution of 0.9% sodium chloride (NaCl) solution kept at 37°C. Reflect the greater omentum backward onto the sponge.

9. Examine the mesentery. Note the distribution of blood vessels and the presence of whitish lacteals.

10. Observe the movements of the small intestine. Note pendular, segmental, and peristaltic movements.

ALTERNATE PROCEDURE

If Exercise 3 is to be done, have your instructor or a laboratory assistant remove a section of jejunum from the rat at this time and immediately immerse it in 37°C Locke's solution.

11. Note the movements of the gastrointestinal tract as the tissues become ischemic.

12. Open the stomach along the greater curvature. Test the pH of the gastric contents with pH paper. Slit open the ileum and test the pH of ileal contents. Record the pH.

13. Dispose of the rat according to the procedure given by your laboratory instructor. *Clean your equipment thoroughly.*

14. Record all your observations in the LABORATORY REPORT RESULTS at the end of the chapter.

What is the purpose of nonpropulsive movements in the gastrointestinal tract? ________

____

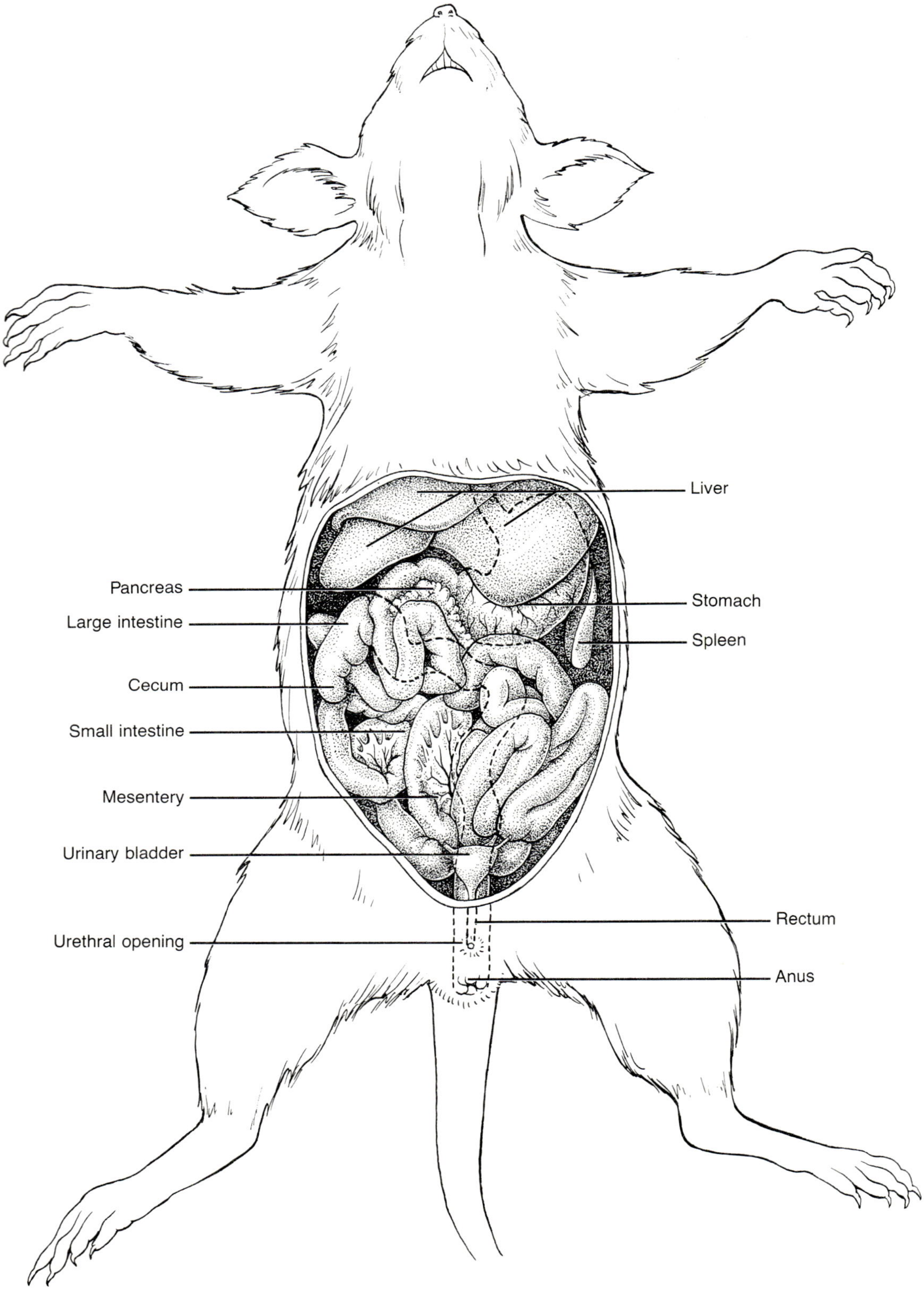

FIGURE 20.2 Abdominal anatomy of the rat.

EXERCISE 3. Physiology of Intestinal Smooth Muscle

OBJECTIVE

To observe the inherent contractile activity in intestinal smooth muscle

To describe the effect of various chemical agents on smooth muscle activity

The muscularis of the small intestine is composed of smooth (involuntary) muscle, arranged in circular and longitudinal layers. Its major nerve supply is from the ***myenteric (Auerbach's) plexus*** located between the layers. This plexus is innervated by both sympathetic and parasympathetic fibers, but its major activity is an intrinsic rhythmic action which is amplified by distension or irritation of the gastrointestinal tract.

MATERIALS

- Small mammal (rat, rabbit, guinea pig) which has not been fed for 24 hours
- Dissection pan or frog board
- Latex gloves
- Thermometer
- Locke's solution in water baths at 18°, 37°, and 43°C
- Six medicine droppers
- Thread
- Two small beakers
- Probe
- L-tube attached to air supply
- Large beaker
- Heat source
- Myograph
- 1:10,000 dilution of acetylcholine
- 1:50,000 solution of norepinephrine
- 1:50,000 solution of atropine
- Locke's solution with $O(Ca)_e$
- Safety goggles
- Laboratory apron or coat

PROCEDURE FOR EXPERIMENTAL SETUP

CAUTION! *Please reread Section C, "Precautions Related to Working With Reagents" in Chapter 1 before you begin any of these exercises.*

1. *Read this entire procedure carefully and examine Figure 20.3 before you begin, so that the muscle does not become ischemic or overstretched as the result of faulty technique.* Also, determine the responsibilities of each member of your group before you begin.
2. Obtain a 2 inch section of jejunum from your instructor. *Do not stretch it.*
3. Immediately immerse the jejunum in 37°C Locke's solution.
4. Fill a medicine dropper with 37°C Locke's solution and gently flush out the luminal contents of the jejunal segment. Cut off the mesentery, and cut the segment into 1 inch pieces.
5. Place the segments in a beaker of clean 37°C Locke's solution.
6. Using a probe, make a small hole in each end of the segment. Tie a 3 inch thread loop through one hole; tie an 8 inch length of thread through the other loop.
7. Slip the small loop over the L-tube. Tie the end of the long thread to the hook.
8. Adjust the tension so that the string is taut but the tissue is not overly stretched. *NOTE*: Depending on the model of the myograph utilized, either turn up the sensitivity or attach the string to the most sensitive arm of the transducer.
9. Adjust the air flow so that a continuous, light stream of air passes across the intestinal segment.
10. Adjust the transducer so that the amplitude of the contractions is from 1.5 to 2.5 cm. If contractions are not observed after oxygen has bubbled through the solution, raise the heat to 39° until contractions commence. If contractions are still not observed, use a medicine dropper to add one drop of 1:10,000 acetylcholine.

ALTERNATE PROCEDURE

Use a muscle bath as diagrammed in Figure 20.4.

EXPERIMENTAL PROCEDURES

All observations are to be recorded in the LABORATORY REPORT RESULTS at the end of the chapter.

A. Inherent Contractile Activity

1. After allowing an initial 5 to 10 minutes for the intestinal segment to stabilize, record its basal activity with the physiograph.

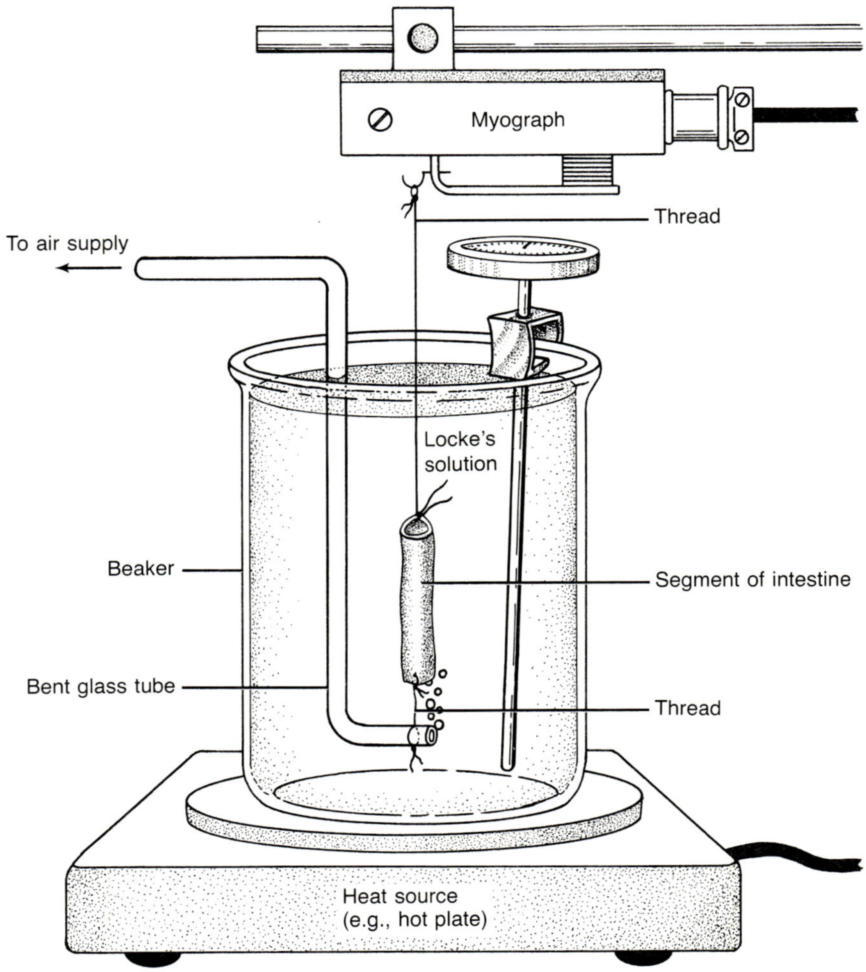

FIGURE 20.3 Experimental setup for the physiology of intestinal smooth muscle.

2. Note the nature and pattern of the baseline activity in the LABORATORY REPORT RESULTS at the end of the chapter.

B. Effect of Oxygen

1. Shut off the oxygen supply until you notice a change in contractile activity. Describe the pattern in the LABORATORY REPORT RESULTS at the end of the chapter.

2. Resupply oxygen and describe recovery.

C. Effect of Temperature

1. Remove the 37°C Locke's solution and replace it with Locke's solution at 18°C.

2. Record any changes in the strength and frequency of contraction and the speed of contraction.

3. Replace the cold Locke's solution with a 43°C solution. Note any changes which occur.

D. Effect of Norepinephrine

1. Place the segment in fresh 37°C Locke's solution for 5 minutes.

2. Using a medicine dropper, add 5 to 8 drops of a 1:50,000 norepinephrine solution to the Locke's solution.

3. Record any changes in basal tone, strength and frequency of contraction, and speed of contraction in the LABORATORY REPORT RESULTS at the end of the chapter.

E. Effect of Acetylcholine

1. Place the segment in fresh 37°C Locke's solution for 5 minutes.

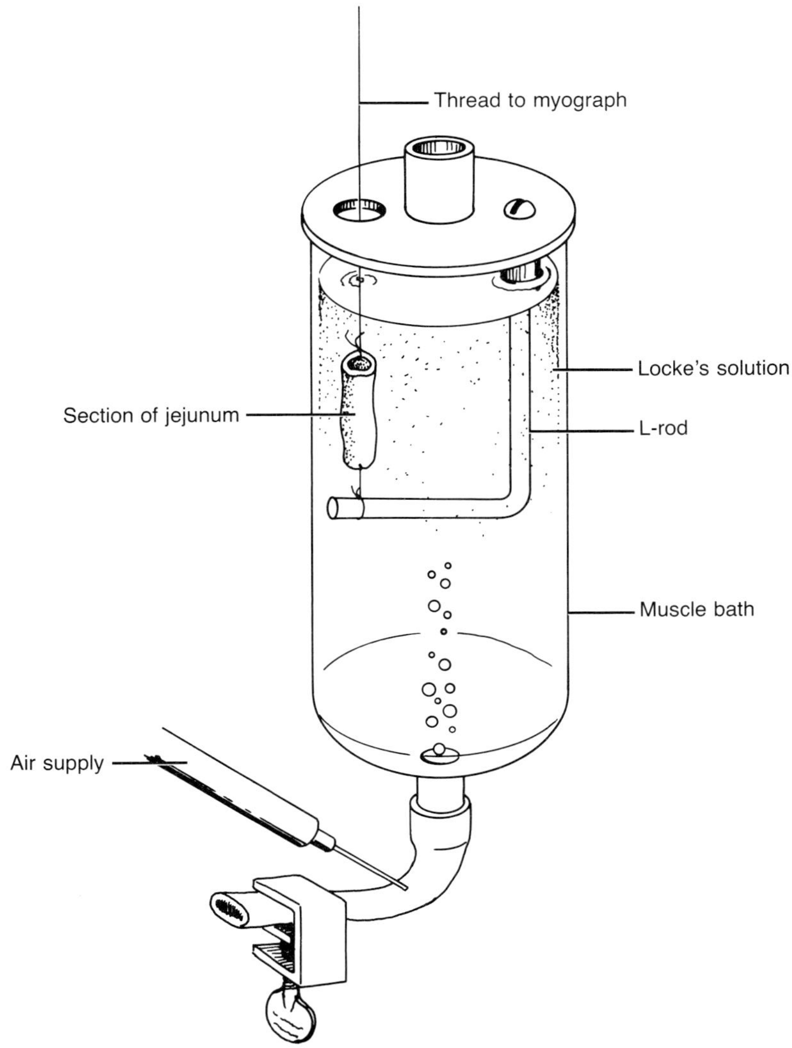

FIGURE 20.4 Muscle bath setup for the physiology of intestinal smooth muscle.

2. Using a medicine dropper, add 1 to 5 drops of a 1:1000 acetylcholine solution to the Locke's solution.

3. Record any changes in basal tone, strength and frequency of contraction, and speed of contraction in the LABORATORY REPORT RESULTS at the end of the chapter.

F. Effect of Atropine

1. Place the segment in fresh 37°C Locke's solution for 5 minutes.

2. Using a medicine dropper, add 5 to 10 drops of a 1:50,000 atropine solution to the Locke's solution.

3. Record any changes in basal tone, strength and frequency of contraction, and speed of contraction in the LABORATORY REPORT RESULTS at the end of the chapter.

G. Effect of Atropine and Acetylcholine

1. Using a medicine dropper, add 1 to 5 drops of a 1:1000 acetylcholine solution to the Locke's solution already containing atropine.

2. After 3 to 5 minutes, record any changes in basal tone, strength and frequency of contraction, and speed of contraction in the LABORATORY REPORT RESULTS at the end of the chapter.

H. Effect of Atropine, Acetylcholine, and Norepinephrine

1. Using a medicine dropper, add 5 to 8 drops of a 1:50,000 norepinephrine solution to the Locke's solution already containing atropine and acetylcholine.

2. After 3 to 5 minutes, record any changes in basal tone, strength and frequency of contraction, and speed of contraction in the LABORATORY REPORT RESULTS at the end of the chapter.

I. Effect of Calcium Removal

1. Place the intestinal segment in fresh 37°C Locke's solution for 5 minutes. To determine if recovery has been complete, record a minute of contractile activity and compare your observations with those in Section A.

2. Replace the Locke's solution with Locke's solution containing $O(Ca)_e$ (no calcium).

3. Record any changes in basal tone, strength and frequency of contraction, and speed of contraction in the LABORATORY REPORT RESULTS at the end of the chapter.

Which substance(s) used in this exercise stimulate (depolarize) intestinal smooth muscle?

____

Which substances used in this exercise inhibit (hyperpolarize) intestinal smooth muscle?

____

EXERCISE 4. Enzymatic (Chemical) Digestion

OBJECTIVES

To describe the basic chemical structure of the major nutrient groups
To demonstrate the action of digestive enzymes
To determine the effect of pH and temperature on enzymatic reactions
To demonstrate emulsification
To describe the absorption of the end products of digestion

In order to be utilized by the body, nutrients must first be absorbed from the gastrointestinal tract. Absorption can occur only if the molecular size is small enough for active or passive transport to move the substance across the lining of the tract. Digestive enzymes catalyze the breakdown of large carbohydrate, protein, and lipid molecules into smaller subunits.

Enzymes are large proteins. As catalysts, they increase the rate of reaction by reducing the activation energy without being changed by the reaction. Digestive enzymes catalyze ***hydrolysis reactions***, those which break chemical bonds with the addition of water.

The digestion of a substance can be diagrammed as

$$\underset{\text{(food)}}{\text{Substrate}} \xrightarrow{\text{enzyme}} \text{Product(s)}$$

The amount and nature of the enzyme do not change in this process. The rate of the reaction can be measured by noting either the disappearance of the substrate or the appearance of the product.

The digestive enzymes are highly specific in that they only hydrolyze certain substrate molecules, and they only function at specific temperatures and pHs. Table 20.1 lists various features of the digestive enzymes.

A. Digestion of Proteins

Proteins are long chains of amino acids. ***Peptidases***, the enzymes that catalyze the digestion of protein, must be secreted in an inactive form, so that they do not digest the tissues of the gastrointestinal tract.

Protein digestion begins in the stomach where pepsin splits peptide bonds between certain amino acids yielding short chain polypeptides, peptones, and proteoses. Most protein digestion occurs in the small intestine, where the pancreatic enzymes ***trypsin***, ***chymotrypsin***, and ***carboxypeptidase*** cleave specific additional peptide bonds. The intestinal juice contains ***aminopeptidase*** and ***dipeptidase*** which complete protein digestion into single amino acids.

Amino acids are absorbed into the capillary blood in intestinal villi.

MATERIALS

Five Pyrex test tubes
Wax marking pencil

Four 10 ml graduated cylinders
0.5% pepsin solution
0.8% HCl
0.5% NaOH
Boiling water bath (hot plate and beaker)
40°C water bath
pH paper
Fibrin
Safety goggles
Laboratory apron or coat

PROCEDURE

CAUTION! *Please reread Section A, "General Procedures and Safety Precautions," and Section C, "Precautions Related to Working With Reagents," in Chapter 1 before you begin any of the following exercises. You should also read the exercises before you perform them to be sure that you understand all of the procedures and safety precautions.*

1. Prepare and number the following five test tubes. For this test, the quantity of each solution must be *measured carefully*.

Tube 1: 5 ml of 0.5% pepsin + 5 ml of 0.8% HCl
Tube 2: 5 ml of 0.5% pepsin + 5 ml of water
Tube 3: 5 ml of 0.5% pepsin, boiled for 10 minutes in a water bath + 5 ml of 0.8% HCl

CAUTION! *Make sure that the mouth of the test tube is pointed away from you and all other persons in the area. Use a test tube holder to remove the test tube from the water bath.*

Tube 4: 5 ml of 0.5% pepsin + 5 ml of 0.5% NaOH
Tube 5: 5 ml of water + 5 ml of 0.8% HCl

2. Determine the approximate pH of each tube with pH paper and record the results in the LABORATORY REPORT RESULTS at the end of the chapter.

3. Using forceps, place the same amount of protein in each tube. Use a piece of fibrin about the size of a pea.

4. *Using a test tube holder*, place the tubes in a 40° water bath and shake occasionally for at least 1½ hours.

5. Watch the change that the protein undergoes. Swelling of the fibrin does not indicate digestion. Digested protein becomes transparent and dissolves as soluble peptides are produced.

6. Record your observations in the LABORATORY REPORT RESULTS at the end of the chapter.

How did boiling affect pepsin? ______________

____

B. Digestion of Fats

Fats are nonpolar (insoluble in water) molecules composed of one molecule of glycerol combined with three molecules of fatty acids. Most ingested fat is in globules which must be emulsified before chemical digestion can occur. ***Emulsification*** is a process that breaks up the globules by separating the fat molecules physically without any chemical digestion. This separation allows lipases to hydrolyze the bonds between the fatty acids and glycerol. ***Bile salts***, soluble in both water and fat, are the substances that bring about emulsification.

Almost all fat digestion occurs in the duodenum through the action of ***pancreatic lipase***. This enzyme splits the bonds between fatty acids and glycerol, yielding monoglycerides (by the removal of two fatty acids) and fatty acids, along with glycerol. These products along with bile salts aggregate into water soluble ***micelles*** (mī-SELZ) which are absorbed into the epithelial cells of the intestinal lumen.

In the epithelial cells, triglycerides are resynthesized. They combine with protein to form ***chylomicrons*** (kī-lō-MĪ-kronz), which are secreted into the lacteals in the intestinal villi. The absorbed fats return to the blood through the lymphatic circulation. In the blood, a plasma lipase hydrolyzes them to glycerol and fatty acids for use by the tissue cells.

In this exercise, litmus, a pH indicator, will be used to test for the presence of digested fats. Undigested fats will not change the pH, so the litmus will remain blue. If fat digestion has occurred, fatty acids will lower the pH, turning the litmus red.

1. Emulsification

MATERIALS

Two Pyrex test tubes with stoppers
Wax marking pencil

Bile solution
Two 10 ml graduated cylinders
Vegetable oil in dropper bottle
Fat-soluble dye
Test tube rack
Safety goggles
Laboratory apron or coat

PROCEDURE

a. Add 5 ml water to a test tube marked "W" and add 5 ml bile solution to a test tube marked "B." Add five drops of oil which has been colored with a fat-soluble dye to each tube.

b. Put a stopper in each tube and shake them *vigorously*. Let them stand in a rack for 10 minutes.

c. Note the difference in the appearance of the two tubes in the LABORATORY REPORT RESULTS at the end of the chapter. If emulsification has not occurred, the fat will lie on the surface of the water. If the fat has been emulsified, fat droplets will be suspended in the water in the form of an ***emulsion***.

2. Action of Lipase on Fats

MATERIALS

Pancreatin
Bile solution
Three 20 ml Pyrex test tubes
Wax marking pencil
Two 10 ml graduated cylinders
Litmus cream (heavy cream to which powdered litmus has been added)
0.1M HCl in a dropper bottle
Three glass rods
40°C water bath
Safety goggles
Laboratory apron or coat

PROCEDURE

a. Obtain three test tubes. Mark one "C" for control, one "L" for lipase, and one "LB" for lipase and bile.

b. Place 5 ml of litmus cream in each tube.

c. While stirring with a glass rod, add 0.1 M HCl to the control tube drop by drop until the litmus turns red (and hence the litmus cream turns pink). This reaction will identify solutions in which fat digestion has released fatty acids which lower the pH.

d. Add 5 ml of pancreatin (a mixture of pancreatic enzymes containing lipase) to tube "L"; add 5 ml of pancreatin and 5 ml bile solution to tube "LB."

e. Stir tubes "L" and "LB" with a glass rod and incubate in a 40°C water bath until a color change occurs.

f. Record your observations in the LABORATORY REPORT RESULTS at the end of the chapter.

Why does litmus cream change color in this exercise? ______________________________

____

C. Digestion of Carbohydrates

Carbohydrates, sugars and starches, contain carbon, hydrogen, and oxygen in a general formula $(CH_2O)_n$. Simple sugars or ***monosaccharides***, such a glucose, galactose, and fructose, are the end products of carbohydrate digestion. ***Disaccharides*** such as sucrose, maltose, and lactose, and complex polysaccharide molecules such as starch and glycogen, must be hydrolyzed into their component monosaccharides before they can be absorbed into the capillaries of the intestinal villi.

Carbohydrate digestion begins in the mouth with the action of ***salivary amylase*** (formerly known as ptyalin). It continues in the small intestine with the action of ***pancreatic amylase*** and the intestinal enzymes, ***lactase***, ***maltase***, and ***sucrase***.

1. Benedict's Test for Sugar

Upon boiling, Benedict's solution reacts with reducing sugars to form an insoluble red precipitate of cuprous oxide. The Benedict's solution turns green, yellow, orange, or red depending on the amount of sugar present, according the following scale.

Blue (−)
Green (+)
Yellow (++)
Orange (+++)
Red (++++)

MATERIALS

- Pyrex or Kimex test tube and test tube holder
- Two pipettes and pipette bulbs
- Maltose solution
- Starch solution
- Benedict's solution
- Boiling water bath (hot plate and beaker)
- Test tube rack
- Safety goggles
- Laboratory apron or coat

PROCEDURE

a. Using separate pipettes, place 2 ml maltose solution and 2 ml Benedict's solution in a test tube.

b. CAUTION! *Using a test tube holder*, place the test tube in a boiling water bath for 5 minutes. *Make sure that the mouth of the test tube is pointed away from you and all other persons in the area*. Note the color change.

c. *Using a test tube holder*, remove the test tube from the water bath and place it in a rack to cool.

d. Repeat steps a to c using starch solution instead of maltose. Notice that the color does not change, because the solution contains no sugar.

2. Lugol's Test for Starch

Lugol's solution is a brown solution which contains iodine and reacts with starch by producing a deep blue to black color. Cellulose, monosaccharides, and disaccharides do not react with Lugol's solution.

MATERIALS

- Spot plate
- Wax marking pencil
- Lugol's solution in dropper bottle
- Starch solution in dropper bottle
- Medicine dropper
- Safety goggles
- Laboratory apron or coat

PROCEDURE

a. Label three spots on the spot plate "W," "M," and "S."

b. Using separate medicine droppers, place a drop of water, maltose solution, and starch solution in the appropriate spot.

c. Add a drop of Lugol's solution to each solution.

d. Note the blue-black color which forms as the Lugol's solution complexes with the starch.

3. Digestion of Starch

Salivary amylase hydrolyzes starch to the disaccharide maltose. This enzyme is pH specific, most effective in a pH range from 6.0 to 7.4. Only about 5% of all the starches ingested are hydrolyzed by salivary amylase because this enzyme is inactivated when it enters the low pH in the stomach. You can experience the effect of this process by chewing a piece of plain bread for a minute and tasting the sweet flavor which arises when the starch is digested.

MATERIALS

- Distilled water
- Paraffin or sugarless chewing gum
- Collection cups
- pH paper
- Starch solution
- Pyrex test tube
- Glass rod
- Stop watch or watch with second hand
- Spot plate
- Lugol's solution
- Boiling water bath (hot plate and beaker)
- Test tube holder
- Benedict's solution
- Safety goggles
- Laboratory apron or coat

PROCEDURE

a. Rinse your mouth with distilled water and chew a small piece of paraffin or sugarless gum to stimulate salivary secretion.

b. Collect 3 ml saliva in a small cup and add an equal amount of water to dilute the saliva. Test the pH of your saliva with pH paper. Record the pH in the LABORATORY REPORT RESULTS at the end of the chapter.

ALTERNATE PROCEDURE: Use commercial amylase solution.

c. Using separate medicine droppers, add 3 ml starch solution and 3 ml saliva to a test tube and mix thoroughly with a glass rod.

d. After 1 minute, record the time. Time: ____ Stir the mixture and using the glass rod, remove one drop to a spot plate depression. Test for starch with Lugol's solution.

e. Repeat step d at 1 minute intervals until the test for starch is no longer positive. Record the elapsed time in the LABORATORY REPORT RESULTS at the end of the chapter.

f. Test the remaining mixture for the presence of sugar by combining it with an equal amount of Benedict's solution and use a test tube holder to place it in a boiling water bath for 5 minutes. CAUTION! *Use the test tube holder to direct the opening of the test tube away from you and from other students*. Record the results in the LABORATORY REPORT RESULTS at the end of the chapter.

Why was paraffin or sugarless gum chewed in this exercise? no ______________________

____

____

4. Effect of Temperature on Starch Digestion

MATERIALS

- Distilled water
- Paraffin or sugarless chewing gum
- Collection cups
- Five constant temperature water baths at 1°C, 10°C, 40°C, 60°C, and 100°C
- Test tube holder
- 10 Pyrex or Kimex test tubes
- Two medicine droppers
- Rubber bands
- Glass marking pencil
- Five glass rods
- Lugol's solution in dropper bottle
- Starch solution
- Spot plate
- Safety goggles
- Laboratory apron or coat

PROCEDURE

a. Rinse your mouth with distilled water and chew a small piece of paraffin or sugarless gum to stimulate salivary secretion.

b. Collect 3 ml saliva in a small cup and add an equal amount of water to dilute the saliva.

ALTERNATE PROCEDURE: Use commercial amylase solution.

c. Prepare 10 test tubes by marking five with "A" for amylase and five with "S" for starch. Using separate medicine droppers, place 1 ml of starch in each "S" tube and 1 ml of saliva in each "A" test tube.

d. Using rubber bands, pair "A" and "S" test tubes and use a test tube holder to place one pair in each water bath for five minutes.

e. Pour the "S" tube into its paired "A" test tube, and replace the mixture back into the water bath at its previous temperature.

f. About 1 minute after the contents of the tubes have been mixed, test all five remaining tubes for the presence of starch by using Lugol's solution and the technique in section C2.

g. Repeat the test every minute to determine the time required for starch digestion at each temperature. If no digestion has occurred within 5 minutes, test every 5 minutes. If no digestion has occurred within 10 minutes, test every 10 minutes.

h. If no digestion has occurred within 30 minutes, return the test tube to the 40°C water bath for 10 minutes. Test this tube again according to steps f and g.

i. Record and graph your results in the LABORATORY REPORT RESULTS at the end of the chapter.

At what temperature was starch digestion most rapid? ____

5. Effect of pH on Starch Digestion

MATERIALS

- Distilled water
- Paraffin or sugarless chewing gum
- Collection cups
- Three Pyrex test tubes
- Wax marking pencil

Buffer solutions at pH 4.0, 7.0, and 9.0 in dropper bottles

Starch solution in dropper bottle

Lugol's solution in dropper bottle

Spot plate

Three medicine droppers

Stop watch or watch with second hand

Safety goggles

Laboratory apron or coat

PROCEDURE

a. Rinse your mouth with distilled water and chew a small piece of paraffin or sugarless gum to stimulate salivary secretion.

b. Collect about 2 ml saliva in a small cup and add an equal amount of water to dilute the saliva.

ALTERNATE PROCEDURE: Use commercial amylase solution.

c. Mark three test tubes "4," "7," and "9," to indicate pH.

d. Use a medicine dropper to place about 2 ml of starch solution in each of the three test tubes. Using the droppers on the bottles, place about 1 ml of a buffer solution at pH 4.0 to tube "4," 1 ml of a buffer solution at pH 7.0 to tube "7," and 1 ml of a buffer solution of pH 9.0 to tube "9."

e. Mark three depressions on a spot plate "4," "7," and "9." Use separate medicine droppers to place one drop from each test tube in the appropriate depression.

f. At 1 minute intervals, use the dropper on the bottle to add a drop of Lugol's solution to each depression. Measure the time required for the blue-black color to disappear.

g. Record your times in the LABORATORY REPORT RESULTS at the end of the chapter.

COMPLETE THE LABORATORY REPORT QUESTIONS AT THE END OF THE CHAPTER

LABORATORY REPORT RESULTS

DIGESTION 20

Student ______________________ Date ______________________

Laboratory Section ______________________ Score/Grade ______________________

EXERCISE 1. Deglutition

1. Tongue movement at beginning of deglutition = ______________________

____

2. Description of swallowing with head below pharynx = ______________________

____

3. Laryngeal movements during pharyngeal deglutition = ______________________

____

4. Time lapse between two sounds of deglutition = __________

EXERCISE 2. Observation of the Rat Gastrointestinal Tract

1. Movement of stomach musculature = ______________________

____

2. Reaction of pyloric sphincter upon mechanical stimulus = ______________________

____

3. Reaction of intestinal musculature upon mechanical stimulus = ______________________

____

4. Reaction of intestine upon tissue ischemia = ______________________

____

5. pH of gastric contents = ____
6. pH of intestinal contents = ____

EXERCISE 3. Physiology of Intestinal Smooth Muscle

	Contractile		
	Strength	Frequency	Speed
Baseline			
O_2 Deprivation			
At 18°C			
Norepinephrine			
Acetylcholine			
Atropine			
Atropine and Acetylcholine			
Atropine, Acetylcholine and Norepinephrine			
Calcium removal			

1. Effect of O_2 deprivation: ____________________
2. Effect of cold: ____________________
3. Effect of norepinephrine: ____________________
4. Effect of acetylcholine: ____________________
5. Effect of atropine: ____________________
6. Which substance used in this exercise is a parasympathetic neurotransmitter? ____________________

Which is a sympathetic neurotransmitter? ____________________

Does intestinal smooth muscle have receptors for both sympathetic and parasympathetic neurotransmitters? _____

Atropine counters the effect of which neurotransmitter substance? ____________________

7. Is calcium required for the contraction of intestinal smooth muscle? _____

LABORATORY REPORT QUESTIONS

DIGESTION 20

Student ______________________ Date ______________________

Laboratory Section ______________________ Score/Grade ______________________

PART I. MULTIPLE CHOICE

_____ 1. Which of the following does NOT occur in the mouth? (a) deglutition (b) chemical digestion (c) absorption (d) mastication (e) mechanical digestion

_____ 2. Which of the following is NOT a part of the gastrointestinal tract? (a) cecum (b) colon (c) jejunum (d) pancreas (e) esophagus

_____ 3. Which is the principal organ of absorption? (a) stomach (b) small intestine (c) large intestine

_____ 4. Which is the principal organ of digestion? (a) stomach (b) small intestine (c) large intestine

_____ 5. Protein digestion begins in the (a) mouth (b) stomach (c) small intestine (d) large intestine

_____ 6. Carbohydrate digestion begins in the (a) mouth (b) stomach (c) small intestine (d) large intestine

_____ 7. During the esophageal stage of deglutition (a) the larynx moves against the epiglottis (b) peristalsis moves the bolus toward the pharynx (c) voluntary (skeletal) muscles move the bolus toward the fauces (d) all of the above (e) none of the above

_____ 8. Nonpropulsive movements in the gastrointestinal tract (a) include peristalsis (b) facilitate absorption (c) include segmentation (d) all of the above (e) none of the above

_____ 9. Chyme (a) is a mixture of gastric juice and food (b) has a low pH (c) is mixed by gastric churning (d) all of the above (e) none of the above

_____ 10. The lowest pH is found in secretions of the (a) mouth (b) stomach (c) small intestine (d) large intestine

_____ 11. Which of the following increases the contractile activity of the intestine? (a) norepinephrine (b) acetylcholine (c) atropine (d) oxygen deprivation (e) cold temperature

_____ 12. Hydrolysis reactions (a) cannot occur unless enzymes are present (b) are anabolic (synthesis) reactions (c) involve breaking chemical bonds with the addition of water (d) all of the above (e) none of the above

_____ 13. The breakdown of fat globules into smaller particles (a) is called emulsification (b) is accelerated by lipase (c) occurs in the gallbladder and liver (d) all of the above (e) none of the above

_____ 14. Chylomicrons are (a) the end products of fat digestion (b) aggregates of fatty acids and glycerol which are absorbed from the lumen into the epithelial cells (c) secreted into the capillary blood of intestinal villi (d) all of the above (e) none of the above

_____ 15. Amylase (a) functions at an optimum pH near neutral (b) catalyzes the conversion of starch to maltose (c) is secreted by the salivary glands and the pancreas (d) all of the above (e) none of the above

PART II. COMPLETIONS

16. Bile salts and the products of fat digestion aggregate into water-soluble structures called ________________, which are absorbed into the epithelial cells of the gastrointestinal tract.
17. A uniform suspension of fat droplets in water is called a(n) ________________.
18. Simple sugars are called ________________.
19. Benedict's solution is used to test for the presence or absence of ________________.
20. Lugol's solution is used to test for the presence or absence of ________________.
21. The end products of carbohydrate digestion are ________________.
22. The end products of fat digestion are ________________.
23. The end products of protein digestion are ________________.
24. Pancreatic enzymes act in the ________________.
25. A ball of food mixed with saliva is called a(n) ________________.

PART III. MATCHING

____ 26. Substrate is lactose
____ 27. Product is amino acids
____ 28. Inactive enzyme
____ 29. Secreted in saliva
____ 30. Products are glucose and fructose
____ 31. Last enzyme in protein digestion pathway
____ 32. Activated by enterokinase
____ 33. Precursor is secreted by stomach glands
____ 34. Substrate is emulsified fat
____ 35. Pancreatic enzyme which acts on polysaccharides
____ 36. Effective at pH of 1.0
____ 37. Products are fatty acids and glycerol
____ 38. First enzyme in protein digestion pathway
____ 39. Activates carboxypeptidase
____ 40. Proteolytic enzyme secreted by intestinal epithelium

A. Amylase
B. Dipeptidase
C. Lactase
D. Lipase
E. Maltase
F. Pepsinogen
G. Procarboxypeptidase
H. Sucrase
I. Trypsin

DISCUSSION: A. What structural property of enzymes makes them pH specific?

DISCUSSION: B. Starch is incubated with an unknown enzyme at 37°C and the mixture is tested with Lugol's and Benedict's solution. Both tests give positive reactions. Explain.

DISCUSSION: C. Trace the pathway of a roast beef sandwich from the mouth to the anus. List all steps of mechanical and chemical digestion. Give the end products and absorption sites. List all hormones involved and their functions.

METABOLISM 21

EXERCISE 1. Body Fat Determination
EXERCISE 2. Indirect Calorimetry

WORD ROOTS

ana- = upward
calor- = heat
kymo- = wave
meta- = change

Collectively, all the chemical reactions that take place within the body are called ***metabolism*** (me-TAB-ō-lizm). Since chemical activities either require or release energy, metabolism can be subdivided into catabolism, an energy-generating process, and anabolism, an energy-requiring process.

Anabolism (a-NAB-ō-lizm) includes all the synthesis reactions of the body, in which small, simple molecules combine to form larger complex molecules. These processes require the expenditure of adenosine triphosphate, a high-energy molecule abbreviated as ATP.

Catabolism (ka-TAB-ō-lizm) includes all the decomposition reactions in the body, in which large, complex molecules are broken down. About 55% of the energy released from the chemical bonds during these reactions becomes heat. The remainder is captured and stored in ATP. As the ATP is utilized by cells, the energy in the ATP is also released as heat.

Heat can be measured as temperature and expressed in units called calories. One ***calorie (cal)*** is the amount of heat energy required to raise the temperature of 1 g of water 1°C. The heat energy in foods is measured in ***kilocalories (kcal)***, equal to 1000 calories and defined as the amount of heat required to raise the temperature of 1000 g of water 1°C.

The metabolic rate is the rate at which heat (kilocalories) is produced by the oxidation of the food we eat. Among the factors that affect metabolic rate are

1. ***Exercise***. Strenuous exercise can increase the normal metabolic rate up to 20 times in well-trained athletes.
2. ***Stress***. During stress, the sympathetic nervous system releases norepinephrine (NE) which can increase the metabolic rate of cells.
3. ***Hormones***. In addition to norepinephrine, epinephrine, male sex hormones, human growth hormone (HGH), and thyroxine all increase metabolic rate.
4. ***Body temperature***. Each 1°C rise in body temperature increases metabolic rate about 10 percent. Fever may increase the metabolic rate substantially.
5. ***Ingestion of protein***. Some of the end products of digestion, particularly amino acids, stimulate cellular metabolism. This is called the ***specific dynamic action (SDA)*** of protein. SDA can raise the metabolic rate as much as 10–20%.
6. ***Age and sex***. Because of differences in body composition, the metabolic rate is higher in males than in females and decreases with age in both sexes (see Table 21.5).

The metabolic rate is studied by measuring the effect of these and other factors on the ***basal metabolic rate (BMR)***, a measure of the rate at which the body catabolizes food (and therefore releases heat) under the baseline conditions of minimal energy use that are described in Exercise 2. In addition, the BMR of an individual can be measured and compared with the mean BMR for individuals of the same height and weight.

EXERCISE 1. Body Fat Determination

> OBJECTIVES
>
> To describe the storage of fats
> To measure subcutaneous fat
> To estimate percent body fat from subcutaneous measurements

When caloric intake (food consumption) exceeds the energy requirements of the body, the excess calories are stored as fat. Proteins, carbohydrates, and fat are all digested before they cross the lining of the gastrointestinal tract; any of the products of their digestion that are not utilized are converted metabolically to body fat. ***Obesity*** is an abnormal increased amount of body fat.

Body fat is stored in the liver and in adipose cells, which can contain about 95% of their volume in fat. Since about 50% of the body fat is subcutaneous, measurement of subcutaneous fat gives a good indication of the total amount of fat in the body. Table 21.1 lists normal and abnormal values for the percent of body weight that is fat.

This exercise involves the measurement of subcutaneous fat at various sites on the body. These measurements are then used in a mathematical formula to determine the percent of fat in the body.

MATERIALS

Fat-O-Meter or other caliper device
Alcohol wipes

PROCEDURE

1. Use the formulas in Table 21.2 to determine the four or five sites that are to be measured on your laboratory partner.
2. Identify the first site to be measured. Using the photographs in Figure 21.1, locate the site carefully because a small error in site location can cause a gross error in results.
3. Take hold of the skin and subcutaneous fat (no muscle) between the left thumb and middle finger and with the right hand, grasp the caliper with the scale facing you.
4. Slide the caliper open and slowly allow it to close around the skin fold. Place the caliper about 1 millimeter (mm) away from the fingers at the crest of the fold.
5. Record the reading to the nearest mm.
6. Reopen the caliper and close it manually. *DO NOT* allow the spring to close the caliper.
7. Repeat steps 2–6 for each additional site to be measured.
8. Wipe the caliper with an alcohol wipe.
9. Calculate your fat density by using the equations in Table 21.2.
10. Calculate your percent fat by using the following formula

$$\text{percent fat} = \frac{457}{\text{density}} - 414.2$$

TABLE 21.1
NORMAL AND ABNORMAL VALUES FOR THE PERCENT OF BODY WEIGHT THAT IS FAT IN ADULTS

Male			Female		
U.S.A. Averages	**Interpreting Results**		**U.S.A. Averages**	**Interpreting Results**	
Under 30	Elite athletes	5–10%*	Under 30	Elite athletes	10–15%*
	Good	11–14%		Good	16–19%
	Acceptable	15–17%		Acceptable	20–24%
Over 30	Too Fat	18–19%	Over 30	Too Fat	25–29%
	Obese	20% & over		Obese	30% & over

*Care should also be taken with respect to the low end of the scale. Individuals should be advised against too low a body fat. For males 5–7% can be considered minimum while 10–12% is a minimum for females. Some medical problems cause low % fat.
Source: Health and Education Services, Addison, IL.

TABLE 21.2
FORMULAS FOR DETERMINING FAT DENSITY

Density Formula for Females

Age group	Equation
15–19	Density = 1.0802 − .0002(Site 2) − .0007(Site 6) − .0003(Site 7) − .0006(Site 8) − .0004(Site 9)
20–24	Density = 1.0861 − .0005(Site 2) − .0011(Site 5) − .0015(Site 6) − .0005(Site 9) + .0006(Site10)
25–29	Density = 1.0757 − .0017(Site 2) − .0008(Site 3) − .0003(Site 5) − .0004(Site 6) − .0005(Site 8)
30–39	Density = 1.0827 − .001(Site 2) + .0012(Site 3) − .0007(Site 5) − .0007(Site 6) − .0012(Site 7)
40–49	Density = 1.0726 − .0005(Site 1) + .0002(Site 5) + .0007(Site 6) − .0003(Site 8) − .0013(Site 9)
50+	Density = 1.0674 − .0003(Site 1) − .0008(Site 3) − .0007(Site 5) − .0002(Site 7) − .0009(Site 8)

Density Formula for Males

Age group	Equation
15–19	Density = 1.0832 + .0006(Site 1) − .0009(Site 2) + .0004(Site 5) + .0021(Site 6) − .0023(Site 7)
20–24	Density = 1.0971 + .0005(Site 1) − .0023(Site 8) − .0005(Site 4) − .0005(Site 5) + .0005(Site 10)
25–29	Density = 1.0862 − .0016(Site 2) + .0016(Site 3) − .0005(Site 4) + .0025(Site 6) − .0009(Site 9)
30–39	Density = 1.0926 + .0008(Site 3) − .0008(Site 6) − .0009(Site 7) − .0010(Site 9)
40–49	Density = 1.0737 − .0012(Site 2) + .0005(Site 3) − .0004(Site 4) − .0015(Site 6) − .001(Site 10)
50+	Density = 1.0639 + .0004(Site 1) + .0003(Site 2) − .0003(Site 5) − .0013(Site 7) − .0002(Site 10)

Source: Health and Education Services, Addison, IL.

Record this figure in the LABORATORY REPORT RESULTS at the end of the chapter.

11. Multiply your percent fat times your weight to determine how many pounds of fat you are carrying. Record the results in the LABORATORY REPORT RESULTS at the end of the chapter.

Would the measurement of muscle mass give an accurate evaluation of obesity? Why? ______

____

EXERCISE 2. Indirect Calorimetry

> OBJECTIVES
>
> To use the spirometer to measure basal metabolic rate (BMR)
> To measure BMR and metabolic rate after exercise and protein ingestion
> To calculate BMR on the basis of oxygen consumption
> To compare a measured BMR with a predicted normal BMR
> To describe some causes of elevated and depressed BMRs

Carbohydrates, proteins, and fats all release a specific amount of heat energy when they are oxidized. This heat can be measured by burning a given foodstuff in a calorimeter.

During oxidation, each foodstuff must combine with a given amount of oxygen, so if the amount of oxygen consumed is known, we can determine the amount of food being burned, that is, the amount of energy being consumed by the body.

Direct calorimetry has determined that glucose releases 5.01 kilocalories when combined with 1 liter of oxygen; starches, 5.06 kilocalories; protein, 4.60 kilocalories; and fats, 4.70 kilocalories. Since the body utilizes a mixture of different foodstuffs as energy sources, we can calculate that an average balanced diet provides 4.825 kilocalories per liter of oxygen consumed.

It is important to know how much energy the body consumes when it is at rest, that is, the basal metabolic rate (BMR). BMR is measured under conditions in which all factors that could affect metabolic rate have been reduced as much as possible. The baseline conditions are

1. Fasting from food for at least 12 hours before testing.
2. Normal body temperature (98.6°F) and comfortable environmental temperature (68° to 80°F). Temperatures below 68°F activate the sympathetic nervous system and increase thyroxine production; temperatures above 80°F

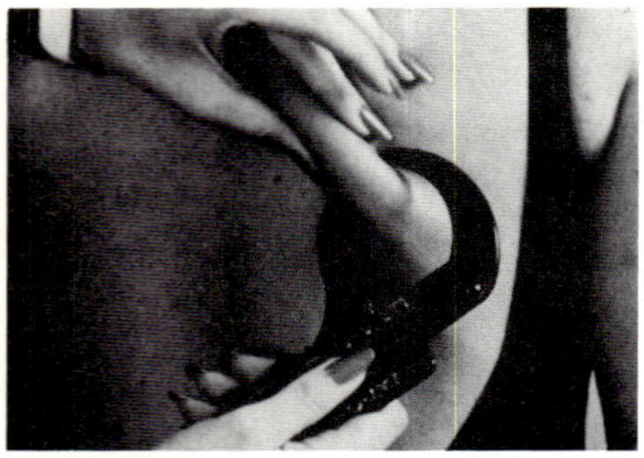

(a) SITE 1
SUBSCAPULAR
Inferior angle of the scapula, following the natural fold of the skin, about 1 cm below the angle.

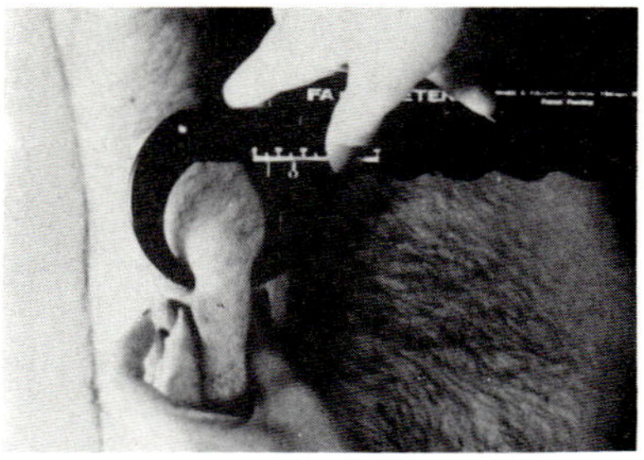

(b) SITE 2
TRICEPS
Halfway between the acromion process of the scapula and olecranon process of the ulna on the dorsum (back) of the arm.

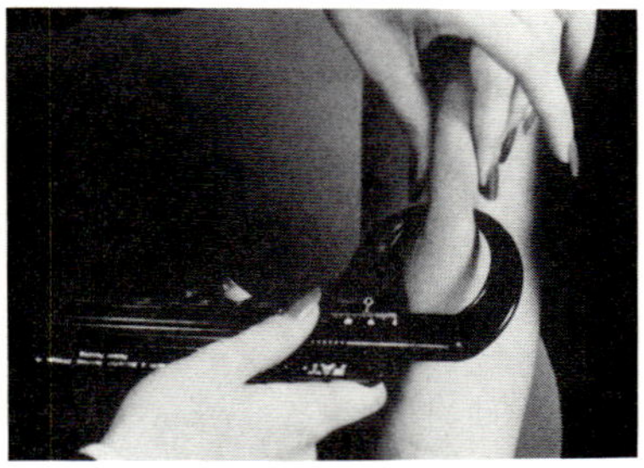

(c) SITE 3
BICEPS
Anterior of the arm, halfway between the greater tubercle of the humerus and the coronoid fossa.

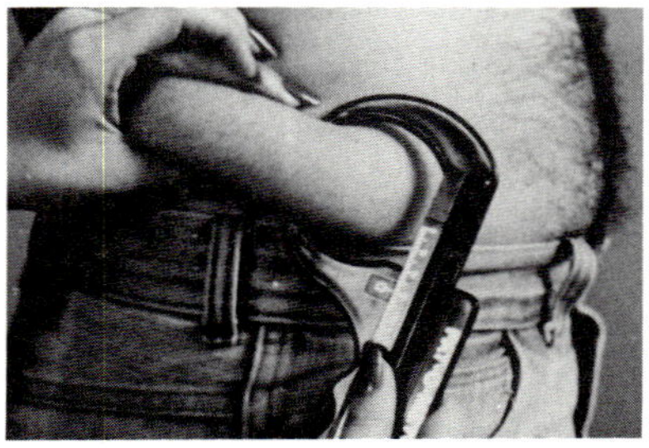

(d) SITE 4
SUPRAILIAC
A diagonal fold immediately above the iliac crest following the natural fold of the skin.

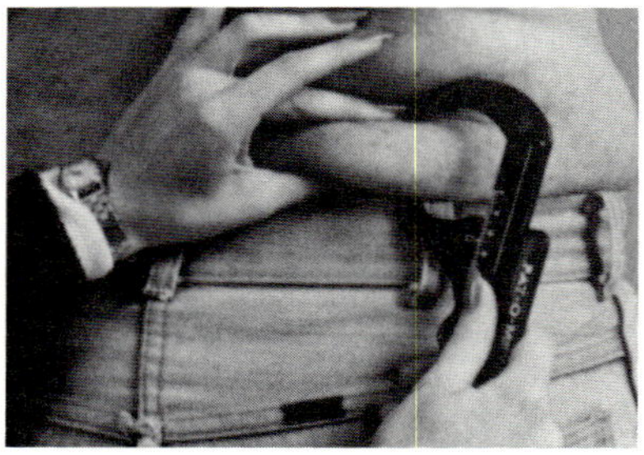

(e) SITE 5
POST SUPRAILIAC
5 cm to the right of the first lumbar spine.

FIGURE 21.1 Sites for measurement of body fat. (a) Site 1: Subscapular. (b) Site 2: Triceps. (c) Site 3: Biceps. (d) Site 4: Suprailiac. (e) Site 5: Post-suprailiac.

cause sweating and agitation due to discomfort.

3. Mental and physical relaxation. The subject must recline in a quiet, semidark environment for 30 minutes before testing. Testing is usually performed in the morning.

Repeated measurement of BMR in the same individual under these conditions shows that BMR remains constant for years with a variance of only 5–10 percent.

The most convenient way to determine BMR is to measure it indirectly by measuring oxygen consumption. If the body is at rest, the amount of oxygen consumed per hour is a measure of the energy requirements under basal conditions.

The ***respirometer*** or ***spirometer*** (see Figure 17.4c) is used to measure oxygen consumption directly; the metabolic rate can be calculated indirectly from knowledge of the amount of oxygen consumed. The respirometer is a device filled with oxygen which is breathed through a mouthpiece. Exhaled carbon dioxide is absorbed by a container of soda lime. As oxygen is consumed, the level of the respirometer bell falls. The top of the bell is connected to a cord running to a stylus that records the level of the gas container on a rotating kymograph. As the level of the bell falls, the level of the stylus rises.

From the record on the kymograph, the amount of oxygen consumed during a given time can be measured. Thus, if 1.8 liters of oxygen are consumed in 6 minutes, 18 liters are consumed per hour. Since 4.85 kilocalories are generated for every liter of oxygen consumed, metabolic rate can be calculated by

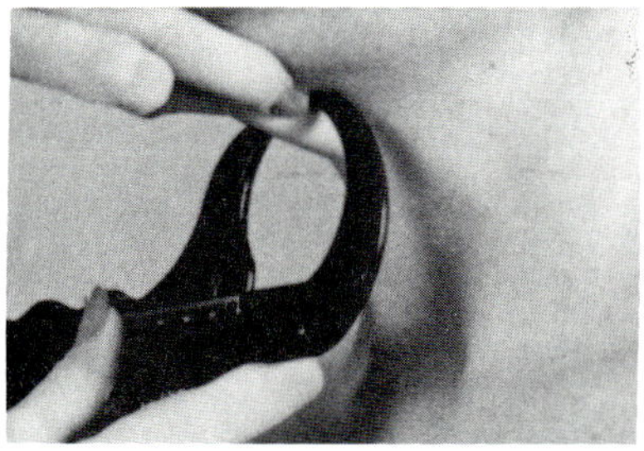

(f) SITE 6
CHIN
Under the chin above the hyoid bone.

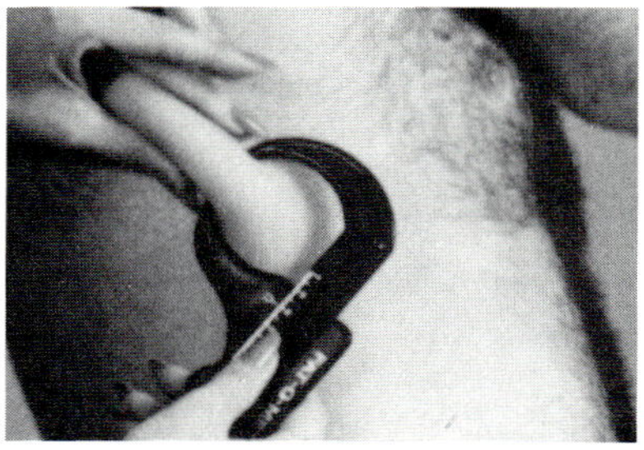

(g) SITE 7
MID AXILLARY
Anterior diagonal fold in the mid axilla at the level of the 5th rib.

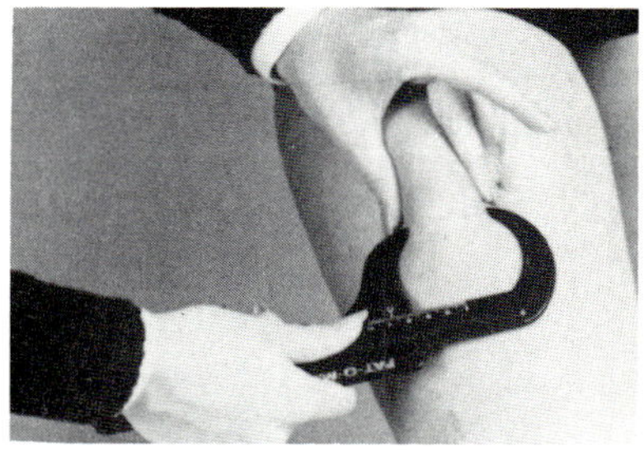

(h) SITE 8
THIGH
Vertical fold on front of the thigh midway between the greater trochanter of the femur and the top of the patella.

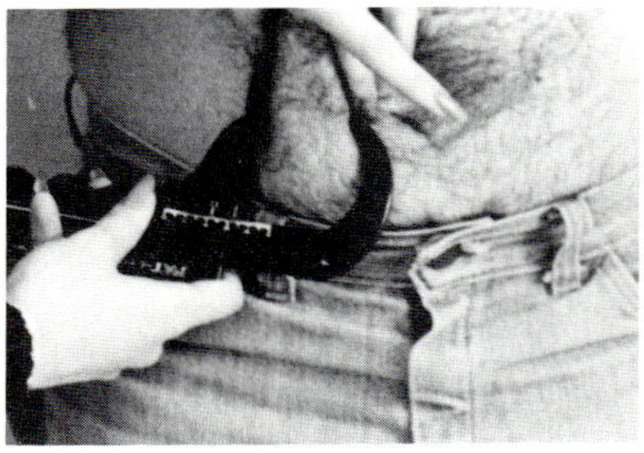

(i) SITE 9
UMBILICUS
A vertical fold to the side of the umbilicus.

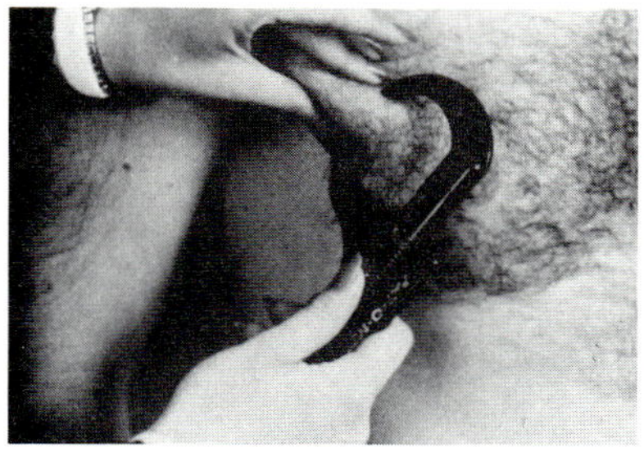

(j) SITE 10
PECTORAL
Midway between the axillary fold and the nipple in a fold parallel to the tendon of pectoralis major.

FIGURE 21.1 ***(Continued)*** Sites for measurement of body fat. (f) Site 6: Chin. (g) Site 7: Mid-axillary. (h) Site 8: Thigh. (i) Site 9: Umbilicus. (j) Site 10: Pectoral.

the formula

metabolic rate =

$$\frac{\text{liters of oxygen}}{\text{hour}} \times \frac{4.85 \text{ kcal}}{\text{liter of oxygen}}$$

In the example just given, the metabolic rate would be 18 liters of oxygen/hour × 4.85 kilocalories/liter of oxygen or 86.85 kilocalories/hour.

Since BMR varies with body size, it is usually expressed as kilocalories per square meter of body surface per hour. Body surface area is derived from a standard table (see Table 21.4). Thus, if the subject described above weighs 75 kg and is 190 cm tall, the body surface area is 2 square meters, and the BMR is 86.85 kilocalories/hour divided by 2 m^2 or 43.43 kilocalories/m^2/hour.

BMRs of a large number of individuals of different ages and sexes have been averaged and these "predicted normal values" are given in Table 21.5. About 85% of normal individuals have BMRs within 10% of these mean values. Thus, a deviation of ±10% is considered normal.

The percent deviation from normal of a given BMR is calculated as follows.

Percent deviation =

$$\frac{\text{Predicted normal value} - \text{Measured value}}{\text{Predicted normal value}} \times 100$$

If the given test result is below normal, it is expressed as a minus value (e.g., −18%). If the given test result is above normal, it is expressed as a plus value (e.g., +24%). Depressed BMRs occur with hypothyroidism, Vitamin B_1 deficiency, Addison's disease, anorexia nervosa, and other diseases. Elevated BMRs occur with hyperthyroidism, hypersecretion of human growth hormone (acromegaly and giantism), pregnancy, some leukemias, polycythemia vera, emphysema, and congestive heart failure. Since BMR is also elevated following exercise, measurement is ideally done in the morning, after a minimal amount of activity.

PROCEDURE FOR SUBJECT PREPARATION

1. Before you come to the laboratory, record your height, unclothed weight, and gender in the LABORATORY REPORT RESULTS at the end of the chapter. If weighing must be done in the laboratory, subtract 1 kilogram for the weight of clothing.
2. Eat a light dinner the night before the test. Get at least eight hours of sleep.
3. Rise and dress slowly. *DO NOT* eat breakfast, drink coffee, tea, or milk, or smoke before the test. If the test is performed in the afternoon, you may eat a light protein-free breakfast, but this will elevate your BMR.
4. Come to the laboratory at least 30 minutes before the test. Rest quietly in a supine position for 30 minutes.

PROCEDURE FOR EQUIPMENT PREPARATION

1. Make sure that the leveling screws are adjusted so that the bell does not rub on the metal body.
2. Feed paper from a roll onto the kymograph and tape it in place OR tape the paper on in a single sheet.
3. Make sure the soda lime is pink (fresh) and not purple (saturated with carbon dioxide).
4. Fill and prime the pen reservoirs.
5. Turn the oxygen control valve to *ON* and push the bell down all the way. Turn the oxygen control valve to *OFF*. Open the oxygen petcock and fill the bell slowly with oxygen. When the bell reaches its top position, shut off the oxygen tank and close the petcock.
6. Position the ventilometer pen (the upper pen, usually with black ink) so that it will begin writing near the center of the spirogram paper.
7. Set the free-breathing valve so that the opening is on the upper surface.
8. Place a *sterile or disposable* mouthpiece in the spirometer.
9. Record the room temperature ____ ° and barometric pressure ____ mm Hg.

MATERIALS

Noseclip
Spirometer
Kymograph paper, pens

PROCEDURE FOR BMR

1. Place the rubber pads of the noseclip on the fleshy part of the subject's nose. Adjust the noseclip so that it prevents exhalation under moderate pressure.
2. Place the mouthpiece in the subject's mouth and have the subject breathe atmospheric air until he or she is comfortable with the apparatus. If the apparatus is uncomfortable, adjust the support arm.
3. When the subject is comfortable, turn the oxygen-control valve to *ON*. At the end of an expiration, and before the next inspiration, close the free-breathing valve so that no opening is seen. The subject will now be breathing pure oxygen.
4. Turn the spirometer on to slow speed and have the subject breathe oxygen for about ten minutes. At this speed, the pen will move the distance between two vertical lines (32 mm) in one minute.
5. At the end of the test, turn off the kymograph, remove the mouthpiece from the subject, and turn the oxygen-control valve to *OFF*. CAUTION! *Dispose of the mouthpiece as directed by your laboratory instructor*, and remove the spirogram from the kymograph.

PROCEDURE FOR CALCULATION OF THE METABOLIC RATE

1. Using Figure 21.2 as a model, delineate a six minute recording cycle, beginning at the first vertical line to the right of the end of the tracing. This will be the leftmost vertical line that intersects the tracing. Label it *6 minutes*. The cycle will end at the sixth vertical line to the right of this line. Label it *0*. This selection eliminates the beginning and immediate end of the test during which respiratory rhythms may be irregular because of stress.
2. Draw the best-fitting straight line which connects the bottom of all respiratory cycles within the six minute period.

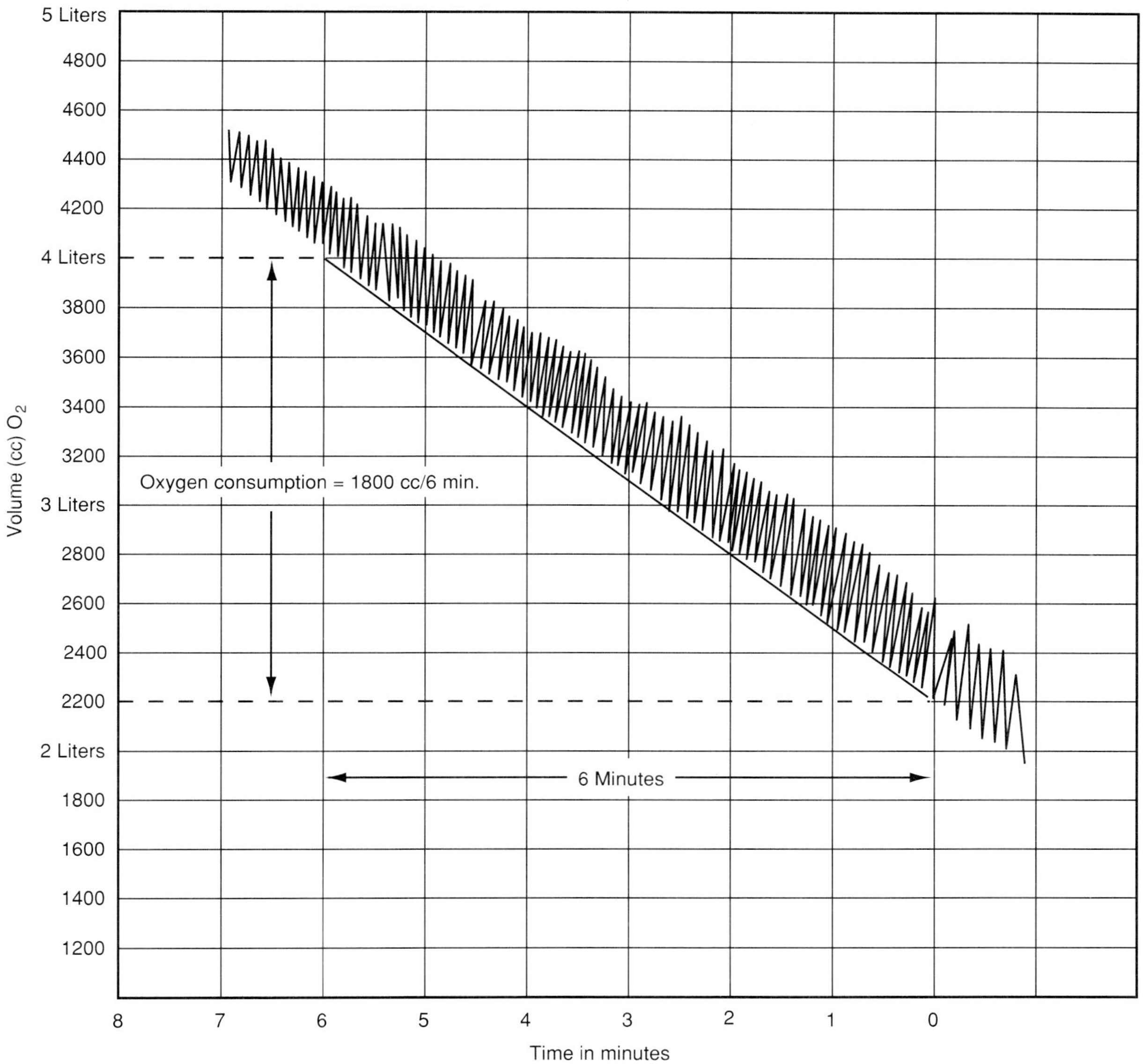

FIGURE 21.2 Measurement of oxygen consumption from the spirogram.

3. Draw a horizontal line from the bottom of the tracing at measured time *0*, to the vertical axis denoting volume.

4. Draw another horizontal line from the bottom of the tracing at measured time *6 minutes* to the vertical axis denoting volume.

5. Record both volumes in the LABORATORY REPORT RESULTS at the end of the chapter. Subtract the beginning volume from the end volume to derive total oxygen consumption for six minutes.

6. Multiply by 10 to derive oxygen consumption per hour.

7. Since metabolic rates are expressed at a standard temperature (0°C) and pressure (760 mm Hg), without the inclusion of water vapor, use Table 21.3 to obtain an appropriate correction factor, and multiply the volume of oxygen consumed by this factor. Record the corrected volume in the LABORATORY REPORT RESULTS at the end of the chapter.

8. Using Table 21.4, calculate the subject's

TABLE 21.3
FACTORS FOR REDUCING VOLUME OF MOIST GAS TO VOLUME OCCUPIED BY DRY GAS AT 0°C, 760 mm Hg

Observed Barometric Reading, Uncorrected for Temperature	15°	16°	17°	18°	19°	20°	21°	22°	23°	24°	25°	26°	27°	28°	29°	30°	31°	32°
700	0.855	851	847	842	838	834	829	825	821	816	812	807	802	797	793	788	783	778
702	857	853	849	845	840	836	832	827	823	818	814	809	805	800	795	790	785	780
704	860	856	852	847	843	839	834	830	825	821	816	812	807	802	797	792	787	783
706	862	858	854	850	845	841	837	832	828	823	819	814	810	804	800	795	790	785
708	865	861	856	852	848	843	839	834	830	825	821	816	812	807	802	797	792	787
710	867	863	859	855	850	846	842	837	833	828	824	819	814	809	804	799	795	790
712	870	866	861	857	853	848	844	839	836	830	826	821	817	812	807	802	797	792
714	872	868	864	859	855	851	846	842	837	833	828	824	819	814	809	804	799	794
716	875	871	866	862	858	853	849	844	840	835	831	826	822	816	812	807	802	797
718	877	873	869	864	860	856	851	847	842	838	833	828	824	819	814	809	804	799
720	880	876	871	867	863	858	854	849	845	840	836	831	826	821	816	812	807	802
722	882	878	874	869	865	861	856	852	847	843	838	833	829	824	819	814	809	804
724	885	880	876	872	867	863	858	854	849	845	840	835	831	826	821	816	811	806
726	887	883	879	874	870	866	861	856	852	847	843	838	833	829	824	818	813	808
728	890	886	881	877	872	868	863	859	854	850	845	840	836	831	826	821	816	811
730	892	888	884	879	875	871	866	861	857	852	847	843	838	833	828	823	818	813
732	895	890	886	882	877	873	868	864	859	854	850	845	840	836	831	825	820	815
734	897	893	889	884	880	875	871	866	862	857	852	847	843	838	833	828	823	818
736	900	895	891	887	882	878	873	869	864	859	855	850	845	840	835	830	825	820
738	902	898	894	889	885	880	876	871	866	862	857	852	848	843	838	833	828	822
740	905	900	896	892	887	883	878	874	869	864	860	855	850	845	840	835	830	825
742	907	903	898	894	890	885	881	876	871	867	862	857	852	847	842	837	832	827
744	910	906	901	897	892	888	883	878	874	869	864	859	855	850	845	840	834	829
746	912	908	903	899	895	890	886	881	876	872	867	862	857	852	847	842	837	832
748	915	910	906	901	897	892	888	883	879	874	869	864	860	854	850	845	839	834
750	917	913	908	904	900	895	890	886	881	876	872	867	862	857	852	847	842	837
752	920	915	911	906	902	897	893	888	883	879	874	869	864	859	854	849	844	839
754	922	918	913	909	904	900	895	891	886	881	876	872	867	862	857	852	846	841
756	925	920	916	911	907	902	898	893	888	883	879	874	869	864	859	854	849	844
758	927	923	918	914	909	905	900	896	891	886	881	876	872	866	861	856	851	846
760	930	925	921	916	912	907	902	898	893	888	883	879	874	869	864	859	854	848
762	932	928	923	919	914	910	905	900	896	891	886	881	876	871	866	861	856	851
764	936	930	926	921	916	912	907	903	898	893	888	884	879	874	869	864	858	853
766	937	933	928	924	919	915	910	905	900	896	891	886	881	876	871	866	861	855
768	940	935	931	926	922	917	912	908	903	898	893	888	883	878	873	868	863	858
770	942	938	933	928	924	919	915	910	905	901	896	891	886	881	876	871	865	860
772	945	940	936	931	926	922	917	912	908	903	898	893	888	883	878	873	868	862
774	947	943	938	933	929	924	920	915	910	905	901	896	891	886	880	875	870	865
776	950	945	941	936	931	927	922	917	912	908	903	898	893	888	883	878	872	867
778	952	948	943	938	934	929	924	920	915	910	905	900	895	890	885	880	875	869
780	955	950	945	941	936	932	927	922	917	912	908	903	898	892	887	882	877	872

Source: Peters and Van Slyke, *Quantitative Clinical Chemistry,* Vol. 11 (Methods). Baltimore: Williams and Wilkins, 1932, reprinted 1956.

TABLE 21.4
BODY SURFACE AREA IN METERS SQUARED (BSA/M²)

Height in centimeters (cm)	Weight in kilograms (kg)																
	25	30	35	40	45	50	55	60	65	70	75	80	85	90	95	100	105
200							1.84	1.91	1.97	2.03	2.09	2.15	2.21	2.26	2.31	2.36	2.41
195						1.73	1.80	1.87	1.93	1.99	2.05	2.11	2.17	2.22	2.27	2.32	2.37
190				1.56	1.63	1.70	1.77	1.84	1.90	1.96	2.02	2.08	2.13	2.18	2.22	2.28	2.33
185				1.53	1.60	1.67	1.74	1.80	1.86	1.92	1.98	2.04	2.09	2.14	2.19	2.24	2.29
180				1.49	1.57	1.64	1.71	1.77	1.83	1.89	1.95	2.00	2.05	2.10	2.15	2.20	2.25
175	1.19	1.28	1.36	1.46	1.53	1.61	1.67	1.73	1.79	1.85	1.91	1.96	2.01	2.06	2.11	2.16	2.21
170	1.17	1.26	1.34	1.43	1.50	1.57	1.63	1.69	1.75	1.81	1.86	1.91	1.96	2.01	2.06	2.11	
165	1.14	1.23	1.31	1.40	1.47	1.54	1.60	1.66	1.72	1.78	1.83	1.88	1.93	1.98	2.03	2.07	
160	1.12	1.21	1.29	1.37	1.44	1.50	1.56	1.62	1.68	1.73	1.78	1.83	1.88	1.93	1.98		
155	1.09	1.18	1.26	1.33	1.40	1.46	1.52	1.58	1.64	1.69	1.74	1.79	1.84	1.89			
150	1.06	1.15	1.23	1.30	1.36	1.42	1.48	1.54	1.60	1.65	1.70	1.75	1.80				
145	1.03	1.12	1.20	1.27	1.33	1.39	1.45	1.51	1.56	1.61	1.66	1.71					
140	1.00	1.09	1.17	1.24	1.30	1.36	1.42	1.47	1.52	1.57							
135	0.97	1.06	1.14	1.20	1.26	1.32	1.38	1.43	1.48								
130	0.95	1.04	1.11	1.17	1.23	1.29	1.35	1.40									
125	0.93	1.01	1.08	1.14	1.20	1.26	1.31	1.36									
120	0.91	0.98	1.04	1.10	1.16	1.22	1.27										

*From DuBois, E.F., *Basal Metabolism in Health and Disease,* 3rd ed. (Philadelphia: Lea & Febiger, 1936). Used by permission.

body surface area in square meters and record the results in the LABORATORY REPORT RESULTS at the end of the chapter.

9. Record the subject's basal metabolic rate in kilocalories/m²/hour in the LABORATORY REPORT RESULTS at the end of the chapter.

10. Using Table 21.5, calculate the percent deviation from normal according to the formula given in the introduction to this exercise. Record this figure in the LABORATORY REPORT RESULTS at the end of the chapter.

What factors can cause inaccurate results in this method of determining the BMR? ________

____

____

How many kilocalories/hour are expended to maintain the BMR in this subject? ____

COMPLETE THE LABORATORY REPORT QUESTIONS AT THE END OF THE CHAPTER

TABLE 21.5
PREDICTED NORMAL VALUES OF MEAN BASAL METABOLIC RATE (BMR) IN KILOCALORIES PER SQUARE METER OF BODY SURFACE PER HOUR

Females		Males	
Age at Last Birthday	Mean	Age at Last Birthday	Mean
6	50.62	6	53.00
6½	50.23	7	52.45
7	49.12	8	51.78
7½	47.84	8½	51.20
8	47.00	9	50.54
8½	46.50	9½	49.42
9–10	45.90	10	48.50
11	45.26	10½	47.71
11½	44.80	11	47.18
12	44.28	12	46.75
12½	43.58	13–15	46.35
13	42.90	16	45.72
13½	42.10	16½	45.30
14	41.45	17	44.80
14½	40.74	17½	44.03
15	40.10	18	43.25
15½	39.40	18½	42.70
16	38.85	19	42.32
16½	38.30	19½	42.00
17	37.82	20–21	41.43
17½	37.40	22–23	40.82
18–19	36.74	24–27	40.24
20–24	36.18	28–29	39.81
25–44	35.70	30–34	39.34
45–49	34.94	35–39	38.68
50–54	33.96	40–44	38.00
55–59	33.18	45–49	37.37
60–64	32.61	50–54	36.73
65–69	32.30	55–59	36.10
		60–64	35.48
		65–69	34.80

Source: American Journal of Physiology, July 1936.

METABOLISM 21

Student ______________________ Date ______________________

Laboratory Section ______________________ Score/Grade ______________________

EXERCISE 1. Body Fat Determination

1. Fat Density = ____
2. Percent Fat = ____
3. Pounds of Fat = ____

EXERCISE 2. Indirect Calorimetry
Subject Preparation

1. Height = ____
2. Unclothed weight = ____
3. Gender = ____

Basal Metabolic Rate (BMR)

1. End volume = ____ cc
   Beginning volume = ____ cc
   Oxygen consumed = ____ cc
2. Oxygen consumption per hour = ____ cc
3. Corrected volume of oxygen consumed per hour = ____ cc
4. Body surface area = ____ square meters
5. BMR = ____ kilocalories/m^2/hour
6. Deviation from normal = ____

LABORATORY REPORT QUESTIONS

METABOLISM 21

Student ______________________ Date ______________________

Laboratory Section ______________________ Score/Grade ______________________

PART I. MULTIPLE CHOICE

_____ 1. The digestion of food is (a) an energy generating process (b) a catabolic process (c) a part of metabolism (d) all of the above (e) none of the above

_____ 2. Anabolism (a) generates heat energy (b) produces ATP (c) refers to synthesis reactions (d) all of the above (e) none of the above

_____ 3. A calorie (a) is the amount of energy needed to raise the temperature of 1 g of water 1°C (b) is the standard measure of heat energy in food (c) is an end product of digestion (d) all of the above (e) none of the above

_____ 4. Metabolic rate is increased (a) by the ingestion of protein (b) when age increases (c) when body temperature falls (d) all of the above (e) none of the above

_____ 5. Obesity is defined as excess (a) weight (b) size (c) fat (d) all of the above (e) none of the above

_____ 6. If we know the amount of oxygen consumed during a given time at rest, we can determine (a) the amount of food being oxidized (b) basal metabolic rate (c) the amount of energy needed to sustain body processes (d) all of the above (e) none of the above

_____ 7. Causes of an elevated basal metabolic rate (BMR) include (a) increased levels of thyroxine (b) pregnancy (c) increased levels of growth hormone (d) all of the above (e) none of the above

_____ 8. The specific dynamic action (SDA) of protein is (a) the amount of kilocalories produced by oxidizing protein (b) the effect of amino acids on metabolic rate (c) the energy released by protein catabolism (d) 4.60 kilocalories

_____ 9. Which of the following is NOT a condition required for measuring basal metabolic rate (BMR)? (a) fasting from food for 12 hours (b) normal body temperature (c) barometric pressure of 760 mm Hg (d) mental and physical relaxation (e) ambient temperature of 68°–80°F

_____ 10. The spirometer is used to compute basal metabolic rate (BMR) by measuring the (a) amount of kilocalories produced (b) amount of calories produced (c) amount of oxygen consumed (d) amount of energy required to maintain a basal state of metabolism (e) amount of food oxidized

PART II. COMPUTATION

A 100 pound, 5 foot tall, 22 year old female consumes a corrected oxygen volume of 12 liters per hour. What is her BMR in kilocalories/m^2/hr? _____ What is her percent deviation from normal? _____

DISCUSSION: Why is basal metabolic rate (BMR) calculated with relation to body surface area?

RENAL PHYSIOLOGY 22

EXERCISE 1. Urine Formation
EXERCISE 2. Physical Urinalysis
A. Color and Transparency
B. pH
C. Specific Gravity
EXERCISE 3. Chemical Urinalysis
A. Chloride and Sodium Chloride
B. Glucose
C. Protein
D. Ketone Bodies
E. Bile Pigments
F. Hemoglobin and Myoglobin
EXERCISE 4. Microscopic Urinalysis

WORD ROOTS

glomerulus = little ball
nephr- = kidney
py-, pyo- = pus
rena-, reni- = kidney

The ***urinary system*** maintains homeostasis by controlling the composition and volume of the blood. This system filters the end products of metabolism from the blood into urine, and it also actively secretes other waste substances into urine. In addition to their primary function of eliminating wastes, the kidneys manufacture ***renal erythropoietic*** (e-rith′-rō-poy-ET-ic) ***factor***, a substance which liberates erythropoietin from its carrier protein. Erythropoietin then stimulates bone marrow to produce red blood cells. The kidneys help to regulate blood pressure through the secretion of ***renin***. Renin initiates a reaction which results in the production of angiotensin II, a potent vasoconstrictor which also stimulates the adrenal cortex to secrete ***aldosterone*** (al-DOS-ter-ōn), a hormone which causes salt and water retention by the kidney. The active form of vitamin D is also produced in the kidneys.

The functional and structural unit of the kidney is the ***nephron*** (NEF-ron); there are about 1,200,000 nephrons in each kidney. The nephron, shown in Figure 22.1, consists of a tuft (knot) of about 50 capillaries, called a ***glomerulus*** (glo-MER-yoo-lus), surrounded by a ***glomerular (Bowman's) capsule*** and a series of tubules. Fluid is filtered from the glomerular blood into the glomerular capsule. This filtrate then passes through the ***proximal convoluted tubule***, the descending and ascending limbs of the ***loop of the nephron (loop of Henle)***, and the ***distal convoluted tubule***. Filtrate from the distal convoluted tubule is received by the ***collecting duct***. From here it passes into the ***renal pelvis, ureters*** (YOO-re-ters), ***urinary bladder***, and ***urethra*** (yoo-RĒ-thra), and is finally excreted as urine.

To review nephron anatomy, label the structures indicated in Figure 22.1.

EXERCISE 1. Urine Formation

OBJECTIVES

To describe the processes by which urine is formed
To measure the effect of osmolarity on urine production
To measure the effect of increased potassium and hydrogen ions on urine production
To demonstrate diuresis

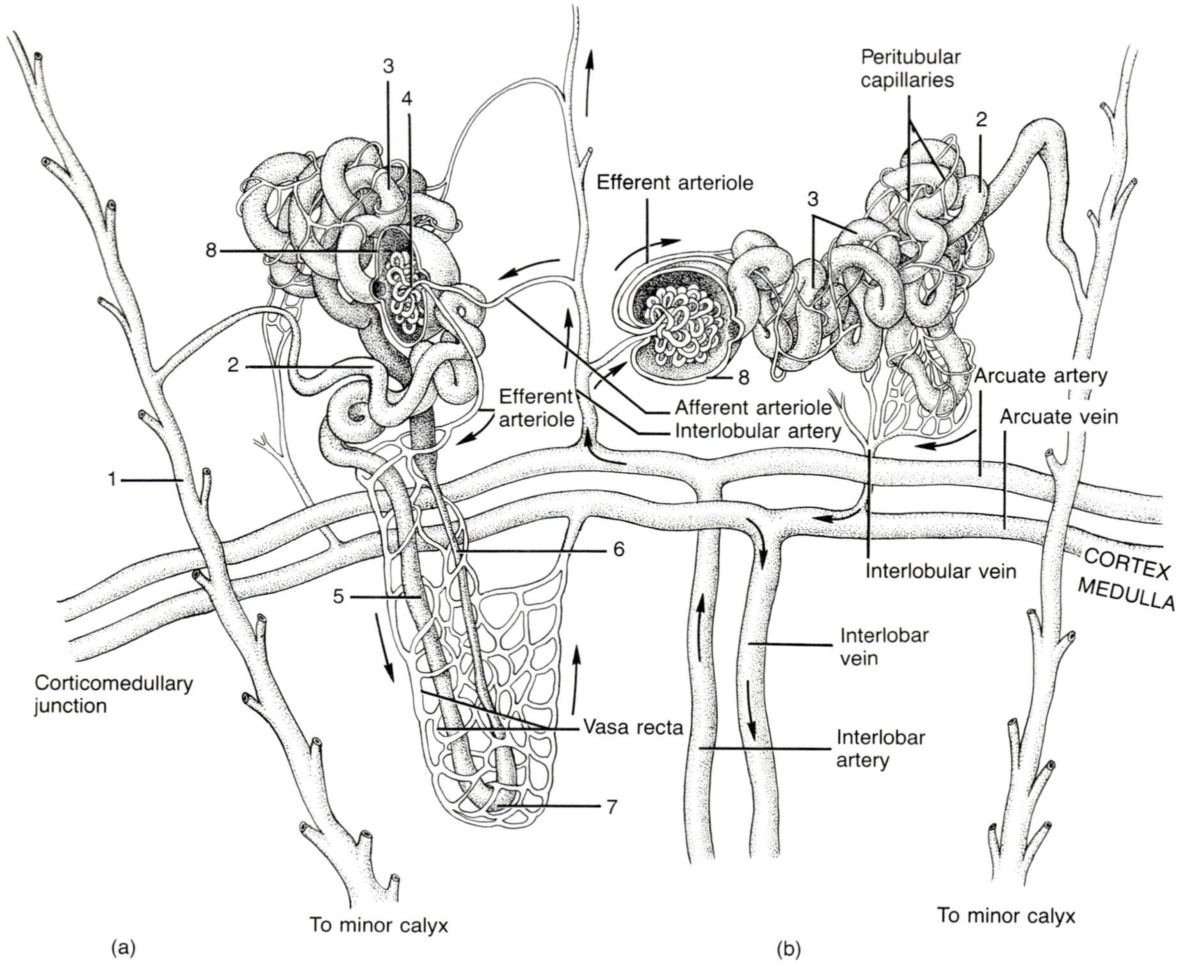

___ Ascending limb
___ Collecting duct
___ Descending limb
___ Distal convoluted tubule
___ Glomerular capsule
___ Glomerulus
___ Loop of the nephron
___ Proximal convoluted tubule

FIGURE 22.1 Nephrons. (a) Juxtamedullary nephron. (b) Cortical nephron.

Urine formation is the result of three processes: (1) ***glomerular filtration***, (2) ***tubular reabsorption***, and (3) ***tubular secretion***. In overview, glomerular blood is filtered into the glomerular capsule. About 99 percent of this filtrate is conserved by being reabsorbed back into the blood; 1 percent of the filtrate is excreted. Small amounts of waste substances are secreted into the filtrate by the tubular cells. Thus, urine is composed mainly of substances filtered from the blood, but it also includes secreted substances.

Glomerular filtration filters about 180 L/day of glomerular blood into the glomerular (Bowman's) capsule. The filtrate must cross the ***endothelial-capsular membrane*** between the glomerular capillaries and the inside of the glomerular capsule. This membrane, shown in Figure 22.2, filters all substances with diameters greater than 7 millimicrons (molecular weights greater than 70,000). Thus blood cells and large proteins remain in the blood, and the filtrate has about the same composition as blood plasma, minus the large plasma proteins. The force of filtration in the glomeruli is measured as the ***effective filtration pres-***

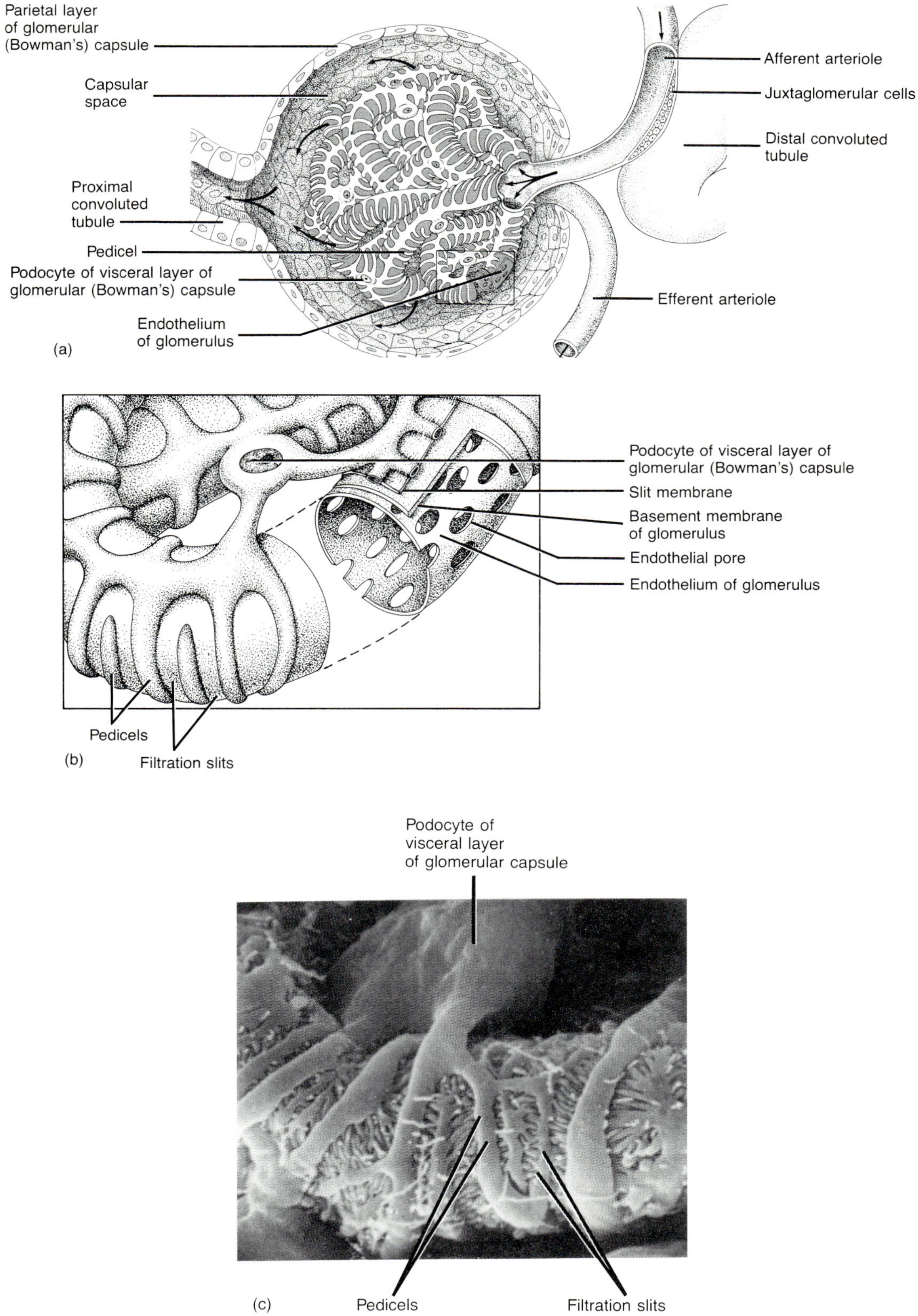

FIGURE 22.2 Endothelial-capsular membrane. (a) Components of glomerulus and glomerular capsule. (b) Details of endothelial-capsular membrane. (c) Scanning electron micrograph of a portion of the membrane at 7800×. (Part (c) from *Tissues and Organs: A Text-Atlas of Scanning Electron Microscopy* by Richard G. Kessel and Randy H. Kardon. W. H. Freeman and Company. Copyright ©1979.)

sure (P_{eff}). The P_{eff} is the sum of the two forces (blood hydrostatic pressure (BHB) and capsular osmotic pressure (COP)) which move fluid out of glomerular blood minus the sum of the two forces which pull fluid into the blood (capsular hydrostatic pressure (CHP) and blood osmotic pressure (BOP)).

$$P_{eff} = (BHP + COP) - (CHP + BOP)$$

Tubular reabsorption selectively removes about 179 L/day of water and solutes from the 180 L/day that are filtered. The reabsorbed substances move from the tubular cells into interstitial fluid and then into peritubular capillaries. This process returns usable substances to the blood, while wastes are retained in the filtrate. Most reabsorption occurs in the proximal convoluted tubule and involves both active and passive transport.

Tubular secretion occurs throughout the tubules of the nephron and in the collecting duct. This process moves substances from the blood of the peritubular capillaries and from the tubular cells into the filtrate. Typically, materials secreted by the nephron are incompletely metabolized compounds, weak acids and bases, ions, and foreign substances. Table 22.1 lists various components of the renal filtrate and of urine. By comparing the four columns, you can see the outcome of the various processes involved in urine formation.

The primary control of urine formation is exerted by two hormones: ***antidiuretic hormone (ADH)*** from the neurohypophysis and ***aldosterone*** from the adrenal cortex. ADH production is regulated by osmoreceptors in the hypothalamus. When the concentration of water in the blood falls below normal levels, ADH is released. ADH increases the permeability of the collecting duct cells to water and thus causes (1) increased water reabsorption ***(facilitated reabsorption of water)***, (2) decreased urine volume, and (3) increased urine tonicity (concentration of solute).

Aldosterone causes (1) increased sodium and water reabsorption by the distal tubule and collecting duct cells, (2) decreased urine volume, and (3) increased potassium excretion. Aldosterone secretion is increased by (1) a decrease in the systemic blood pressure, (2) a decrease in plasma sodium levels, (3) an increase in plasma potassium levels, and (4) increased ACTH (adrenocorticotropic hormone) levels.

This exercise will investigate how urine is affected by the consumption of (1) excess water, (2) excess sodium chloride, (3) excess potassium, and (4) caffeine. Caffeine exerts a diuretic (dī'-yoo-RET-ik) effect by inhibiting sodium reabsorption in the proximal convoluted tubule. Diuresis is the production of large volumes of urine. Note that the reabsorption of chloride is directly related to the reabsorption of sodium, since Na^+ is actively reabsorbed by the renal tubules, Cl^- follows passively by electrostatic attraction.

TABLE 22.1
CHEMICALS IN PLASMA, FILTRATE, AND URINE DURING 24-HOUR PERIOD*

Chemical	Plasma	Filtrate Immediately After Glomerular (Bowman's) Capsule	Reabsorbed from Filtrate	Urine
Water	180 liters	180 liters	178–179 liters	1–2 liters
Proteins	7,000–9,000	10–20	10–20	0
Chloride (Cl^-)	630	630	625	5
Sodium (Na^+)	540	540	537	3
Bicarbonate (HCO_3^-)	300	300	299.7	0.3
Glucose	180	180	180	0
Urea	53	53	28	25
Potassium (K^+)	28	28	24	4
Uric acid	8.5	8.5	7.7	0.8
Creatinine	1.4	1.4	0	1.4

*All values, except for water, are expressed in grams/24 hours. The chemicals are arranged in sequence from highest to lowest concentration in plasma.

MATERIALS

Graduated urine collecting and measuring cups

Graduated drinking cups

Gatorade®

Unsweetened orange juice

Strong coffee or tea

pH paper

Urinometer and cylinder

Pyrex or Kimex test tube

Medicine dropper

20% potassium chromate solution with dropper

2.9% silver nitrate solution with dropper

Safety goggles

Laboratory apron or coat

CAUTION! *Please reread Section A, "General Procedures and Safety Precautions," and Section C, "Precautions Related to Working With Reagents," in Chapter 1 before you begin any of the exercises in this chapter. You should also read the exercises before you perform them to be sure that you understand all of the procedures and safety precautions.*

PROCEDURE

1. Try not to void during the two hours preceding the laboratory period.

2. At the beginning of the laboratory period, take a collection cup to the restroom. Use the Urine Collecting Procedure described at the end of the chapter to collect a midstream sample. Consider this sample as your control sample.

3. Work in groups of five. Immediately upon returning to the laboratory, one member of each group should drink one of the following solutions. CAUTION! *If any member of your group has cardiovascular or renal disease or is pregnant, they should participate only by drinking solution a.*

a. 500 ml of water

b. 500 ml of Gatorade®

c. 500 ml of unsweetened strong coffee or tea

d. 500 ml of unsweetened orange juice (a potassium source with an acidic pH)

4. Every 30 minutes after drinking, until the end of the period, completely empty the urinary bladder into a graduated collection cup.

5. For the control sample and for each subsequent sample, measure and record the volume, specific gravity, pH, and sodium chloride (NaCl) concentration. The instructions for measuring specific gravity and pH are in Exercise 2; the instructions for measuring sodium chloride concentration are in Exercise 3.

6. Determine the rate of urine excretion by dividing the number of ml in each sample by 30. Your answer will be in ml excreted per minute.

7. Record your results in the LABORATORY REPORT RESULTS at the end of the chapter.

8. Plot the following four parameters against time: (a) volume excreted, (b) specific gravity, (c) sodium chloride concentration, and (d) pH. Compare the results derived from each of the five members of the group. Your instructor may ask you to combine and average the results for all groups in your laboratory section before you plot your results.

9. Compare your results with those derived by the other four members of your group.

Drinking which solution produced the highest volume of urine? ______________________

the lowest volume? ______________________

the highest specific gravity? ______________________

the lowest specific gravity? ______________________

the the lowest pH? ______________________

the highest sodium chloride concentration?

____

the lowest sodium chloride concentration?

____

Explain these results on the basis of your knowledge of urine formation. ______________________

____

____

____

____

EXERCISE 2. Physical Urinalysis

OBJECTIVES

To determine physical characteristics of normal and abnormal urine

To describe causes of various abnormalities in the urine

Urinalysis is the physical, chemical, and microscopic analysis of urine. The composition of urine varies with the physiological status of the individual and the needs of the internal environment. Temperature, fluid balance, and physical activity all affects its composition.

In certain pathological conditions, normal constituents of urine may increase in amount, and abnormal constituents may be present. These constituents are described in the following section on urinalysis. Before beginning, read the following instructions on collecting urine and on the general procedures used in performing a urinalysis.

URINE COLLECTION PROCEDURE

Urine may be collected at any time for routine tests; urine voided within three hours after meals, however, may contain abnormal constituents. The first void in the morning is preferred for this reason and because it is the most concentrated sample.

1. Obtain a clean (sterile, if possible) container. Void a small amount of urine; collect a midstream sample in the container; finish emptying the urinary bladder. This procedure avoids contamination by leucocytes and bacteria normally found in the urethra and by material present on the external genitalia.
2. If the specimen is not to be tested immediately, refrigerate it to prevent bacterial growth which can lower the pH and/or ammonia production which can raise pH.

GENERAL PROCEDURES FOR URINALYSIS

1. Before testing *always* mix urine by swirling or stirring with a clean stick or rod.
2. *Discard all disposable sticks, stirs, and containers in a plastic garbage bag.*
3. Rinse all glassware with *cold* water; if the glassware is hot, do not rinse it until it has cooled.
4. Dispose of urine in lab sinks and flush the drains well with cold water.

A. Color and Transparency

Normal urine is a straw yellow to amber transparent liquid with a characteristic odor. The color varies considerably according to the diet and to the ratio of solute to water. Cloudy urine sometimes reflects the secretion of mucin from the urinary tract lining and is not necessarily pathological. Cloudiness may also result from the precipitation of phosphate salts by an alkaline urine. Most of the color of urine is due to the presence of small amounts of urochrome, urobilin, and other breakdown products of bilirubin. Some causes of anomalous colors are

Color	Possible Cause
Pale	Increased urine volume (polyuria) or diabetes insipidus
Silvery, milky	Pus, bacteria, epithelial cells
Smoky brown, rust	Blood
Orange, green, blue, red	Medications or liver disease

MATERIALS

Clean clear container

Glass rod

Safety goggles

Laboratory apron or coat

PROCEDURE

1. Obtain a urine sample and note the color.
2. Evaluate the transparency of your sample by stirring and noting any cloudiness.
3. Record your observations in the LABORATORY REPORT RESULTS at the end of the chapter.

How would sickle-cell anemia affect urine color? ______________________________

____

____

B. pH

Although the normal pH range of urine is between 5.0 and 7.8, its mean pH is usually slightly acidic. Because normal metabolic activity produces more acid than base, hydrogen ions (H^+) must be continually secreted. Their presence accounts for the difference between the normal urine mean pH of about 6.0 and the normal arterial blood pH of about 7.4. A high protein diet increases urine acidity while a vegetarian diet increases alkalinity. Urine voided in the daytime usually has a higher pH than that voided after sleep. Upon standing, urine becomes alkaline because urea is converted to ammonia.

MATERIALS

Clean urine container

pH paper or Dipstix®

PROCEDURE

1. Test the pH of your urine with Dipstix® or with pH paper by placing the indicator strip in the urine and shaking off any excess urine.
2. Compare the color with the indicator color chart.
3. Record the pH in the LABORATORY REPORT RESULTS at the end of the chapter.

How would the ingestion of antacids such as sodium bicarbonate affect the pH of urine?

____

C. Specific Gravity

The ***specific gravity*** of a substance is the ratio of the weight of a volume of that substance to the weight of an equal volume of distilled water. By definition, water has a specific gravity of 1.000. The specific gravity of urine depends on the concentration of solute and normally varies from 1.003 to 1.030. The greater the concentration of solute, the higher the specific gravity. Solutes normally present in urine are shown in the right-hand column of Table 22.1.

MATERIALS

Urinometer

Urinometer cylinder

PROCEDURE

1. Familiarize yourself with the scale on the urinometer neck. Determine the change in specific gravity represented by each calibration.
2. Allow your urine to reach room temperature. Urinometers are calibrated to read the specific gravity at 15°C (69°F). If the temperature differs, add or subtract 0.001 for each 3°C above or below 15°C.
3. Fill the cylinder three-fourths full of urine and insert the urinometer. Make sure that it is free floating; if not, spin the neck gently.
4. Read the scale at the bottom of the meniscus when the urinometer is at rest.
5. Record the specific gravity in the LABORATORY REPORT RESULTS at the end of the chapter.
6. Rinse the urinometer and cylinder. *Follow your instructor's directions for cleaning them.*

How would dehydration affect the specific gravity of urine? ______________________________

____

____

EXERCISE 3. Chemical Urinalysis

OBJECTIVES

To analyze some chemical characteristics of urine

To describe causes of chemical abnormalities of urine.

Chemical analyses may be performed by mixing urine with various reagents or reagent tablets, or by the use of plastic Dipstix® to which paper squares impregnated with reagent are affixed. The Dipstix® may be specific for one urine constituent or they may test for many constituents at once. Several different methods for testing for each constituent are given. Your instructor will tell you which procedure to use. If you have been instructed to use a form of Dipstix®, use the following method.

Use of Dipstix®

1. Determine which component(s) of urine are measured by the Dipstix® you are using. If you are using a stick which tests for multiple substances, determine which squares measure

which substances. Locate the color chart used to read the results. Note the appropriate time for reading each test.

2. Remove a test strip from the vial and *replace the cap*.

3. Dip the test strip into the urine for 1 second, being sure that all reagents on the strip are immersed.

4. Remove any excess urine from the strip by drawing it along the rim of the urine container.

5. Compare the reagent blocks on the test strip to the colors on the color chart.

6. Record your results in the LABORATORY REPORT RESULTS at the end of the chapter.

A. Chloride and Sodium Chloride

Most of the sodium chloride (NaCl) present in the renal filtrate is reabsorbed; a small amount remains as a normal component of urine. The mean of the normal values for chloride (Cl^-) is 476 mg/100 ml; for sodium (Na^+) it is 294 mg/100 ml.

MATERIALS

- Urine collecting cup
- Medicine dropper
- Test tube
- Medicine dropper (20 drops per ml)
- 20% potassium chromate solution with dropper
- 2.9% silver nitrate solution with dropper
- Glass rod
- Safety goggles
- Laboratory apron or coat

PROCEDURE

1. Using a medicine dropper, place 10 drops of urine into a Pyrex test tube.

2. Use a medicine dropper to add one drop of 20% potassium chromate and *gently* agitate the contents of the tube with a glass rod. It should be a yellow color.

3. Use a medicine dropper to add 2.9% silver nitrate solution *one drop at a time*, counting the drops and agitating the test tube during the time the solution is being added.

4. Count the number of drops needed to change the color of the solution from bright yellow to brown.

5. Determine the chloride and sodium chloride concentrations of the sample. Each drop of silver nitrate added in step 4 is equivalent to (1) 61 mg of Cl^- per 100 ml of urine, and (2) 100 mg of NaCl per 100 ml of urine.

Thus, to determine the chloride concentration of the sample, multiply the number of drops times 61 to obtain the number of mg of Cl^- per 100 ml of urine.

To determine the sodium chloride concentration of the sample, multiply the number of drops times 100 to obtain the number of mg of NaCl per 100 ml of urine.

What could a high NaCl content in the urine indicate? ____________________

____

____

B. Glucose

Detectable levels of glucose are not normally present in urine because all of it is reabsorbed from the filtrate (see Table 22.1). The process of reabsorption requires a carrier-mediated transport system, which has a typical maximum capacity of 180 mg/dl. Normal blood glucose level is 60–120 mg/dl, so glycosuria (the presence of glucose in urine) indicates a significant defect, i.e., the level of glucose in the blood and hence in the filtrate must exceed 180 mg/dl before the system fails to reabsorb it by transporting it into the peritubular capillaries. Glycosuria is typical in diabetes mellitus.

Clinitest® Reagent Method

MATERIALS

- Urine collecting cup
- Pyrex or Kimex test tube
- Test tube rack
- Clinitest® tablet
- Two medicine droppers
- Forceps
- Test tube holder
- Safety goggles
- Laboratory apron or coat

PROCEDURE

1. Using medicine droppers, place 10 drops of water and 5 drops of urine in a Pyrex test tube.

CAUTION! *Place the tube in a test tube rack because it will become too hot to hold.*

2. With forceps, add one Clinitest® tablet to the test tube and close the bottle. CAUTION! *The concentrated NaOH in the tablet generates enough heat to make the liquid in the test tube boil. Make sure the mouth of the test tube is pointed away from you and all other persons in the area.*

3. Fifteen seconds after boiling has stopped, use a test tube holder to shake the test tube *gently*. CAUTION! *Make sure the mouth of the tube is pointing away from you and others.* Evaluate the color according to the table below. Disregard any color change which occurs after 15 seconds.

Color	Glucose concentration
Blue	0–100 mg/100 ml
Greenish yellow	100–500 mg/100 ml (1+)
Olive green	500–1400 mg/100 ml (2+)
Orange-yellow	1400–2000 mg/100 ml (3+)
Brick red	>2000 mg/100 ml (4+)

4. Record your results in the LABORATORY REPORT RESULTS at the end of the chapter.

How would a high sugar diet affect the urine?

Explain. ______________________________

____

____

C. Protein

Normally, the glomerular filtrate has only traces of very small proteins although strenuous physical exercise may cause increased permeability of glomerular capillaries and hence leakage of small proteins into the filtrate. ***Proteinuria*** (prō′-tē-in-YOO-rē-a), the presence of excess protein in urine, also results from hypertension and kidney disease such as ***glomerulonephritis*** (glō-mer′-yoo-lō-nef-RĪ-tis). Albumin is the first protein detected in the urine because it is the most abundant serum protein and it is relatively small (molecular weight = 69,000).

Exton's® Reagent Method

MATERIALS

Urine collecting cup
Pyrex or Kimex test tube
Medicine dropper
Exton's® reagent in dropper bottle
Safety goggles
Laboratory apron or coat

PROCEDURE

1. Using separate medicine droppers, place equal volumes (about 3–5 ml) of urine and Exton's® reagent in a test tube.

2. *Gently*, roll the tube between your palms to mix the two fluids.

3. If a precipitate is formed, the liquid will appear cloudy because of the presence of albumin.

4. Record your results in the LABORATORY REPORT RESULTS at the end of the chapter.

Albutest® Reagent Method

MATERIALS

Urine collecting cup
Paper towel
Albutest® tablet and color chart
Forceps
Two medicine droppers
Safety goggles
Laboratory apron or coat

PROCEDURE

1. Using forceps, place an Albutest® tablet on a clean paper towel and use a medicine dropper to add one drop of urine.

2. After the urine drop has been absorbed, use a medicine dropper to add two drops of water and allow these to penetrate the tablet.

3. Compare the color (in daylight or fluorescent light) on the top of the tablet with the color chart provided.

4. If albumin is present in the urine, a blue-green spot will appear on the surface of the tablet. The amount of protein is indicated by the intensity of the blue-green color. If no protein is present, the tablet color will not change.

5. Record your results in the LABORATORY REPORT RESULTS at the end of the chapter.

Why is protein not normally present in urine?

____

____

D. Ketone (Acetone) Bodies

When carbohydrates are not available as an energy source, the body shifts to fat as an energy source. After the hydrolysis of lipids to fatty acids and glycerol, the liver begins the degradation of fatty acids by converting them to ketone bodies: acetone, acetoacetic acid, and beta-hydroxybutyric acid. When produced in normal quantities, these ketone bodies are oxidized in peripheral tissues. When there is an excess of ketone bodies they spill into the urine. Causes of ketosis are starvation (inadequate carbohydrate supply), diabetes mellitus (inadequate utilization of carbohydrates), and a high fat diet.

MATERIALS

Urine collecting cup
Acetest® tablet and paper towel
Forceps
Medicine dropper
Safety goggles
Laboratory apron or coat

PROCEDURE

1. Use forceps to place an Acetest® tablet on a paper towel and use a medicine dropper to place one drop of urine on the tablet.
2. If acetone or ketone is present, a lavender-purple color develops within 30 seconds. If the table becomes cream-colored from wetting, the results are negative.
3. Record your results in the LABORATORY REPORT RESULTS at the end of the chapter.

Why would starvation cause ketosis? ________

____

____

E. Bile Pigments

Over 200 billion erythrocytes are destroyed by the reticuloendothelial system each day. The liberated hemoglobin is broken down, and the heme is converted to bilirubin. Most of the bilirubin is excreted in the bile. A very small amount of bilirubin is converted by intestinal bacteria to urobilinogen which is reabsorbed into the blood and excreted in the urine. Bilirubin appears in the urine only when there is excess destruction of erythrocytes (as in hemolytic diseases), obstruction of the bile ducts, or liver disease such as cirrhosis and hepatitis.

Shaken Tube Test for Bilirubin

MATERIALS

Urine collecting cup
Test tube and stopper
Safety goggles
Laboratory apron or coat

PROCEDURE

1. Fill a Pyrex test tube half full of urine, stopper the tube, and shake it vigorously, being careful to keep the tube stoppered.
2. The presence of foam of an intense yellow color indicates the presence of conjugated bilirubin.
3. Record your results in the LABORATORY REPORT RESULTS at the end of the chapter.

Icotest® for Bilirubin

MATERIALS

Urine collecting cup
Paper towel
Icotest® tablet and mat
Forceps
Two medicine droppers
Watch with second hand
Safety goggles
Laboratory apron or coat

PROCEDURE

1. Place an Icotest® mat onto a paper towel and use a medicine dropper to place 10 drops of urine onto the mat.
2. Use a forceps to place one Icotest® reagent tablet in the center of the moistened area. CAUTION! *Do not touch the tablets with your fingers. Recap the bottle.*
3. Add one drop of water directly to the tablet; after 5 seconds, add another drop of water to the tablet so that the water runs off onto the mat.

4. Observe the color of the mat around the tablet at 60 seconds. The presence of bilirubin will turn the mat blue or purple. A slight pink or red color is negative for bilirubin.

5. Record your results in the LABORATORY REPORT RESULTS at the end of the chapter.

Why would a transfusion reaction cause bilirubin to be present in the urine? ______________

____

F. Hemoglobin and Myoglobin

When erythrocytes are destroyed, the liberated hemoglobin is phagocytized by reticuloendothelial cells and split into its heme and globin portions. If the amount of red blood cell destruction increases beyond the limits of the reticuloendothelial system, free hemoglobin appears in the urine. This condition, ***hemoglobinuria***, occurs in hemolytic disease, burns, malaria, transfusion reactions, and exposure to toxins in such things as snake venom and poisonous mushrooms.

Myoglobin is a protein similar to hemoglobin in its ability to combine with oxygen. It is found in slow (red) muscle. Myoglobin is not present in urine unless muscle destruction has occurred as the result of trauma, strenuous exercise, muscle disease, and so forth.

There is no simple test for the presence of hemoglobin and myoglobin other than the use of Dipstix®.

What is the relationship between bilirubinuria and hemoglobinuria? ______________

____

____

EXERCISE 4. Microscopic Urinalysis

OBJECTIVES

To perform a microscopic examination of urine
To identify some contents of urinary sediment
To describe causes of abnormalities in urine seen upon microscopic examination of urine

To examine the materials suspended in urine, you can let it stand for several hours to allow the substances to settle, or you can centrifuge a urine sample for five minutes. A centrifuge is pictured in Figure 22.3. The microscopic examination of urinary sediment may reveal any of the following substances, which are illustrated in Figure 22.4.

a. ***Casts***. Casts are tiny masses of various organic and inorganic substances which have hardened and assumed the shape of the tubule where they were formed. Casts usually have square ends and the same diameter for their entire length. Since the various constituents of casts are usually bound by albumin, their presence may indicate a kidney disease which causes proteinuria.

b. ***Erythrocytes***. ***Hematuria*** is a condition in which red blood cells are seen in the urine in appreciable amounts; it is indicative of a pathological condition such as ***urinary calculi*** (kidney stones), glomerular infection, and tumor. Red blood cells are also seen when a urine sample is contaminated by menstrual flow.

c. ***Leucocytes***. ***Pyuria*** is a condition in which white blood cells and other components of pus are found in the urine. It is indicative of a urinary tract infection.

d. ***Epithelial cells***. Cells sloughed off from the lining of the urinary tract are seen in normal urine.

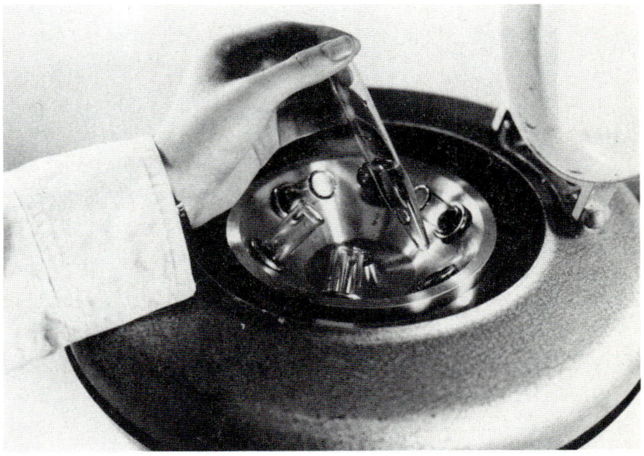

FIGURE 22.3 Tabletop centrifuge for obtaining urine sediment for microscopic analysis.

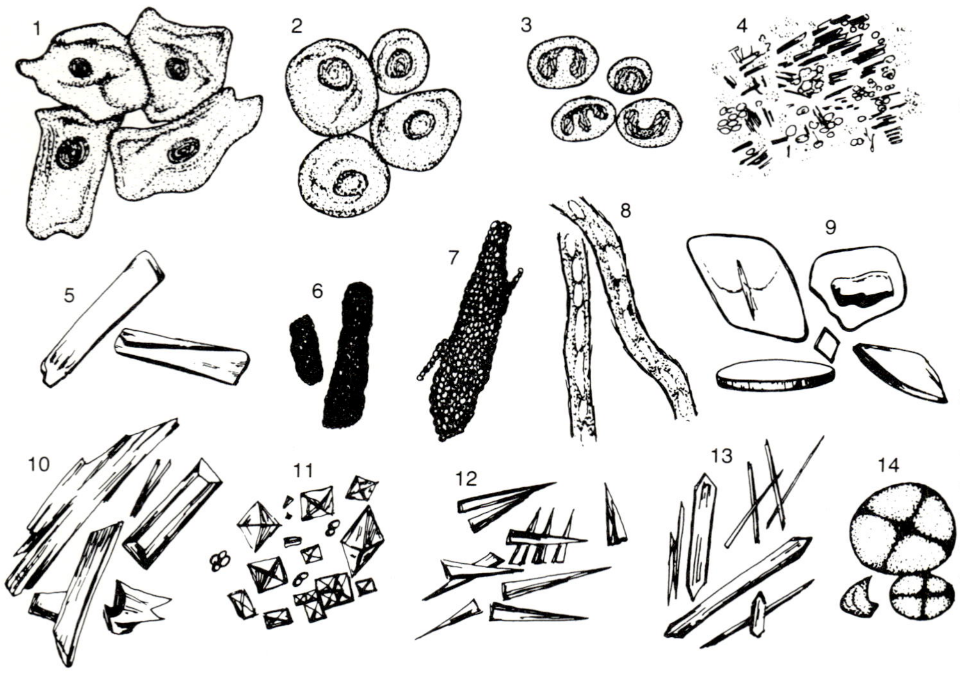

FIGURE 22.4 Diagram of microscopic elements in urine.

e. ***Bacteria***. Bacteria are not normally present in urine. However, if the specimen has not been obtained by a sterile technique (catheterization), and if it has been left at room temperature, bacterial growth can be rapid.

f. ***Crystals***. A few crystals may be present in normal urine; a large number indicates a tendency to form kidney stones. Uric acid crystals precipitate out in gout. Crystals may be identified as follows.

Calcium oxalate. Dumbbell and octahedral shapes.

Calcium phosphate. Pointed, wedge shaped crystals which may occur individually or in rosette groupings.

Cholesterol. Spherical crystals with a cross-like configuration inside.

Hippuric acid. Long needlelike crystals.

Triple phosphates. Prisms or feathery forms.

Uric acid. Rhombic prisms, wedges, dumbbells, rosettes, irregular crystals. Their color varies from yellow to dark reddish brown.

MATERIALS

Urine collecting cup
10 ml graduated cylinder
Centrifuge and centrifuge tube
Long medicine dropper or Pasteur pipette and bulb
Microscope slide and cover glass
Immersion oil
Sedi-stain™ or methylene blue
Safety goggles
Laboratory apron or coat

PROCEDURE

1. Place 5 ml fresh urine in a centrifuge tube. Follow the directions of your instructor to centrifuge the tube for 5 minutes at a slow speed (1500 rpm).

2. Dispose of the supernatant (the clear urine) and mix the sediment by shaking the test tube.

3. Use a long medicine dropper or a Pasteur pipette to place a small drop of sediment on a

clean glass slide, add one drop of Sedi-stain™ or methylene blue, and place a cover glass over the specimen.

4. Using low power and reduced light, examine the sediment for any of the microscopic elements pictured in Figure 22.4.

5. Increase the light and use high power or oil immersion to look for crystals.

6. Record your results in the LABORATORY REPORT RESULTS at the end of the chapter.

Why might some red blood cells in urinary sediment be crenated? ____________________

____

____

Why might yeast be seen in the urine of a person with diabetic mellitus? ____________________

____

____

COMPLETE THE LABORATORY REPORT QUESTIONS AT THE END OF THE CHAPTER

LABORATORY REPORT RESULTS

RENAL PHYSIOLOGY 22

Student ______________________ **Date** ______________________

Laboratory Section ______________________ **Score/Grade** ______________________

REABSORPTION

SOLUTION CONSUMED: ______________________

	Control	+ 30 Min.	+ 1 Hour	+ 1½ Hours	+ 2 Hours
Volume					
Specific gravity					
pH					
NaCl					

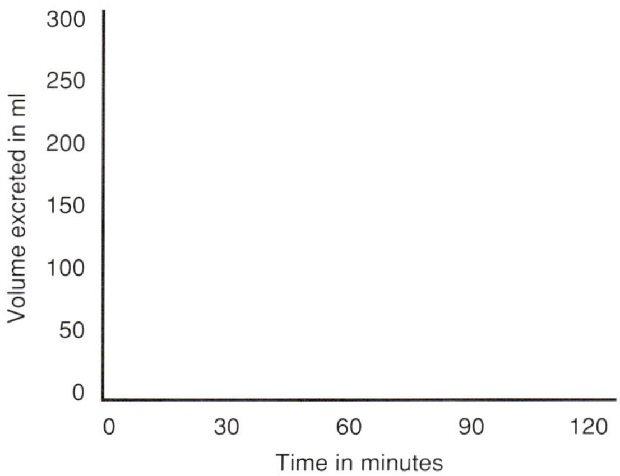

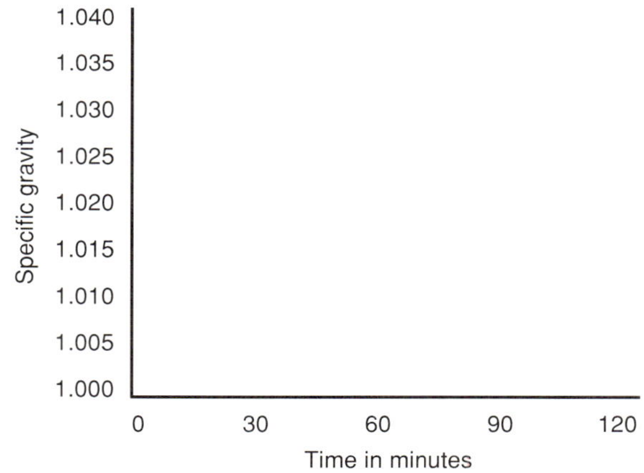

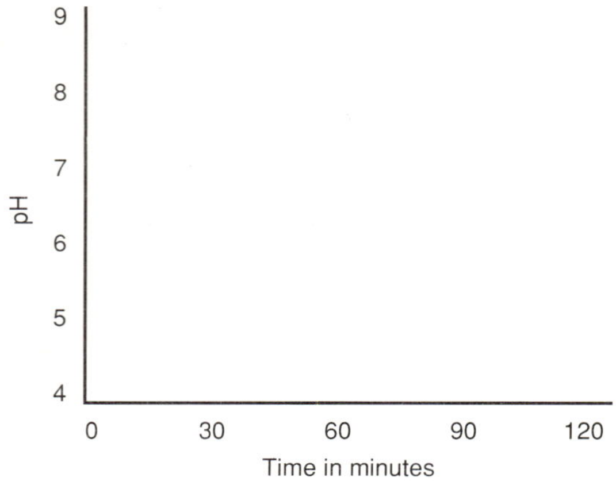

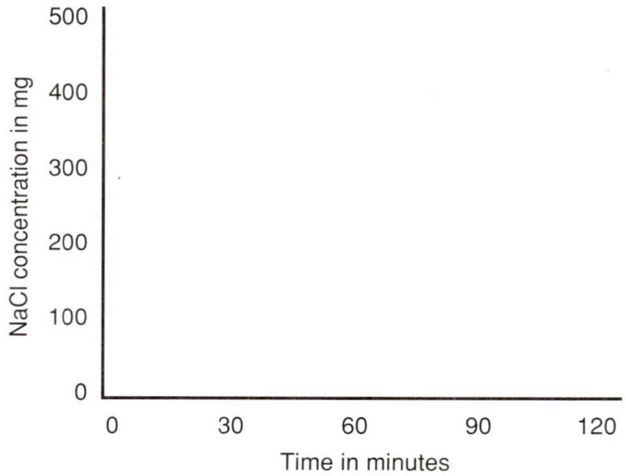

Urinalysis

Color	
Transparency	
pH	
Specific Gravity	
Chloride Concentration	mg/100 ml
Sodium Chloride Concentration	mg/100 ml
Glucose	
Protein	
Ketone Bodies	
Bile Pigments	
Hemoglobin	
Casts	
Erythrocytes	
Leucocytes	
Epithelial Cells	
Bacteria	
Crystals	

LABORATORY REPORT QUESTIONS

RENAL PHYSIOLOGY 22

Student ______________________ Date ______________________

Laboratory Section ______________________ Score/Grade ______________________

PART I. MULTIPLE CHOICE

_____ 1. Which of the following is NOT a function of the urinary system? (a) regulation of blood pressure (b) regulation of acid-base balance (c) activation of vitamin D (d) red blood cell formation (e) regulation of cellular metabolism

_____ 2. Filtration (a) occurs at the glomerular (Bowman's) capsule (b) is a function of blood pressure (c) produces 180 L of filtrate per day (d) all of the above (e) none of the above

_____ 3. Which of the following substances does NOT have the same concentration in the glomerular filtrate and in the blood plasma? (a) glucose (b) urea (c) sodium (d) water (e) protein

_____ 4. Reabsorption (a) occurs mostly in the distal convoluted tubule (b) is a means of conserving plasma proteins (c) is mostly a process of active transport (d) all of the above (e) none of the above

_____ 5. Tubular secretion (a) is the passive transport of hydrogen ions into the filtrate (b) is a means of excreting excess water into the filtrate (c) is the active transport of solute into the tubular filtrate (d) all of the above (e) none of the above

_____ 6. Antidiuretic hormone (ADH) (a) is secreted when blood becomes more hypotonic (b) decreases the permeability of the distal convoluted tubule and the collecting duct to water (c) causes increased reabsorption of water (d) all of the above (e) none of the above

_____ 7. Aldosterone (a) causes increased active transport of sodium (b) causes increased reabsorption of water (c) both of the above (e) neither of the above

_____ 8. The normal pH range of urine is (a) 3.0 to 7.0 (b) 5.0 to 7.8 (c) 5.8 to 7.0

_____ 9. The normal mean pH of urine is (a) 7.0 (b) 6.0 (c) 5.0

_____ 10. The normal specific gravity of urine is (a) 1.000 (b) 1.003 to 1.0003 (c) 1.3 to 1.03 (d) .03 to .003 (e) 1.03 to 1.003

_____ 11. The specific gravity of urine would increase in (a) proteinuria (b) dehydration (c) glycosuria (d) all of the above (e) none of the above

_____ 12. Hypertension could cause (a) proteinuria (b) increased urine volume (c) both of the above (d) neither of the above

_____ 13. Ketosis could be caused by (a) a high protein diet (b) hypertension (c) dehydration (d) all of the above (e) none of the above

_____ 14. Hemolytic anemia would NOT necessarily cause which of the following? (a) hemoglobinuria (b) bilirubinuria (c) erythrocytes in the urine

_____ 15. Crystallized urinary salts are called (a) casts (b) renal calculi (c) glomeruli

DISCUSSION: A. Compare the renal function of two individuals, (1) a severely dehydrated individual, and (2) an individual who has just consumed 2 oz of alcohol. Describe the effects on urine volume, pH, specific gravity, ADH production, and aldosterone production.

DISCUSSION: B. Why is the measurement of blood glucose a better diagnostic tool than the measurement of glucose levels in the urine of a diabetic?

APPENDIX A: PITHING OF FROGS

By definition, *pithing* is destruction of the central nervous system by piercing the brain or spinal cord. This procedure is used in animal experimentation to render the animal unconscious so that it feels no pain. A single-pithed frog is one in which only the brain is destroyed, whereas a double-pithed frog has its spinal cord destroyed too. Usually the double-pithing procedure is used.

1. Hold the frog in a paper towel with its dorsal side up and with the index finger pressing the nose down so that the head makes a right angle with the trunk.
2. Locate the slight depression formed by the first vertebra and the skull about 3 mm behind the line joining the posterior borders of the tympanic membrane. This groove represents the area of the foramen magnum.
3. To single-pith the frog, carefully insert a long sharp-tipped needle or probe into the foramen magnum and direct it forward and a little downward (see Figure A-1).
4. Exert a steady pressure and rotate it, moving it from side to side in the cranial cavity to destroy the brain.
5. To double-pith the frog, insert the needle into the vertebral canal, directing it downward until it has reached the end of the canal. Move the needle from side to side as you go (see Figure A.1).

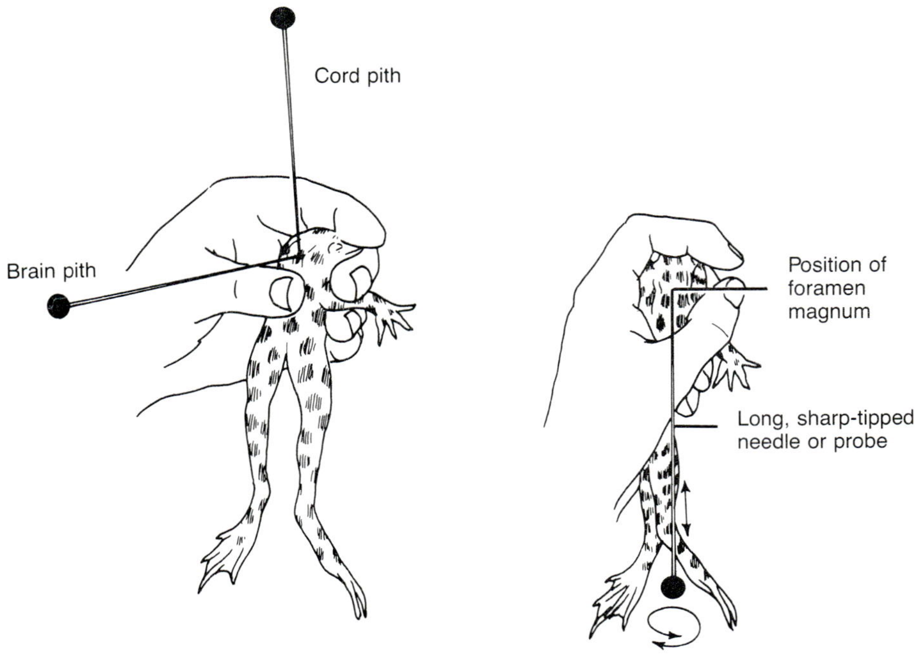

FIGURE A.1 Procedure for pithing a frog.

FIGURE CREDITS

2.1 Courtesy of Fisher Scientific, an Allied Company, and S.T.E.M. Laboratories, copyright ©1975.

4.1 Courtesy of Cambridge Instruments, Inc., Optical Systems Division, Buffalo, NY.

5.5 Courtesy of Joseph Kurantsin-Mills, George Washington University.

6.6 (a)–(f) By James R. Smail, Macalester College.

7.3 Adapted from Sylvia L. Mader, *Biology: Evolution, Diversity, and the Environment*. Dubuque, IA: Wm. C. Brown Publishers, 1985.

9.6 Adapted from Warren D. Dolphin, *Biology Laboratory Manual*. Dubuque, IA: Wm. C. Brown Publishers, 1983.

9.7 Courtesy of Narco BioSystems, Inc., Houston, TX.

11.2 Biomedical Graphics Department, University of Minnesota Hospitals.

11.3 By Hope H. Adams.

11.8 Adapted from Marks, Dobelle, and MacNichol, Jr.: *Science*, 143: 1181, 1964; and from Brown and Wald: *Science*, 144: 45, 1964. Copyright © 1964 by the American Association for the Advancement of Science.

12.3 Courtesy of Special Instruments Division, Beltone Electronics Corp., Chicago, IL.

15.1, 15.2, 15.4 Courtesy of Dr. Robert J. Sullivan.

15.5 (a) Supplied by Carolina Biological Supply Company, Burlington, NC.

15.5 (b) Courtesy of March of Dimes Birth Defects Foundation, New York, NY.

16.1 (a)–(c) Courtesy of Fisher Scientific, an Allied Company, and S.T.E.M. Laboratories, copyright © 1975.

16.4 By James R. Smail, Macalester College.

16.5 Courtesy of Fisher Scientific, an Allied Company.

16.7 (a)–(d) Courtesy of Cambridge Instruments, Inc., Optical Systems Division, Buffalo, NY.

16.8 Courtesy of Lenni Patti.

17.8 Copyright © 1983 by Gerald J. Tortora, courtesy of Geraldine C. Tortora and Matt Iacobino.

18.4 (a) Courtesy of Kinetics, Upper Saddle River, NJ.

18.4 (b) By Hope H. Adams, courtesy of Jeannie Martz.

18.4 (c) Courtesy of Warren E. Collins, Inc., Braintree, MA.

19.1 By Hope H. Adams, courtesy of Bruce H. Adams.

21.1 (a)–(j) Courtesy of Novel Products, Inc., Health and Education Services, Addison, IL.

22.2 (c) From *Tissues and Organs: A Text-Atlas of Scanning Electron Microscopy* by Richard G. Kessel and Randy H. Kardon. Copyright © 1979, W. H. Freeman and Company.

23.12 By James R. Smail, Macalester College.

INDEX

A

A band, 116
ABO blood groups, 230, 249
Accommodation, 155, 158
Acetylcholine (ACh), 117
Achalasia, 314
Acid, 24
Acid-base balance, 24
Acidosis, 24
Acrosome, 201, 207
Activation energy, 21, 23
Active transport, 46, 55
Adaptation, 137, 141, 143
Adenohypophysis, 180
Adenosine triphosphate (ATP), 118
Adrenal (suprarenal) gland, 184
Adrenocorticotropic hormone (ACTH), 183
Aerobic fitness, 305
Afferent nervous system, 93
Afterimage, 137
Agglutinin, 249
Agglutinogen, 249
Agranulocyte, 241, 244
Albumin, test for, 50
Aldosterone, 186, 347, 350
Alimentary canal, 311
Alkalosis, 24
All-or-none principle, 81, 118, 127
Allantois, 210
Allele, 219
Amniocentesis, 210
Amnion, 210
Ampulla, 167, 172
Anabolic reaction, 21
Anabolism, 333
Anemia, 244, 247
Anosmia, 97
Anterior cavity, 152
Antibody, 249
Antidiuretic hormone (ADH), 183, 350
Antigen, 187, 249
Antrum, 207
Aorta, 262
Aqueous humor, 152
Astigmatism, 155, 157
Atrial natretic factor (ANF), 188
Atrioventricular node, 263
Audiometry, 171
Auditory (Eustachian) tube, 167
Auricle, 262
Auscultation, 272
Autonomic nervous system, 93
Autosome, 219
Axon, 116

B

B cell, 187
Babinski reflex, 101
Barany test, 173
Baroreceptor (pressoreceptor), 138
Barr body, 222
Basal metabolic rate (BMR), 333
Base, 24
Basilar membrane, 167
Basophil, 241, 244
Bell's palsy, 98
Benedict's test, 322
Beriberi, 5
Bile, 321, 356
Binocular vision, 159
Bipolar neuron, 151
Blastocoel, 209
Blastocyst, 209
Blastomere, 209
Blind spot, 157
Blood, 241
Blood pressure, 274
Blood typing, 230, 251
Bowman's capsule, 347
Boyle's Law, 283
Bradycardia, 273
Brain sand, 186
Brain stem, 93
Brownian movement, 46
BTSP factor, 294
Buccal smear, 223
Buffer system, 25
Bulbourethral (Cowper's) gland, 195
Bundle branch, 263

C

Calcitonin (CT), 183
Calculi, 357
Calorie, 333
Calorimetry, 335
Canal of Schlemm, 151
Carbohydrate, 322
Cardiac cycle, 266
Cast, 357
Catabolic reaction, 22
Catabolism, 333
Catalyst, 23
Celsius scale, 15
Central nervous system, 93
Centromere, 73, 220
Cerebellar ataxia, 93
Cerebellum, 93
Cerebrum, 93
Chemical reaction, 21
Chemoreceptor, 138
Chiasma, 198
Cholecystokinin (CCK), 187
Chordae tendineae, 263
Chorion, 210
Chorionic villi, 209
Choroid, 151
Chromaffin cell, 184
Chromatin, 72
Chromosome, 73, 219
Chylomicron, 321
Chyme, 315
Ciliary body, 151
Ciliary muscle, 151
Ciliospinal reflex, 103
Cleavage, 209
Cleavage furrow, 73
Clotting factors, 248
Clotting time, 250
Coagulation, 248
Cochlea, 167
Codominance, 230
Codon, 66
Colloid, 54
Color blindness, 231
Complementary base pairing, 65
Compound light microscope, 31
Conduction myofiber, 263
Conductive deafness, 170
Cone, 151
Conjunctiva, 151
Consensual response, 103
Contractility, 115
Contralateral reflex, 100
Convergence reflex, 159
Corona radiata, 207
Coronary sinus, 262
Corpus albicans, 207
Corpus luteum, 207
Cortisol (hydrocortisone), 186
Cranial nerves, 93
Crenation, 52
Cri du chat syndrome, 220
Crossed extensor reflex, 101
Crystalloid, 54
Cupula, 168
Cytogenetic defect, 220
Cytokinesis, 72

D

Dead air volume, 288
Decidua functionalis, 207
Decomposition reactions, 22
Deflection wave, 263
Deglutition, 312
Deletion, 220
Deoxyribonucleic acid, 63
Depth perception, 159
Diabetes mellitus, 185, 188, 352, 356
Dialysis, 49
Diastole, 266
Diencephalon, 93
Diffusion, 46
Digestive enzymes, 313
Dihybrid cross, 229
Diploid number, 72, 196
Diplopia, 159
Disaccharide, 322
Dissecting microscope, 31
Dominance, 220
Down's syndrome, 220
Ductus (vas) deferens, 195
Dynamic equilibrium, 168, 172

E

Eardrum, 167
Ectoderm, 209
Effective filtration pressure (P_{eff}), 350
Efferent nervous system, 93
Eijkman, Christiaan, 5
Elasticity, 115
Electrocardiograph (ECG, EKG), 263
Electron microscope, 31
Embolism, 250
Embryo, 210
Emmetropia, 155
Emulsification, 321
Endergonic reaction, 21
Endocardium, 261
Endocrine system, 179
Endocytosis, 56
Endoderm, 209
Endolymph, 167
Endometrium, 207
Endomysium, 116
Endothermic reaction, 21
Endurance, 303
Enterocrinin, 187
Eosinophil, 241, 244
Epididymis, 195
Epimysium, 116
Epinephrine, 186
Epithalamus, 93
Equatorial division, 196
Equilibrium, 46, 138, 172
Ergograph, 128
Erythroblastosis fetalis, 254
Erythrocyte, 241, 243, 357
Erythropoietin, 188, 347
Estrogens, 186, 205, 208
Exchange reaction, 22
Excitability, 115
Excitatory postsynaptic potential, 82
Exercise 301, 333
Exergonic reaction, 21
Exocrine glands, 179
Exocytosis, 56
Exothermic reaction, 21
Expiratory reserve volume, 288
Extensibility, 115
External auditory canal (meatus), 167
External ear, 167
Exteroceptor, 138
Extracellular fluid, 45
Extrinsic eye muscles, 98, 151

F

Facilitated diffusion, 55
Facilitation, 82
Fahrenheit scale, 15
Fascicle, 116
Fat, 321, 334
Fatigue, 126
Fauces, 313
Fertilization, 195
Fetus, 210
Fibrillation, 264
Fibrin, 250
Fibrinogen, 250
Field size, 38
Filtration, 54, 350
Finger puncture procedure, 256
Flexibility, 303
Flexor reflex, 101
Follicle-stimulating hormone (FSH), 183, 201, 205
Foramen ovale, 262
Forced expiratory volume (FEV_T), 289
Fossa ovalis, 262
Frequency, 170
Functional residual capacity, 288
Fundus, 153

G

Gamete, 195
Ganglion neuron, 151
Gastric inhibitory peptide, 187
Gastrin, 187
Gastrointestinal (GI) tract, 311
Gastrulation, 209
Gene, 219
Genetics, 219
Genome, 220
Genotype, 220
Glomerular (Bowman's) capsule, 347
Glomerular filtration, 350
Glomerulonephritis, 355
Glomerulus, 347
Glucagon, 185–186
Glucocorticoids, 186
Glucosuria, 188
Glycogenolysis, 188
Glycosuria, 354
Gonad, 185, 195
Gonadocorticoids, 186
Gonadotropin releasing hormone (GnRH), 201, 205
Graafian follicle, 207
Granulocyte, 241, 244
Growth hormone (GH), 183
Gustation, 142

H

H zone, 116
Haploid number, 72, 196
Hardy-Weinberg principle, 228
Haustral churning, 314
Heart, 261
Heart conduction system, 261
Hematocrit, 245
Hematuria, 357
Hemizygosity, 231
Hemoglobin, 241, 247
Hemoglobinometer, 248
Hemoglobinuria, 357
Hemolysis, 52
Hemolytic disease of the newborn, 254
Hemopoiesis, 255
Heterocrine gland, 180
Heterozygosity, 220
Homozygosity, 220
Hormone, 179, 333
Human chorionic gonadotropin (HCG), 187, 208
Human chorionic somatomammotropin (HCS), 188
Hyaluronidase, 207
Hydrolysis reaction, 320
Hydrometer, 15
Hyperglycemia, 188
Hyperinsulinism, 188
Hyperopia (hypermetropia), 155
Hypertonic solution, 52
Hypoinsulinism, 188
Hypothalamus, 93, 180
Hypothesis, 5
Hypotonic solution, 52

I

I band, 116
Immunoassay, 208
Implantation, 209
Incomplete dominance, 229
Incus, 167
Inferior vena cava, 262
Infundibulum, 180
Inhibin, 201
Inner ear, 167
Inspiratory capacity, 288
Inspiratory reserve volume, 288
Insulin, 185–186
Intensity, 170
Intercalated disc, 115
Interstitial endocrinocyte (cell of Leydig), 185, 201
Intracellular fluid, 45
Ion, 24
Ipsilateral reflex, 100
Isometric contraction, 122
Isometric strength, 305
Isotonic contraction, 122
Isotonic solution, 52
Isotonic strength, 305

K

Karyokinesis, 72
Karyotype, 220
Kilocalorie, 333
Kinetic energy, 23
Kleinfelter's syndrome, 225
Kymograph, 122

L

Laboratory procedures and safety precautions, 2
Labyrinth, 167
Latent period, 122
Law of Segregation, 199
Le Chatelier's Principle, 23
Leucocyte, 241, 243, 357
Leucocytosis, 2
Leucopenia, 244

Light microscope, 31
Liminal stimulus, 81
Linear measurement, 11
Locus, 219
Lugol's test, 323
Luteinizing hormone (LH), 183, 201, 207, 208
Lymphocyte, 187, 241, 244
Lyonization, 223

M

M line, 116
Macula, 168, 172
Macula lutea, 151
Magnification, 38
Malleus, 167
Mass, 14
Mastication, 310
Measurement, 11
Mechanoreceptor, 138
Mediastinum, 261
Medulla, 93
Meiosis, 72, 196
Melanocyte-stimulating hormone (MSH), 183
Membrane (resting) potential, 81
Menarche, 205
Menstrual cycle, 205
Mesoderm, 209
Metabolism, 333
Metric system, 11
Micelle, 321
Microscope, 31
Microtubule, 73
Midbrain, 93
Middle ear, 167
Mineralocorticoids, 186
Minimal volume, 288
Mitochondrion, 116
Mitosis, 72
Mitotic spindle, 73
Modality, 137
Modiolus, 167
Mole, 24
Monocyte, 241, 244
Monohybrid cross, 229
Mononucleosis, 244
Monosaccharide, 322
Monosomy, 220
Monosynaptic reflex, 100
Morula, 209
Multiple alleles, 230
Muscle contraction, 116
Muscle fiber (cell), 116
Muscle spindles, 142
Muscle tissue, 115
Myenteric (Auerbach's) plexus, 314, 317
Myocardium, 261
Myofibril, 116
Myofilaments, 117
Myoglobin, 357
Myogram, 122
Myopia, 155

N

Nephron, 347
Nerve action potential (nerve impulse), 81
Nervous system, 93
Neurohypophysis, 180
Neuromuscular (myoneural) junction, 117
Neuron, 116
Neurotransmitter, 117
Neutrophil, 241, 244
Nociceptor, 138
Nondisjunction, 222
Norepinephrine (NE), 186
Nucleic acids, 63
Nucleoside, 65
Nucleotide, 65
Nystagmus, 98, 173

O

Obesity, 334
Olfaction, 142
Oogenesis, 203
Oogonium, 203, 210
Ophthalmoscopy, 153
Optic (II) nerve, 97, 152
Optic chiasma, 97, 152
Optic disc, 152
Ora serrata, 151
Oscilloscope, 83
Osmoreceptor, 138
Osmosis, 51
Ossicle, 167
Otolith, 168, 172
Otoscopy, 169
Oval window, 167
Ovary, 186, 195
Ovulation, 207
Ovum, 195, 205
Oxytocin (OT), 183

P

P wave, 263
P-R interval, 263
Packed cell volume (PCV), 245
Pain, 141
Pancreas, 185
Papillary muscle, 263
Parathyroid gland, 184
Parathyroid hormone (PTH), 185
Passive transport, 46
Pendular movement, 314
Peptidase, 320
Perceptive deafness, 170
Pericardium, 261
Perilymph, 167
Perimysium, 116
Peripheral nervous system, 93
Peristalsis, 314
pH, 24, 352
Phagocytosis, 56
Phantom pain, 141
Phenotype, 220
Phenylthiocarbamide (PTC), 228
Pheochromocytoma, 185
Philadelphia chromosome, 221
Photoreceptor, 138
Physical fitness, 303
Physiograph, 122
Pineal gland (epiphysis cerebri), 186
Pitch, 170
Pituitary gland (hypophysis), 180
Placenta, 210
Plasma, 241–242, 250
Plasma membrane, 45
Platelet, 241, 244
Pleural membrane, 261
Pneumograph, 287
Pneumothorax, 285
Polar body, 205
Polarity, 81
Polycythemia, 244
Polydypsia, 188
Polysynaptic reflex, 100
Polyuria, 188
Pons, 93
Posterior cavity, 152
Precautions for blood and body fluids, 3
Precautions for reagents, 3
Precautions related to dissection, 4
Pregnancy testing, 208
Presbyopia, 155, 158
Pressure, 140
Primary follicle, 207
Primary oocyte, 203
Primary spermatocyte, 201
Principle, 5
Probability, 231
Progesterone (PROG), 186, 205, 208
Projection, 137
Prolactin (PRL), 183
Pronunciation guide, 1
Proprioception, 95
Proprioceptor, 138, 141
Prostate gland, 195
Protein, 320
Protein synthesis, 66
Proteinuria, 355
Prothrombin, 250
Ptosis, 97
Pulmonary artery, 262
Pulse, 272
Pulse pressure, 274
Punctate distribution, 138
Punnett square, 226
Pupil, 151
Pupillary reflex, 103
Purine, 64
Purkinje fiber, 263
Pyrimidine, 65
Pyuria, 357

Q

QRS wave (complex), 263

R

Reabsorption, 347, 350
Receptor, 99, 137
Recessivity, 220
Reduction division, 196
Referred pain, 141
Reflex, 99
Refractive index, 36
Refractory period, 82, 271
Regulating hormone (factor), 180
Relaxin, 186
Renal erythropoietic factor, 188, 347
Renin, 347
Residual volume, 288
Resolving power, 31
Respiratory rate, 288
Respirometer, 289, 294, 336
Retina, 151
Reversible reactions, 23
Rh factor, 227, 251, 254
Rhodposin, 160
Ribonucleic acid, 63, 66
Rinne's test, 170
Rod, 151
Round window, 167

S

S-T segment, 263
Saccule, 167, 172
Salivary reflex, 103
Sarcolemma, 116
Sarcomere, 116
Sarcoplasmic reticulum, 116
Satellite, 220
Scala tympani, 167
Scala vestibuli, 167
Scientific method, 4
Sclera, 151
Scleral venous sinus, 151
Secondary follicle, 207
Secondary oocyte, 205

Secondary spermatocyte, 201
Secretin, 187
Secretion, 347, 350
Sedimentation rate, 248
Segmentation, 314
Semen, 195
Semicircular canal, 167, 172
Seminal vesicle, 195
Seminiferous tubule, 201
Sensation, 137
Serum, 250
Sex chromosome, 219
Sex inheritance, 222
Sickle-cell anemia, 229
Sinoatrial (SA) node, 263
Sliding filament theory, 118
Sodium chloride, test for, 50
Sodium-potassium pump, 81
Solute, 45
Solvent, 45
Somatic nervous system, 93
Somatic reflex, 100
Sound wave, 170
Specific dynamic action (SDA), 333
Specific gravity, 15, 274
Spermatid, 201
Spermatocyte, 201
Spermatogenesis, 201
Spermatogonium, 201, 210
Spermatozoan, 195, 201
Spiral organ (Organ of Corti), 168
Spirometer, 289
Stapedius, 167
Stapes, 167
Starch, test for, 50
Starling's Law, 270
Static equilibrium, 168, 172
Stereopsis, 159
Stimulus, 137
Strength, 303
Stretch reflex, 101
Subthreshold (subliminal) stimulus, 82
Sugar, test for, 50
Summation, 127
Superior vena cava, 262
Surfactant, 285
Suspensory ligament, 152
Sustentacular (Sertoli) cell, 185, 201
Synapsis, 198
Synthesis reactions, 21
Systole, 266

T

T (transverse) tubule, 116
T cell, 187
T wave, 263
Tachycardia, 273
Target cells, 179
Taste, 142
Tectorial membrane, 168
Temperature measurement, 15
Tendon organs, 142
Tensor tympani, 167
Testis, 185, 195
Testosterone, 201
Tetanus (tetany), 120, 127
Tetrad, 198
Thalamus, 93
Theory, 5
Thermoreceptor, 138, 140
Threshold stimulus, 81, 120, 125
Thrombin, 250
Thrombocyte, 242, 244
Thrombocytopenia, 244
Thromboplastin, 250
Thrombus, 250
Thymic factor (TF), 187
Thymic humoral factor (THF), 187
Thymopoietin, 187
Thymosin, 187
Thymus, 187
Thyroid gland, 184
Thyroid-stimulating hormone (TSH), 183
Thyroxine (T_4), 183
Tidal volume, 288
Total lung capacity, 288
Touch, 138–140
Trabeculae carneae, 261
Transcription, 66
Transducer, 123
Translation, 66
Translocation, 220
Treppe, 120
Triad, 116
Triiodothyronine (T_3), 183
Triple-X syndrome, 225
Trisomy, 220
Trophoblast, 209
Tropic hormone, 180
Turner's syndrome, 225
Twitch, 120, 125
Tympanic membrane, 167

U

U.S. system, 11
Urethra, 195
Urinalysis, 352
Urinary system, 347
Uterine (Fallopian) tube, 195
Utricle, 167, 172

V

Vagina, 195
Variable, 5
Vascular tunic, 151
Ventricular filling, 266
Vertigo, 98
Vesicular follicle, 207
Vestibular nystagmus, 98, 173
Vestibule, 167
Vibration, 140
Visceral (autonomic) reflex, 100, 102
Visceroceptor, 138
Visual pathway, 97, 152
Visual reflexes, 158
Vital capacity, 288
Vitamin D, 188
Vitreous humor, 152
Volumetric measurement, 13
Vulva, 195

W

Warm-up, 303
Weber's test, 170
Weight measurement, 14
Withdrawal reflex, 101
Working distance, 34

X

X-linked inheritance, 230
XYY syndrome, 225

Y

Yolk sac, 210

Z

Z line, 116
Zona pellucida, 207
Zygote, 195, 207